Reconstructive Surgery of the Oesophagus and Stomach

Muntzer Mughal

Reconstructive Surgery of the Oesophagus and Stomach

Springer

Muntzer Mughal
Cleveland Clinic London
London, UK

University College London
London, UK

ISBN 978-3-031-66845-6 ISBN 978-3-031-66846-3 (eBook)
https://doi.org/10.1007/978-3-031-66846-3

This Springer imprint is published by the registered company Springer Nature Switzerland AG
The registered company address is: Gewerbestrasse 11, 6330 Cham, Switzerland

Acknowledgements

I am grateful to my colleagues, Mr Borzoueh Mohammadi, Mr Sacheen Kumar, Mr David Monk, Dr Rehan Haidry, and Mr Andrew Jenkinson, for their invaluable assistance in managing many of the cases discussed in this book.

I would also like to express my appreciation to Mr Joe Curry and Professor Paolo De Coppi, consultant paediatric surgeons at Great Ormond Street Hospital in London, and Mr Tarek Abdel Aziz, consultant endocrine surgeon at University College London Hospitals, for inviting me to assist them with oesophageal reconstruction. Furthermore, I am grateful to Mr David Lawrence and Mr Nikolaos Panagiotopoulos, consultant thoracic surgeons, for their help with many of the cases involving aero-digestive fistulae.

I am deeply indebted to Mr John Bancewicz for sparking my interest in oesophago-gastric surgery, and to Professor Sir Miles Irving for his guidance and mentorship, which has played a central role in my career and for demonstrating and teaching me the importance of decision-making in surgery.

My wife Shameela and children Zahra, Farah, and Waheeda have been a constant source of encouragement and support, and for that, I am truly grateful.

Finally, I would like to thank the team at Springer for their hard work in transforming the manuscript into a finished book.

Introduction

The purpose of this book is to share my experience of oesophageal reconstruction, for which I have been assisted by many trainees and colleagues, including those contributing to this book. My experience has spanned four decades, during which techniques and technology have changed enormously. The reader must consider this when going through the case summaries. Understandably, some may disagree with my treatment decisions. Still, I wanted to convey the difficulties in decision-making in this area of complex work and the thoughts guiding those decisions, albeit supported by the Multidisciplinary Team (MDT) and colleagues. In many cases, we had to 'think outside the box'. Indeed, if I encountered the same cases today, I might treat some differently based on accumulated experience and the emergence of new interventions and techniques.

I have applied a broad definition of reconstruction, which includes not just replacement of the oesophagus and stomach but bypass and corrective surgery. I believe any procedure that modifies the anatomy of the oesophagus and the stomach can be described as reconstruction. By that definition, many reconstructive procedures are now carried out endoscopically, but this is not my area of expertise, and this is a book about surgical procedures.

I hope the chapter on 'bridging strategies' will be helpful to Upper Gastrointestinal (or Foregut) Surgeons in their day-to-day practice, even if they do not specialise in oesophageal reconstruction. For those who do, I have described the steps of the operations I have learned, modified and refined over the years.

The cases presented have been chosen to illustrate the complexities of decision-making and technical challenges. Each case summary is followed by 'learning points'. This is based on contemporaneous notes I made as part of reflective learning. These notes included diagrams I drew describing technical aspects of the operations. I have chosen to use those diagrams in this book, clarifying some, but maintaining the authenticity of my originals. I found the the process of reflective learning helpful in improving my practice. It honed my decision-making and I applied the learning to subsequent cases, including changing my surgical technique and operative strategy. I hope that sharing this experience will be of some value to readers.

Contents

Chapter 1
Multidisciplinary Decision-Making

Abstract This chapter underscores the essential role of collaborative expertise in optimising patient outcomes. Emphasising historical principles of patient well-being and non-maleficence, it advocates for dedicated Multidisciplinary Team Meetings (MDT) involving specialists from various fields. From thoracic surgeons to interventional endoscopists, each specialty contributes crucial insights, ensuring comprehensive case assessment. Effective meeting management and systematic feedback mechanisms drive continuous improvement within the MDT framework. Importantly, the chapter delineates the distinction between MDT deliberations and surgical planning meetings, highlighting their respective roles in recommending management strategies and addressing operative logistics post-patient decision-making. Ultimately, a patient-centered approach guided by multidisciplinary collaboration ensures the successful navigation of complex oesophagogastric reconstructions, leading to optimal outcomes and patient satisfaction.

Keywords Oesophagogastric reconstruction · Multidisciplinary decision-making · Surgical outcomes · Multidisciplinary team meeting (MDT) · Upper GI surgeons · Patient management · Surgical planning meeting · Preoperative preparation · Perioperative care

Oesophagogastric reconstruction is challenging and requires careful decision-making regarding when and how to perform the reconstruction, and the best outcomes are obtained by multidisciplinary working. Mikulicz, who first reported oesophageal reconstruction in 1886 using skin flaps from the neck to bridge a cervical defect, was a proponent of surgical outcomes and abided by the maxims: "salus aegroti suprema lex" (the well-being of the patient is the most important law) and "primum non nocere" (first, do no harm) [1]. These should be the guiding principles of all medical care but are particularly important in the context of potentially complex reconstructive surgery.

Ideally, these cases are discussed in a dedicated multidisciplinary team meeting (MDT). Apart from Upper GI surgeons, it is important to have the expertise of thoracic surgeons, Head and Neck surgeons and plastic surgeons, as required. The assistance

M. Mughal, *Reconstructive Surgery of the Oesophagus and Stomach*,
https://doi.org/10.1007/978-3-031-66846-3_1

of thoracic surgeons is invaluable to enter the chest safely when there has been previous surgery or extensive sepsis. Their involvement is also critical in surgery for oesophageal fistulation to the airways, lung, or chronic empyema. The team should include interventional endoscopists and radiologists as well as gastroenterologists, including those specialising in neurogastroenterology when dealing with conditions such as achalasia and gastroparesis secondary to complications of previous surgery, dietician and clinical nurse specialist. In cases involving adolescents, paediatric surgeons will also form an important part of the team.

It is important that all the information required to properly discuss the case is available for the multidisciplinary team to consider and appropriate time is set aside for the discussion. Needless to say, the meeting needs to be chaired and properly minuted. The chair should manage the discussion, ensuring all members are encouraged and allowed to contribute. It is his or her task to reach a consensus on and formulate recommendations on how the case should be managed. The function of the MDT is to consider the various options for management and recommend the best option, setting out the pros and cons of each so that these can be put to the patient and their relatives in as easily understandable way as possible.

A decade ago, I brought together like-minded colleagues to set up an MDT to discuss benign complex Upper GI cases at University College Hospitals London. Once our MDT meetings had been running for some time and we had started to apply treatment recommendations, the first part of the meeting was reserved for feedback to the team on the outcomes of those recommendations. This was crucial in developing the MDT, providing valuable learning and calibration of the decision-making process. It also led to an increase in the number of referrals by a tangible demonstration of the value of the MDT, drawing in ever more complex cases that further added to the experience of the team. I have continued that practice at Cleveland Clinic London.

It should be stressed that the MDT discussion and outcome is separate from a surgical planning meeting. Whereas the MDT discussion sets out recommendations, the surgical planning meeting addresses the operative strategy, including preoperative preparation and perioperative care, once the patient has decided which option to take.

Reference

1. Cai L, Barrera J, Ma I, Lee G (2020) Multi-disciplinary surgical approach to esophageal reconstruction: the role of the plastic surgeon. Med Res Arch. 2020;8(5). https://doi.org/10.18103/mra.v8i5.2090.

Chapter 2
Investigations

Abstract This chapter delineates the pivotal role of various imaging modalities in understanding anatomy, planning surgeries, and selecting conduits when necessary. It stresses the importance of tailored imaging protocols, collaboration with radiologists, and utilising intravenous contrast for optimal visualization. Emphasising the complementary nature of endoscopy, it highlights the significance of direct mucosal assessment and endoscopic interventions. Additionally, oesophageal function studies are deemed crucial, especially in conditions like achalasia or after anti-reflux surgery complications. Through a comprehensive approach integrating cross-sectional imaging, endoscopy, and functional studies, this chapter underscores the essential diagnostic foundations essential for successful oesophagogastric reconstruction.

Keywords Radiological imaging · CT scan · Intravenous contrast · Luminal contrast · CT angiography · 3-D reconstructions · Endoscopy · Endoscopic interventions · Laparoscopy · Oesophageal function studies

2.1 Radiological Imaging

Appropriate imaging is vital to understanding the current anatomy and planning surgery and selecting a conduit if required.

The exact imaging requirements will vary from case to case. A CT scan of the neck, chest, abdomen and pelvis is invaluable in providing anatomical information. However, it is important to liaise closely with the radiologist and explain exactly what information is sought so that the scan can be protocolised appropriately. Intravenous contrast is almost always required to provide sufficient enhancement and is essential to determine the vascularity of the relevant part of the gastrointestinal tract. In some cases this will be combined with the administration of luminal contrast to provide additional information in cases of suspected perforations and anastomotic leaks. CT angiography may also be necessary to assess the vascularity of the stomach or colon if

M. Mughal, *Reconstructive Surgery of the Oesophagus and Stomach*,
https://doi.org/10.1007/978-3-031-66846-3_2

these are to be used as conduits, particularly if previous surgery might have disrupted the normal vasculature.

Radiologists can also provide bespoke images such 3-D reconstructions which can provide a further level of detail for surgical planning, e.g. the size of a hiatal defect and the quality of the crura, the geometry of a complex hiatus hernia or the detailed anatomy of an aero-digestive fistula.

A barium or gastrografin study can be valuable in assessing strictures, fistulae, and transit. A timed barium swallow is also an extremely helpful study for assessing oesophageal emptying and is, in my experience, not used often enough. It provides an objective, semiquantitative measurement of oesophageal transit, which can be correlated with the patient's symptoms. It is also helpful to perform this as a baseline before interventions to improve oesophageal emptying in treating achalasia and complex strictures.

In some cases, it may be necessary to carry out an endoscopy simultaneously with imaging, particularly if a difficult stricture is being assessed. It is important to record both endoscopic and radiological images for the medical records and an MDT.

Isotope scans are helpful in assessing gastric emptying and excluding metastatic or recurrent disease when reconstruction is being considered in a case where the initial operation was for cancer. Gastric emptying studies help plan treatment, particularly for re-operative hiatal or anti-reflux surgery. Previous surgery may have resulted in vagal injury, significantly affecting gastric emptying. This needs to be considered in planning further surgery and managing patient expectations.

2.2 Endoscopy

Endoscopic assessment is essential and complementary to cross-sectional imaging. Endoscopy allows the direct assessment of the mucosa and is particularly valuable in assessing strictures and the anatomy and dimensions of fistulae. It also enables biopsy of suspicious areas and can be used for interventions such as the application of clips for bleeding and closing small defects, suturing and the placement of stents and the EsoSponge or VAC-stent.

EUS is valuable for assessing luminal, mural and extra luminal lesions as well as enabling targeted biopsies.

Endoscopy combined with cross-sectional imaging with luminal contrast is valuable in the diagnosis and assessment of anastomotic leaks. Even when a leak has been confirmed on imaging endoscopy is important to determine the vascularity of the conduit. This can have a vital bearing on the management of a leak. If the conduit is well-vascularised, and the leak is small and well-controlled, conservative management will most likely succeed. On the other hand, if there is significant ischaemia of the conduit, the leak is unlikely to heal even if it is small.

Endoscopic interventional procedures, including dilatation, stenting, POEM, G-POEM, clipping of anastomotic defects and bleeding vessels, are important adjuncts to the armamentarium of reconstructive surgery.

In the UK, GI surgeons are trained to carry out diagnostic endoscopy, and many Upper GI surgeons choose to perform endoscopy for tumour staging together with laparoscopy, if indicated, and the assessment of an anastomotic leak. Having performed the operation helps guide the scope and interpret the findings, particularly with a complex reconstruction. If the procedure is to be performed by the endoscopy team, it is important to liaise closely with them to ensure they are provided all the relevant information about the anatomy of the reconstruction and whether endoscopic interventions should be carried out at the same time if indicated.

2.3 Oesophageal Function Studies

These are particularly important where the reconstruction is for conditions such as achalasia or reoperation after failure or complication of anti-reflux surgery.

The studies include high-resolution manometry as well as oesophageal pH monitoring. It is important to fully understand the anatomy before requesting these studies. For instance, if there is a high-grade peptic structure, it may not be possible to place the manometry catheter or the pH probe into the oesophagus beyond and across the gastro-oesophageal junction. Similarly, with a capacious, tortuous oesophagus in achalasia, it may not be possible to position the manometry catheter to assess the lower oesophageal sphincter.

Oesophageal pH monitoring can be carried out using pH probes or the Bravo capsule. The latter requires endoscopic placement of the capsule into the oesophagus but is much better tolerated than a pH probe tethered to a tube inserted through the nose. Furthermore, it provides pH data for a period of up to five days rather than 24 hours and, therefore provides a more accurate reflection of the oesophageal pH environment. However, it cannot measure non-acid reflux, which is better assessed with a combined pH and impedance probe.

Chapter 3
Counselling and Consenting of Patients for Complex Oesophagogastric Reconstruction

Abstract This chapter highlights the critical role of informed consent and thorough patient counselling in the preoperative phase. It emphasizes covering essential topics such as the nature of surgery, risks, expected outcomes, and available alternatives, particularly in cases lacking published evidence for risks and benefits. Utilizing radiological images and diagrams aids patient understanding, followed by detailed written communication and ample time for questions. Exploring alternatives to surgery and promoting shared decision-making are highlighted, ensuring patient involvement in treatment planning and consideration of their goals and concerns for optimizing outcomes and quality of life.

Keywords Informed consent · Counselling · Oesophagogastric reconstruction · Patient education · Postoperative outcomes · Quality of life · Patient communication · Multidisciplinary team (MDT) · Management options

Obtaining informed consent and providing appropriate counselling are integral aspects of the preoperative process for patients undergoing complex oesophagogastric reconstruction.

Patient counselling should cover several key topics, including the nature and purpose of the surgery, potential risks and complications, expected postoperative outcomes, and available alternatives. It is crucial to discuss the short-term and long-term complications associated including anastomotic leakage, infection, stricture formation, and potential impact on the quality of life. Furthermore, a thorough explanation of the postoperative recovery process, including possible requirements for nutritional support, should be provided.

However, in many complex cases, there may not be published evidence to quantify the risks and benefits, and even less so for innovative procedures designed for a particular patient and pathology.

After the MDT meeting, I usually see the patient and relatives to explain the recommendations. Showing the relevant radiological images and using diagrams to describe the current situation and the planned reconstruction can aid the patient's understanding. It is important to put aside enough time for the patient and relatives to

M. Mughal, *Reconstructive Surgery of the Oesophagus and Stomach*,
https://doi.org/10.1007/978-3-031-66846-3_3

be able to ask questions when considering a complex and high-risk procedure. I follow this with a letter detailing the management options with the MDT recommendation and set out the risks, benefits and recovery time. The letter ends with an invitation for the patient to ask any questions that have come to mind they may not have been able to ask or thought of asking during the consultation. The Clinical Specialist Nurse (CNS) member of the MDT has an important role in this regard as well supporting the patient and their family throughout their journey.

It is essential to discuss the available alternatives to surgery, including best supportive care, medical treatment and endoscopic interventions. In some cases, these alternatives could be part of a bridging strategy to improve the patient's general condition before they can be considered for a reconstruction. In other cases, the benefits of surgery may be uncertain and a complex procedure with significant and serious risks cannot be justified. In any case, the patient should be offered a second opinion from other experts in the field even if they have not requested it. I have found that patients appreciate that, as they may have been considering that but were afraid to ask.

A central pillar of counselling is shared decision-making as a collaborative process between the patient and the treating team, and should incorporate the patient's goals, expectations, concerns, as well as the potential impact of surgery on the quality of life.

Chapter 4
Preparation and Timing for Reconstructive Surgery

Abstract This underscores the importance of comprehensive patient evaluation, preoperative management, and strategic timing for optimal outcomes. Patient suitability for surgery is determined through thorough assessments, including medical history, physical exams, and tests assessing fitness for surgery. Preoperative management focuses on optimising patient condition through interventions like nutritional optimisation and prehabilitation. Timing of surgery is critical, influenced by factors such as patient clinical status, primary disease, and complexity of reconstruction, with considerations for neoadjuvant treatments and emergency situations. Team briefing and operation planning are essential for coordinating complex surgeries, ensuring clear communication and anticipation of challenges throughout the procedure.

Keywords Reconstructive surgery · Oesophagus · Stomach · Patient evaluation · Psychological well-being · Operation plan · Preoperative management · Surgical outcomes · Postoperative complications · Operation plan · Multidisciplinary approach · Risk assessment

Reconstructive surgery of the oesophagus and stomach can be complex and requires thorough preparation and optimal timing to ensure successful outcomes.

4.1 Patient Evaluation

A comprehensive assessment is necessary to determine the patient's suitability for reconstructive surgery. This evaluation typically includes a detailed medical history, physical examination, and tests to assess fitness for surgery which may involve a thoracotomy, such as CPEX (cardiopulmonary testing), lung function studies and tests of cardiac function. Additionally, nutritional status and psychological well-being assessment are crucial in determining the patient's readiness for surgery.

M. Mughal, *Reconstructive Surgery of the Oesophagus and Stomach*,
https://doi.org/10.1007/978-3-031-66846-3_4

4.2 Preoperative Management

Preoperative management is essential in optimising outcomes once a patient is deemed eligible for reconstructive surgery. This may involve nutritional optimisation, smoking cessation, and management of comorbidities. Prehabilitation, a concept involving physical, nutritional, and psychological preparation, has been shown to improve surgical outcomes and reduce postoperative complications.

4.3 Timing of Reconstructive Surgery

The timing of reconstructive surgery is a critical factor that influences outcomes. Several factors should be considered, including the patient's clinical condition, the primary disease or condition and the complexity of the planned reconstruction. For primary reconstruction in cases of malignancy, neoadjuvant treatment, such as chemotherapy and/or radiotherapy, is likely to have been administered before surgery. The ideal time for surgery following neoadjuvant treatment varies depending on the specific protocol and patient response. However, typically, surgery is usually planned four to six weeks after completing treatment and this interval can be used to further optimise the patient's condition.

In cases requiring emergency surgery, depending on the patient's condition, comorbidity and the operative findings, the principles of 'damage control surgery' should be applied. The primary aim is to deal with any life-threatening issues, leaving reconstruction until the patient is fit to undergo complex surgery. Resection and reconstruction do not have to be carried out at the same time and this is illustrated in some of the case studies presented in this book.

4.4 Team Briefing and Operation Plan

Team briefing is now carried out routinely in the U.K. It is particularly important in complex surgery with multiple phases, and the involvement of different specialists and the use of different equipment and techniques for the various stages. It is important to share and explain the steps of the procedure clearly to the whole team, including anticipated difficulties and mitigations. Because it may be challenging to remember all the steps of the operation that might take the best part of a day, it is helpful to write a plan which can be drawn on a theatre whiteboard for all to see. It can also serve as a checklist to ensure that the various steps have been completed and make contemporaneous brief notes about difficulties encountered that will help with the sign-out and debrief at the end of the operation.

Table 4.1 is a typical plan that describes the phases of surgery, the teams and special equipment required for each phase and the concerns and risks.

Table 4.1 Operation plan

Phase, duration & preparation lor next phase	Addition team Members	Special Equipment	Concerns/Risks
Chest (Closure of TOF & resection of oesophagus) ~ 2 hours Chest closed and patient repositioned supine, with head ring and shoulder support. Neck, chest and abdomen prepared and draped	Thoracic surgeon—Mr P	-Double-lumen ET - Lung set with 2 x Finichietto rib retractors - ? bronchial blocker ? high frequency jet ventilation - Articulated stapler with cartridges for lung, airways and vessels -2 x 28 Fr chest drains - Fibrin glue - Head ring and shoulder support for re-positioning after completion	Temporary air-leak during closure of tracheal defect Air leak on re-inflating right ling
Abdomen (Mobilisation of the stomach to use as a retrosternal conduit for oesophageal replacement) ~ 1,5 hours Abdomen left open and covered	Nil	- Table-mounted retractor with UGI attachments - Staplers for making the gastric conduit - Jejunostomy tube	? need to use colon if stomach unsuitable, therefore need bulldog clips
Neck (Preparing cervical oesophagus) ~1 hour Neck left open and covered ~ 45 minutes	Nil	- Neck set with handheld energy device - bipolar diathermy - nerve stimulator - if IONM to be used, double lumen tube exchanged for NIM tube	Injury to RLN
Retrosternal tunnel & transposition of conduit ~ 30 minutes	Nil	- long, flat, malleable retractor, nylon tape, sterile plastic camera sheath, sterile jelly - sternal saw assembled with blade, tested and ready for use	- Bleeding from injury to brachiocephalic vein - pleural/lung injury
Cervical anastomosis ~ 45 minutes	Nil	- nil else	
Closure of neck and abdomen ~ 45 minutes	Nil	- drains for neck & abdomen	Reconciliation of swab and instrument count

Chapter 5
Chapter Environment and Equipment for Complex Reconstruction

Abstract This chapter highlights the essential elements necessary for safe and effective surgery across multiple body regions. It emphasises the need for a well-equipped operating theatre with appropriate lighting, vision aids like operating loupes, and specialised surgical instruments tailored to the complexity of the procedures involved. Retractors play a crucial role in providing optimal exposure of the surgical field, particularly in challenging areas like the neck, chest, and abdomen. Access to advanced devices for hemostasis, anastomosis, and endoscopic interventions are vital for successful outcomes. Additionally, the availability of materials such as sutures, staplers, and sealants ensures comprehensive support throughout the surgical process, contributing to the overall success of complex reconstructive procedures.

Keywords Oesophagogastric reconstruction · Operating theatre · Surgical instruments · Endoscopic instruments · Lighting · Visual aids · Surgical equipment · Surgical environment

Complex oesophagogastric reconstruction often necessitates operating in multiple body regions, including the neck, chest, and abdomen. Surgeons must have access to a comprehensive set of equipment to perform these procedures safely and effectively.

Apart from equipment, it is vital to have appropriate assistance, whether from other Upper GI colleagues or other specialists in other fields, such as thoracic surgeons, endoscopists, etc.

5.1 The Operating Theatre

The operating theatre must be appropriate for the planned operation, including the space to accommodate ancillary equipment to facilitate simultaneous laparoscopy and endoscopy for planned hybrid procedures. The operating table should be capable of being 'broken' and tilted as needed for optimum access and visualisation of the operative field. This should include the bolt-ons for stabilising the patient, and

M. Mughal, *Reconstructive Surgery of the Oesophagus and Stomach*,
https://doi.org/10.1007/978-3-031-66846-3_5

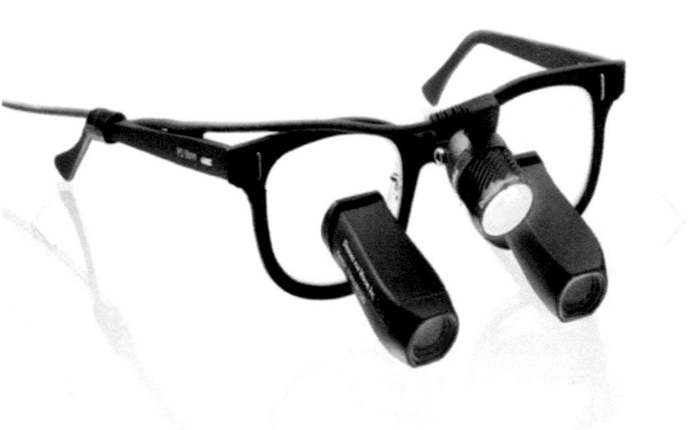

Fig. 5.1 Operating loupes

optimum positioning may require 'bean bags', head rings and pressure relieving gel pads.

5.2 Lighting

Ceiling lights should be easily directable at the field of dissection and headlights are especially useful when operating in a deep cavity through a limited aperture, such as the apex of the chest or the diaphragmatic hiatus.

5.3 Vision

For open surgery, I believe that operating loupes are not only helpful in greatly improving the identification of small vital structures and tissue planes, but can enhance the accuracy of dissection, minimise collateral damage, speed up the operation and improve outcomes (Fig. 5.1).

5.4 Surgical Instruments

A variety of specialised surgical instruments are required for complex oesophagogastric reconstruction. Apart from what could be described as 'standard surgical sets' a comprehensive set of instruments will be required for thoracic and neck surgery. This includes appropriate retractors and dissection instruments. Long dissecting instruments are particularly useful in the chest. For neck dissection, intraoperative nerve monitoring can be very helpful in locating and safeguarding the recurrent laryngeal nerve, particularly for re-operations.

Bulldog clamps of various sizes and Silastic sloops should be available for the temporary isolation of vascular bundles in preparing a colon or jejunal conduit.

5.5 Devices for Haemostasis

Monopolar and bipolar diathermy should be available for use as dictated by the field of dissection, as well as energy devices such as the Thunderbeat and harmonic scalpel. I use bipolar diathermy for most of the dissection in the neck once I am through the muscle layers. Liga clips are also helpful, particularly in areas where space is limited and when dissecting around structures susceptible to injury from heat, such as close to the airways or in the neck close to the course of the recurrent laryngeal nerve.

5.6 Retractors

Retractors are critical for providing adequate exposure of the surgical field, whether in the neck, chest or abdomen. A range of retractors may be required, including self-retaining retractors, handheld retractors, and table-mounted fixed retractors (Fig. 5.2). The correct application of table-mounted retractors, with appropriate attachments, can transform access and make a difficult operation easier.

Access to the hiatus and the left upper quadrant of the abdomen can be challenging, particularly for re-operative surgery. Good exposure can make possible what initially seems unachievable by providing safe and optimal access to the hiatus. I find a combination of retractors to lift the rib cage and retract the liver useful in this situation. Good access to the hiatus is not only necessary for the dissection but vital for enabling a high anastomosis to the oesophagus within the mediastinum.

For the chest, I often use two rib retractors to provide optimum access, particularly when dissection of the whole of the oesophagus is required, from the apex of the chest to the diaphragm.

5.7 Laparoscopic & Endoscopic Instruments

Laparoscopy and thoracoscopy (for instance, for a combined VATS procedure) are adjuncts for open oesophagogastric reconstruction. The ready availability of an endoscope can be valuable for intraluminal inspection in some circumstances. The

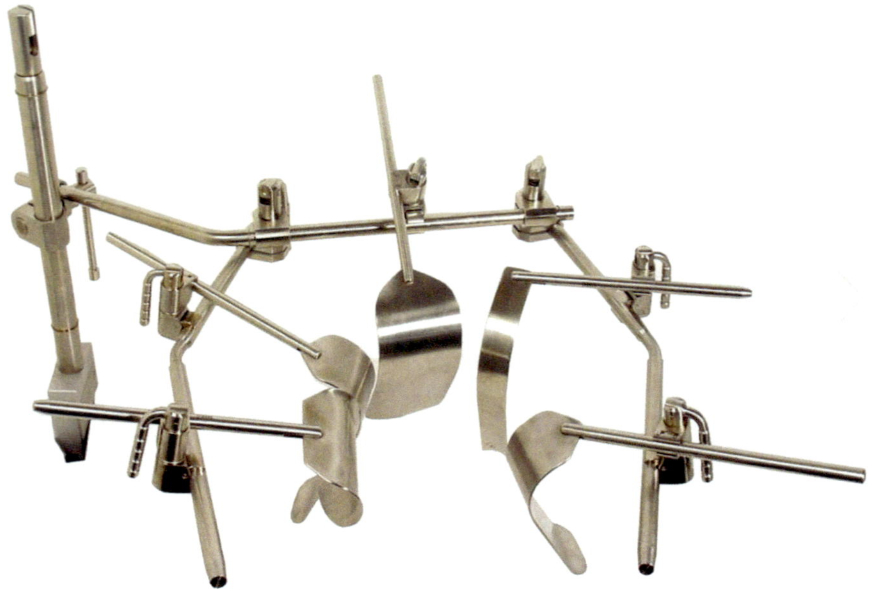

Fig. 5.2 Table-mounted frame with attached retractors

appropriate equipment should be available with the teams trained to set them up for use.

5.8 Anastomotic Devices

Anastomotic devices, such as surgical staplers, are often required, and the anticipated selection should be available.

5.9 Other Instruments

For creating a retrosternal tunnel, I use a long, narrow (30 x 5 cm) malleable retractor (Fig. 5.3) is useful, and I use a sterile plastic sleeve (Fig. 5.4) to protect the conduit during the transposition. I also have a sternal saw available, in case of bleeding, for the creation of a retrosternal tunnel (Fig. 5.5).

The sternal saw, with the blade mounted, should be available and tested before creating the retrosternal tunnel.

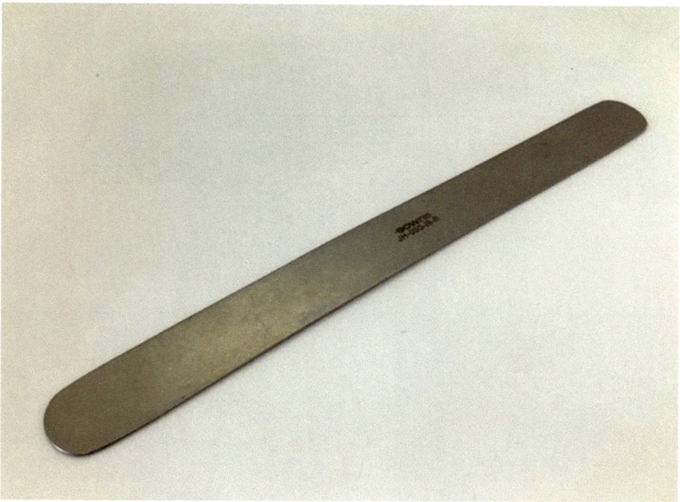

Fig. 5.3 Malleable retractor

Fig. 5.4 Sterile plastic camera sleeve to protect conduit during transposition

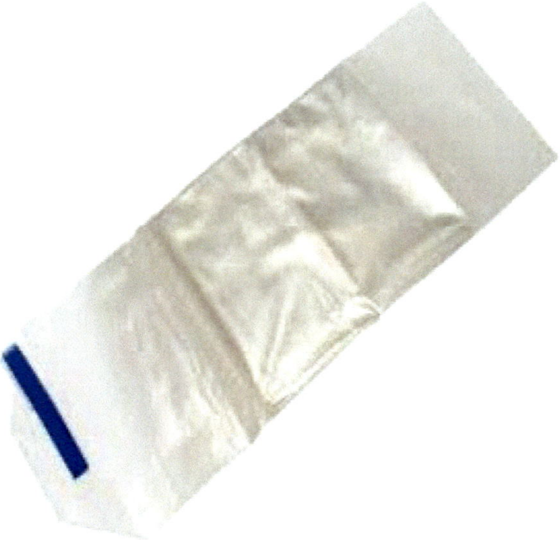

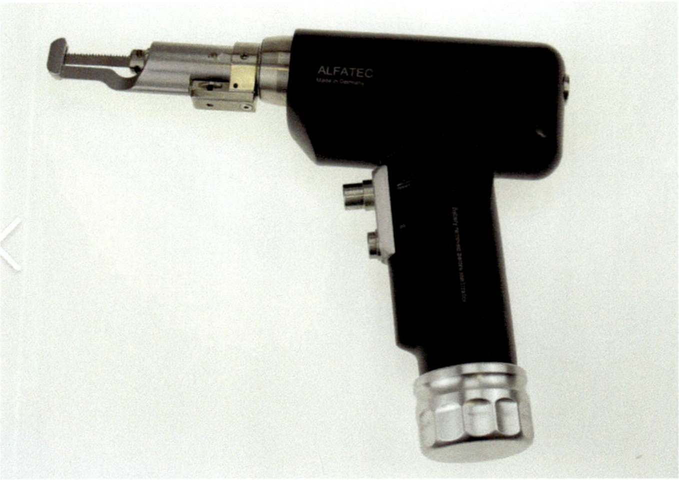

Fig. 5.5 Sternal saw

5.10 Sutures, Staplers and Materials

Apart from sutures for the anastomoses, vascular sutures, e.g. double-ended 4/0 Prolene may be required for vascular repair. Other materials, such as pericardial patches, PTFE pledgets, and biological mesh should be available for buttressing repairs of the airway and repairing the diaphragm and the oesophageal hiatus. Appropriate staplers should also be available for lung resection and transection of the airways and segmental pulmonary vasculature, if needed.

Haemostatic gauze and sealants should also be available.

If retrosternal routing of a conduit is anticipated, sterile plastic sleeve (Fig. 5.4) should be available to protect the conduit.

Chapter 6
Training and Skills for Complex Reconstruction

Abstract This chapter underscores the demanding nature of oesophageal and gastric reconstruction, often necessitating surgical intervention in challenging anatomical regions and complex scenarios. The acquisition of requisite skills is emphasised through training and hands-on experience, highlighting variances in training programs across different countries. While specialised training equips surgeons for certain procedures, gaps may exist in handling intricate cases like neck access and managing aerodigestive fistulae. Collaborative efforts with head and neck surgeons and thoracic surgeons are advocated to optimise patient outcomes. Anatomical knowledge emerges as pivotal for planning safe access and understanding pathophysiological nuances, with a call for enhanced training opportunities and accredited centres to foster expertise in complex oesophagogastric surgery.

Keywords Oesophagogastric reconstruction · Complex surgeries · Surgical skills · Multidisciplinary approach · Surgical training

Complex oesophageal and gastric reconstruction is a demanding procedure often involving operating in the neck, chest, or abdomen in adverse conditions, such as previous failed surgery or sepsis. The skills required for managing these complicated cases are acquired by training and experience. The training for oesophagogastric surgery and professional boundaries vary between countries. In the U.K. training of specialist oesophagogastric surgeons equips them to carry out oesophageal and gastric resections as well as performing hiatal hernia repairs and antireflux surgery.

However, most oesophagogastric surgeons will not have either the training or the experience of operating on the oesophagus in the neck, or in complex re-operative surgery requiring reconstruction using conduits other than the stomach. Even experienced oesophagogastric surgeons may lack the expertise and experience in dealing with aerodigestive fistulae, which are rare and require complex, multi-specialty interventions. Therefore, depending on the circumstances of the case, even experienced surgeons should collaborate with Head and Neck surgeons and thoracic surgeons for complex reconstruction to ensure the best outcomes. In the USA, however, thoracic

M. Mughal, *Reconstructive Surgery of the Oesophagus and Stomach*,
https://doi.org/10.1007/978-3-031-66846-3_6

surgeons operate on the oesophagus, and therefore it would be perfectly reasonable for them to deal with aerodigestive fistulae without involving GI surgeons.

In my opinion, oesophagogastric surgeons in the UK who want to develop a practice in reconstructive oesophagogastric surgery should receive training to access the cervical oesophagus and hypopharynx safely and effectively through the neck. Because endocrine surgery is no longer part of general surgery in the UK, few oesophagogastric surgeons are trained in surgery of the neck. As the vast majority of oesophageal resections carried out in the UK are two-stage Ivor-Lewis operations, surgeons do not develop familiarity with the anatomy of the neck, necessary to carry out difficult anastomoses to the cervical oesophagus and the hypopharynx. Expertise in neck access is even more important for re-operative surgery. Working closely with Head and Neck surgeons is important if one lacks expertise in neck dissection, but I believe that Upper GI surgeons who specialise in oesophageal reconstruction should have the training and expertise to safely access and operate on the entire oesophagus, including the hypopharynx. The ability to mobilise and reflect the thyroid and identify and dissect the recurrent laryngeal nerve are important skills to fully access the cervical oesophagus and operate on cervical tracheo-oesophageal fistulae.

6.1 Anatomical Knowledge

An in-depth understanding of the anatomy of the neck, chest, and abdomen is crucial for successful oesophageal and gastric reconstruction. Anatomical knowledge is important in not only planning safe access to the oesophagus in the neck, chest and abdomen but on the relationship of adjacent structures and understand the pathophysiology of conditions such as aerodigestive and aortoesophageal fistula, as well as being able to safely dissect in these areas. Furthermore, a knowledge of muscle flaps that can be raised to interpose or buttress repairs in the neck and chest is important so that access can be planned, maintaining the integrity of tissue that might be needed and how best to harvest such flaps.

Even so, there should be no hesitation in seeking both the advice and technical help of appropriate subspecialists, such as Head & Neck surgeons and thoracic surgeons for complex cases. I have learned a huge amount from working with colleagues specialising in thoracic surgery, Head and Neck surgery and paediatric surgery.

6.2 Advanced Training and Fellowships

I am unaware of any accredited fellowships in oesophagogastric reconstruction in the UK. This is not surprising because there are no accredited oesophagogastric reconstruction units, although some high-volume oesophagogastric centres have developed a reconstruction practice. I think there is an unmet need for a centre for oesophagogastric reconstruction and have addressed this in Chap. 33. Apart from improving patient outcomes, I believe that concentrating this highly complex work in a few accredited centres will also ensure appropriate training for the future generation of surgeons who wish to specialise in this area of oesophagogastric surgery.

Chapter 7
Surgical Access

Abstract This chapter elucidates the critical techniques and considerations essential for optimal access to the cervical oesophagus and surrounding structures. Emphasising patient positioning, meticulous incision, and dissection strategies, it underscores the significance of avoiding injury to vital structures, particularly the recurrent laryngeal nerve. Techniques such as nerve monitoring are highlighted for minimising nerve injury risks, especially in complex cases. Detailed descriptions of lateral and anterior approaches, along with insights into accessing the cervical oesophagus in previously operated necks, and offer valuable procedural guidance. Moreover, the chapter discusses challenging cases, providing case summaries and learning points to navigate difficulties encountered during surgery, ensuring safe and effective outcomes. Additionally, it touches on abdomen access techniques, offering a comprehensive overview of surgical access considerations for cervical and abdominal surgeries.

Keywords Surgical access · Anatomical knowledge · Cervical oesophagus · Patient positioning · Incisions · Dissection strategies · Lateral neck approach · Anterior neck approach · Retrosternal approach · Difficult thoracic access

7.1 Neck

Optimal access to the cervical oesophagus is achieved by appropriate positioning to extend the neck and making the best incision to provide adequate exposure. Operating in the neck, particularly in previously operated cases, requires meticulous dissection to avoid injury to important adjacent structures, particularly the recurrent laryngeal nerve.

M. Mughal, *Reconstructive Surgery of the Oesophagus and Stomach*,
https://doi.org/10.1007/978-3-031-66846-3_7

7.1.1 Patient Positioning

Proper patient positioning is crucial for optimal access to the cervical oesophagus. The patient should be placed supine with the neck extended, supported by a shoulder roll. The head is draped so that the neck can be rolled to one side or the other.

Venous congestion and bleeding can be minimised by putting the patient in a head-up position during the dissection.

I have used intraoperative nerve monitoring with increasing frequency in recent years, recognising its benefits in minimising recurrent laryngeal nerve injury, particularly in re-operations on the neck. I have found it particularly beneficial in situations such as previous radiotherapy, fistulation and prolonged sepsis or other situations where the anatomy of the neck may be difficult to identify. The anaesthetists and the theatre team need to understand how to set up the equipment and, most of all, the surgeon should be fully trained in the use of the nerve stimulator and interpretation of the signals.

7.1.2 Incision and Dissection

In most cases, for approaching the hypopharynx and the cervical oesophagus to perform a high anastomosis, an incision along the anterior border of the sternocleidomastoid is sufficient. I do not think it matters whether the neck is approached from the left or the right side. However, when the operation also involves a right thoracotomy, and the anaesthetist has therefore chosen to place neck lines on the right side, the left-sided approach is more appropriate. If more extensive exposure is required, it is best achieved through a collar incision, in which case the anaesthetist should use a subclavian approach to place central lines.

I now routinely use magnification loupes, which I have found extremely helpful for neck dissection and when assisting paediatric surgeons with operations on children.

7.1.3 Lateral Approach

I usually start the incision about 3 cm below the mastoid process at the level of the angle of the jaw. The incision follows the anterior border of the sternomastoid and curves across to the other side of the neck just above the sternal notch. After dividing the platysma, dissection is kept close to the anterior border of the sternomastoid and deepened to reveal the omohyoid muscle. If the omohyoid is not required for a muscle flap, I divide it for better access. I also divide the strap muscles on the side of the dissection, conserving the muscles on the other side of the midline for use as a muscle flap, if needed.

Dissection continues anterior to the internal jugular vein and then the carotid sheath, deepening it to reveal the areolar tissue between the vessels and the thyroid lobe medially. The middle thyroid veins are then divided, and the dissection is deepened until the vertebral column is reached (Fig. 7.1). If the neck has not been operated on previously, this is the easiest and safest plane to find and develop. A pledget can then be used to develop the avascular plane between the spine and the oesophagus. This can be carried proximally to get behind the hypopharynx and distally to free up the oesophagus well into the mediastinum. I have found this to not only enable dissection of a good length of cervical oesophagus, but this step enables the safe encircling of the oesophagus. Next, I develop the plane between the oesophagus and the trachea. I locate and display the recurrent laryngeal nerve along its course in the field of dissection. Even when using the nerve stimulator, I rely on dissection to identify the nerve or what I think is the nerve. The stimulator is then used to confirm whether it is indeed the nerve and is particularly useful in tracing the nerve through an area of fibrosis. Once the nerve has been located, it is kept out of the way on the tracheal side while encircling the oesophagus. The plane between the oesophagus and trachea is developed by sharp dissection aided by bipolar diathermy (Fig. 7.2).

In my experience, it is important to start separating of the oesophagus from the trachea for a distance of 4 or 5 cm before developing the depth. Simply trying to get to the other side of the oesophagus through a narrow tunnel of dissection between the trachea and oesophagus is not safe and risks injury to the contra-lateral recurrent laryngeal nerve. Furthermore, without visual confirmation that the whole width of

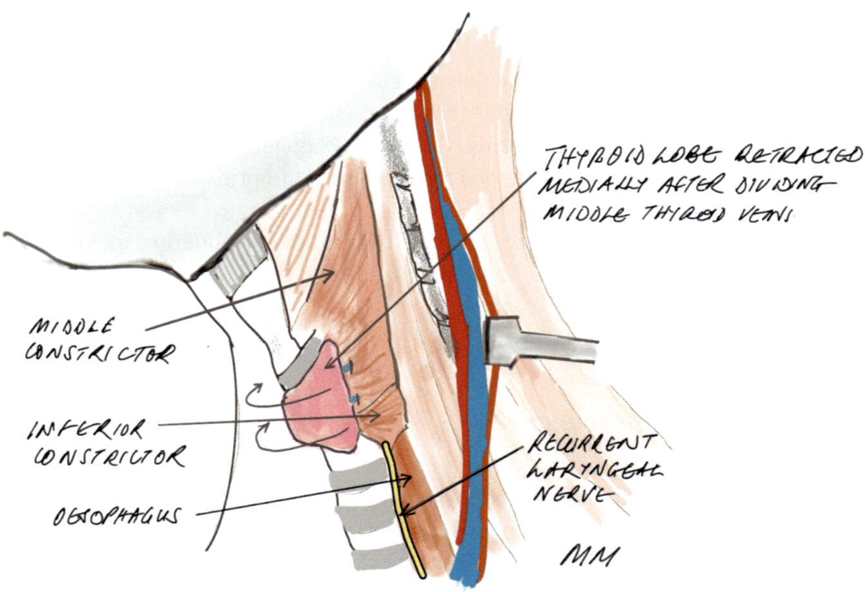

Fig. 7.1 Diagram showing retraction of the sternomastoid to expose the vascular sheath and division of the middle thyroid veins to fully expose the constrictor muscles and the cervical oesophagus

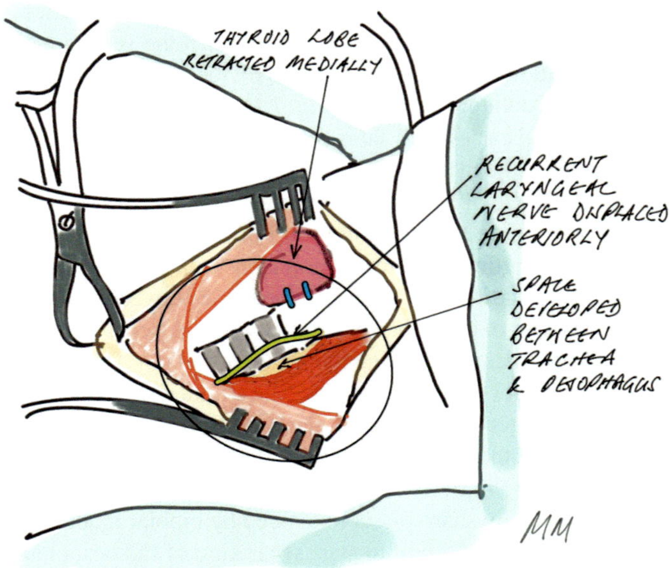

Fig. 7.2 Diagram illustrating separation of the oesophagus from the trachea

the oesophagus has been dissected, trying to pass a Lahey around the oesophagus carries the risk of going through the wall because it has not been fully encircled. Gradually deepening the dissection between the trachea and oesophagus over a 4 to 5 cm length provides better visualisation of the depth of the dissection and results in easier and safer encircling of the oesophagus. During this dissection, tiny blood vessels are usually encountered between the trachea and oesophagus and can be easily dealt with by bipolar diathermy. Once the oesophagus has been encircled, a nylon tape can be passed around it, and by applying appropriate traction, the rest of the dissection can be carried out easily.

By mobilising the oesophagus as far down into the superior mediastinum as possible, a good length can be obtained for a subsequent anastomosis or oesophagectomy.

7.1.4 Anterior Approach

For the anterior approach, I use a collar incision centred midway between the hyoid and the sternal notch. The length of the incision is dictated by the degree of exposure required. After dividing the platysma, the superior and inferior flaps are raised liberally and can either be held apart using a Joll retractor or sutured to the skin. In order to maintain the strap muscles until it is known whether they will be required for interposition or buttressing, I usually start by deepening the dissection in the

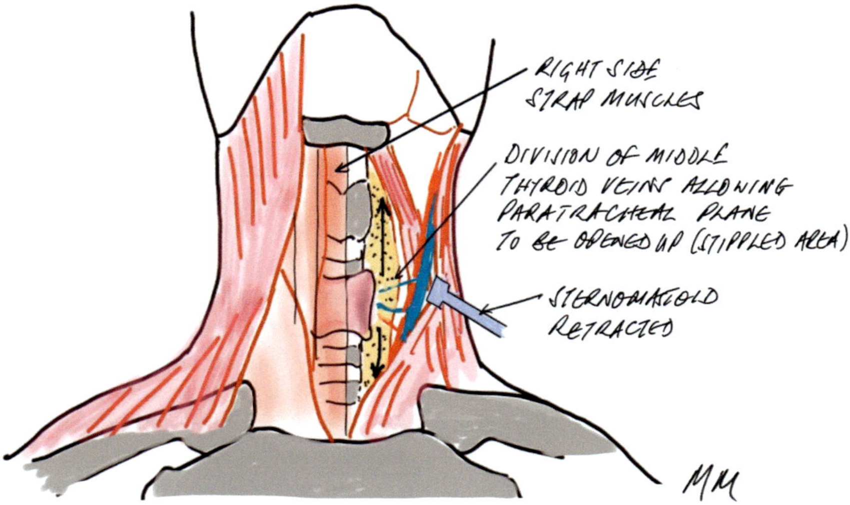

Fig. 7.3 Diagram showing the exposure of the space between the trachea and the vascular sheath to enable wide access to the oesophagus

midline between the strap muscles. This is usually a bloodless plane but anterior jugular veins often cross the midline and are ligated and divided. I like to use an energy device such as the hand-held bipolar or ultrasonic instrument for this as well as all the dissection through the muscle planes. Once the sub-platysma flaps have been reflected widely, it is possible to separate the strap muscles through their entire length in the neck. They are then retracted laterally, providing excellent exposure without the need for transection (Fig. 7.3). From that point on, the approach to and dissection of the oesophagus is identical to the lateral approach.

Accessing the Cervical Oesophagus in Previously Operated Necks

Re-operating in the neck can be challenging because of fibrosis and altered anatomy. The principles of dissection are the same as described above, but there is an even greater need to use every tool and instrument to facilitate safe dissection, as well as engaging the assistance of an appropriate specialist surgical colleague.

7.2 The Chest

7.2.1 Lateral Thoracotomy

The patient is positioned on the side with the upper arm rotated upwards and extended to rotate the scapula and provide access posteriorly. The lower leg is flexed, and the upper leg is kept straight, with a pillow between the two. It helps to break the table to improve access to the thoracic cavity. It is important to properly secure the patient to the table using appropriate attachments and straps so that the table can be tilted in various planes without the danger of the patient slipping or changing position.

The incision is as long as is necessary. After dividing the latissimus dorsi and the serratus anterior and lifting the scapula off the chest wall, the ribs are exposed and the rib space for entering the chest can be chosen. The level depends on which part of the chest requires optimum access, but, as a rule, it is better to keep higher than lower. However, it should be noted that the higher rib spaces provide less length because of the conical sshape of the thoracic cavity. I usually make a long incision from the sternum extending back to almost the level of the sympathetic chain. The longer the incision, the less chance of breaking a rib during retraction. It is important to determine before the operation whether an intercostal flap will be required as this dictates the way that the chest is opened and the level of entry.

If more access is required once the retractors have been placed, a small segment of the rib can be removed as far posteriorly as possible. Access can also be enhanced by placing two retractors, one anteriorly and the other posteriorly (Fig. 7.4).

Re-operation on the chest, particularly within two weeks of the original thoracotomy, can be difficult due to adherence of the lung to the rib cage. In the first instance, I try and go through the same intercostal space as the original operation. However, if the lung is densely adherent, I enter the chest through the adjacent intercostal space where there might be a better plane and the lung can then be more safely separated from the chest wall. The use of diathermy on a low power setting is useful for separating lung adhesions. Blunt dissection should be kept to a minimum to avoid bleeding and air leaks.

It is important to approximate the ribs properly, particularly if a rib has been divided, resected or fractured during retraction. Inadequate closure can result in an incisional hernia, although these are rare. If the table has been "broken", then it should be put back into a neutral position before closing the ribs. Using figure-of-eight sutures ensures that the neurovascular bundle is avoided.

Fig. 7.4 Diagram showing the use of two rib retractors

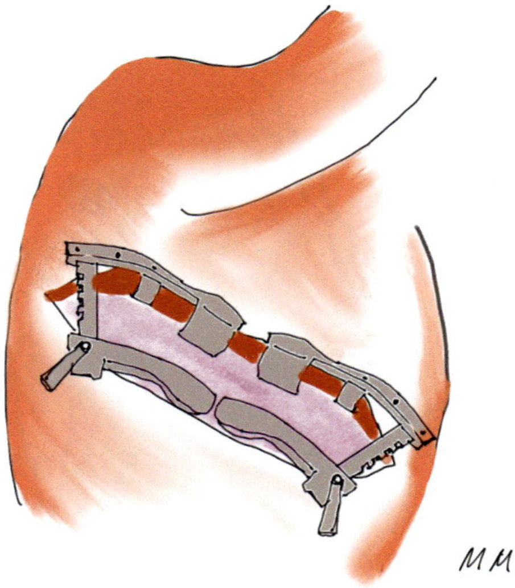

7.2.2 *Creating the Retrosternal Tunnel*

7.2.2.1 Technique

This is a very useful route for a conduit which avoids opening the chest cavity. However, some important technical points need to be emphasised to ensure that the retrosternal space can be created as safely as possible without damage to structures that lie closely apposed to the sternum. Furthermore, it is important to maximise the space so that the blood supply to the conduit is not compromised through being constricted, particularly at the thoracic inlet.

It is easiest to start the dissection from the abdominal side. Whether it is a midline or a rooftop incision, the xiphoid process must be reached. Dissection is then started underneath the xiphoid by first dividing the attachments of the diaphragm to the sternum so that at least four fingers can be comfortably accommodated in this space (Figs. 7.5 and 7.6). The rest of the dissection is done bluntly using the fingers, keeping them in the midline and hugging the back of the sternum as far as the distance the fingers can reach. Unless there has been previous thoracic surgery, this space is easy to develop, and only flimsy adhesions are usually encountered. I usually ask the anaesthetist to stop ventilating the patient whilst carrying out this dissection to avoid breaching the pleura.

If I have made a collar incision, I enlarge it by making a longitudinal extension centrally over the trachea and onto the sternal notch. This is a critical manoeuvre for two reasons. Exposing the notch is important as a landmark in case a sternotomy is required. Secondly, direct visualisation of the important structures is very important to enter the correct, safe plane for starting to create the retrosternal tunnel from the neck (Figs. 7.7 and 7.8).

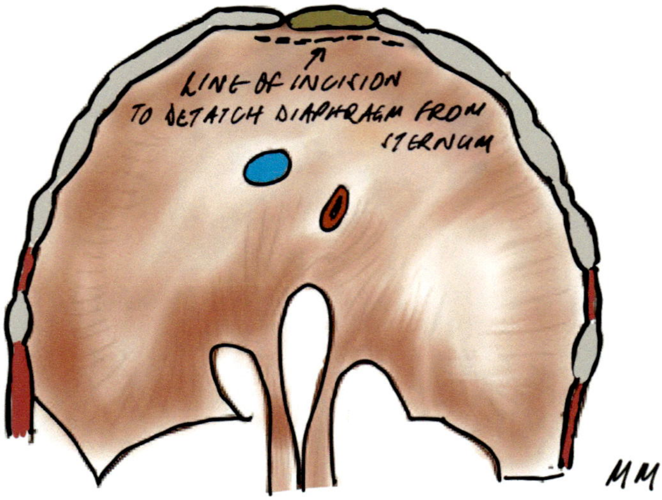

Fig. 7.5 Diagram showing the line of division of the diaphragm to detach it from the sternum to commence the creation of the substernal tunnel

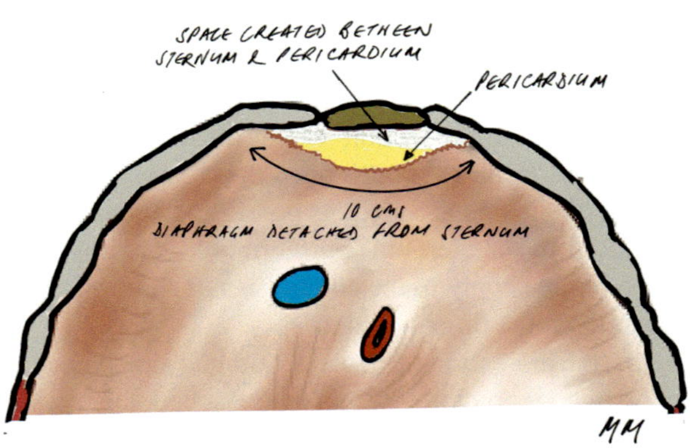

Fig. 7.6 Diagram showing the plane developed from the abdomen into the chest behind the sternum and anterior to the pericardium

Starting and developing the retrosternal plane from the neck is both more difficult and hazardous. Inexperienced surgeons may try to follow the same rules as in developing the plain inferiorly, i.e. hugging the back of the sternum. However, as is shown in Fig. 7.8, the strap muscles are attached to the manubrium and the plane to be developed is behind the strap muscles and in front of the thymus. I start developing this plane by sharp dissection under vision and do not insert my fingers until I am certain I am satisfied that I am in the correct plane. The danger here is damage to the great veins, particularly the brachiocephalic. Venous bleeding can be torrential, and

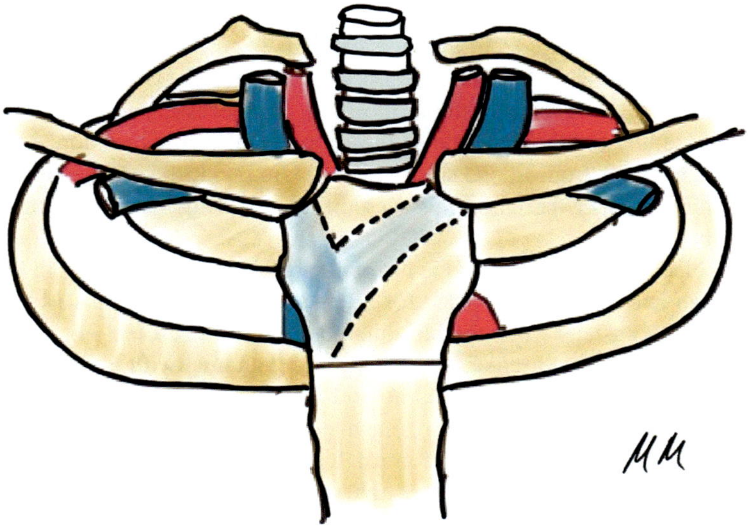

Fig. 7.7 Diagram showing the thoracic inlet and the proximity of the major vessels to the manubrium

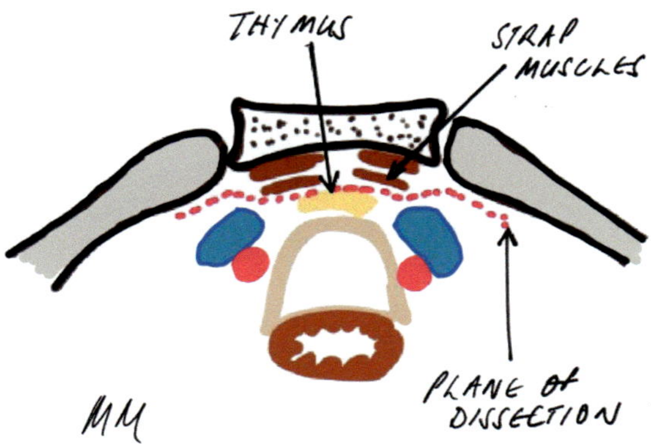

Fig. 7.8 Diagram showing the correct plane (dotted line) for creating the retrosternal tunnel from the neck

therefore I always have the sternal saw available, assembled and tested before I start this dissection.

Once I am satisfied that I am in the right plane coming down from the neck, I insert a long narrow flat, malleable retractor from below, directing it to the neck and keeping it strictly in the midline and hugging the sternum (Figs. 7.9 and 7.10). To avoid damaging the lung or pleura, I ask the anaesthetist to pause ventilation whilst I progressively push the retractor up in short strokes. As the dissection proceeds cranially, resistance is usually encountered from fibrous tissue that needs to be disrupted. It is important to keep the retractor in the midline to avoid damage to the internal mammary vessels. Progress is made by gradually pushing the retractor towards the neck, with pauses to resume ventilation. Eventually, the retractor will reach the neck and emerge from the incision. This is guided visually and with the fingers inserted through the plane developed from the neck. Once the retrosternal space has been fully traversed without bleeding, it is necessary to enlarge it to the maximum width at the thoracic inlet. I have found that this is best done by gently pushing the retractor from side to side, whilst keeping it closely applied to the back of the sternum. In my experience, this is crucial in achieving maximum space at the thoracic inlet.

A little bleeding from the tunnel is inevitable and is easily controlled by pushing down a swab and leaving it in place for a few minutes. Usually, this is all that is necessary. On occasions when the bleeding has been troublesome, but not considered to be due to major vascular injury, packing the tunnel with a swab soaked in a solution of 1:200,000 adrenaline is helpful in achieving haemostasis. However, serious bleeding can occur from tearing the major vessels, particularly the veins, and this usually requires a sternotomy to control. It is important that any bleeding should be stopped before the tunnel is used for transposition.

Some groups have reported using a laparoscope to assist in creating the tunnel, but I have not needed to use this technique.[1] I have never needed to perform a sternotomy to route the conduit. I can see that this technique may be helpful if 'blind' dissection of the retrosternal space was not possible for some reason.

Some surgeons carry out a sternotomy to enable substernal placement of the conduit. During my training, I saw two patients who had undergone a retrosternal

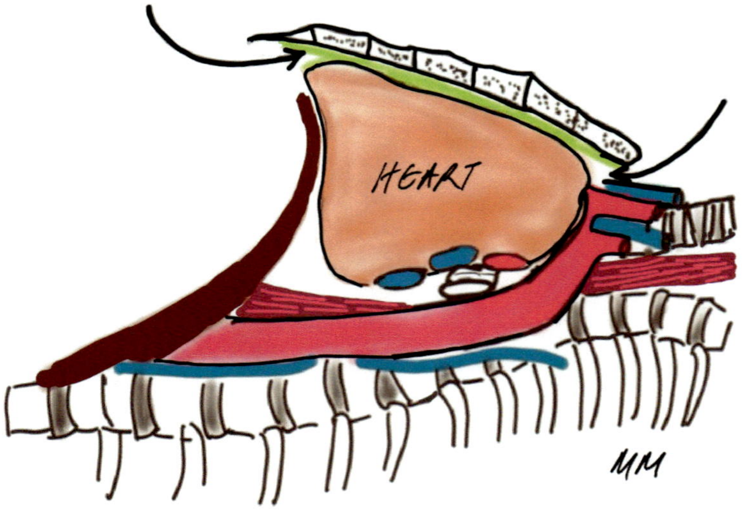

Fig. 7.9 Diagram showing a sagittal section through the midline of the chest. The plane to be developed is shown in green. Inferiorly, this is in front of the heart, but at the level of the neck, the major vessels are in close relationship to the manubrium and space is limited

[1] Manabu et al. [1].

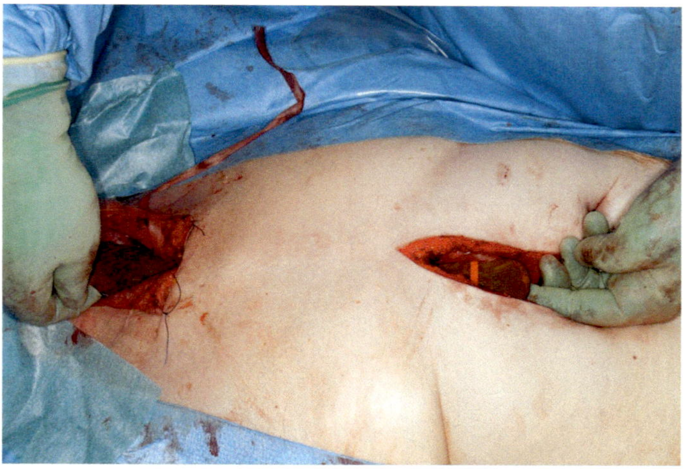

Fig. 7.10 Using a malleable retractor to complete the creation of a substernal tunnel

colonic conduit with a sternotomy and had leaked from the anastomosis. The leak caused a serious and prolonged osteomyelitis of the sternum. The excision of the manubrio-clavicular joint to make space at the thoracic inlet has also been advocated to create more space at the thoracic inlet. I have only performed this on one occasion for a patient who had previously undergone a sternotomy twice for cardiac surgery.

7.2.3 Thoraco-Abdominal Incision

In my experience, this has rarely been necessary for reconstructive surgery.

7.3 Difficult Chest Access

7.3.1 Case Summary

A man in his 60s with T3 N1 M0 adenocarcinoma of the lower third of the oesophagus was referred after resection was abandoned for technical reasons.

The patient was in good general health and did not have a significant past medical history other than that of a serious road traffic accident 15 years ago, causing multiple right-sided rib fractures and haemopneumothorax, for which he was hospitalised for a prolonged period.

He had been treated with neoadjuvant chemotherapy with good response and surgery was commenced with a laparoscopic mobilisation of the stomach, which

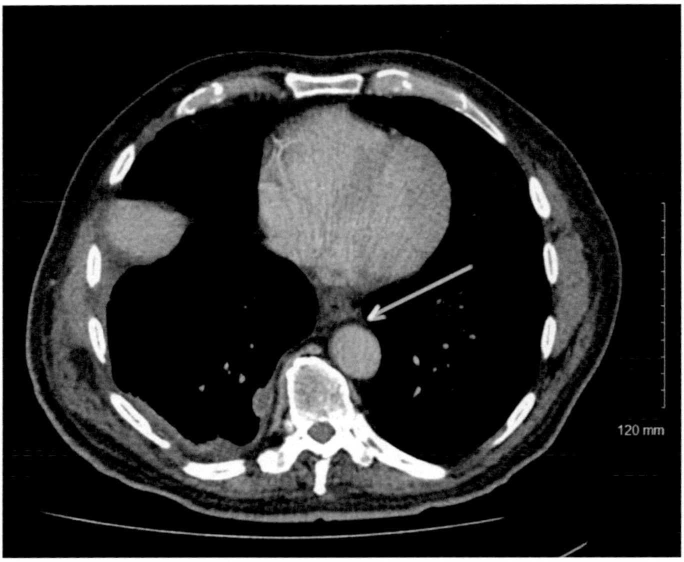

Fig. 7.11 CT section at the level of the tumour with arrow indicating clear fat planes around it

was uneventful. He was repositioned, and a right thoracotomy was attempted but the chest cavity could not be entered because of dense adhesions to the lung. The initial entry had been through the fifth interspace. An opinion and assistance were sought from the thoracic team who attempted entry through a higher space but were also unsuccessful.

He was seen a few weeks after his surgery from which he had recovered well. His imaging was reviewed (Figs. 7.11 and 7.12), and it was decided to carry out a three-stage oesophagectomy approaching the oesophagus from the left chest.

The operation commenced with a left thoracotomy through the sixth intercostal space. Entry into the chest was straightforward, and the oesophagus and the tumour were mobilised below the aortic arch (Fig. 7.13). The normal oesophagus above the arch was mobilised with a combination of blunt and sharp dissection, and the chest closed with a drain.

The patient was repositioned supine and the stomach, which had previously been mobilised, was easily re-mobilised through a midline laparotomy. The cervical oesophagus was approached through a left neck incision and divided 5 cm below the cricopharynx. The distal oesophagus with the tumour was then pulled down into the abdomen and resected. A gastric conduit was created and pulled up through the mediastinum into the neck and anastomosed to the cervical oesophagus (Figs. 7.14 and 7.15).

The patient made an uneventful post-operative recovery.

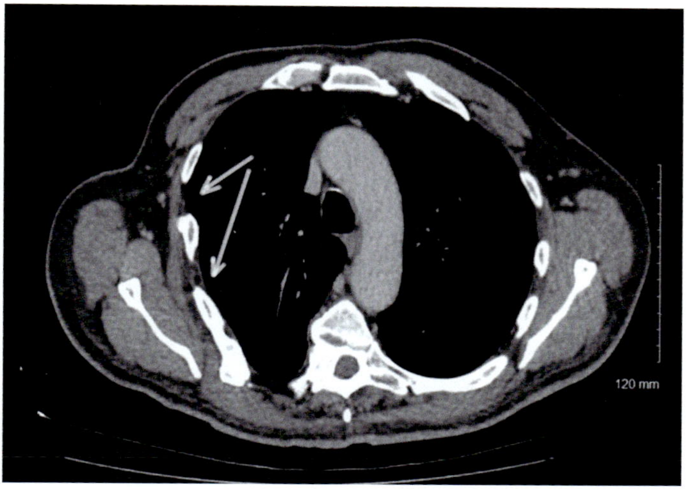

Fig. 7.12 CT section of lower chest with arrows showing right-sided chest wall deformity

Fig. 7.13 Left thoracotomy view showing the oesophagus mobilised up to and under the aortic arch. The upper limit of the tumour is indicated by the tip of the forceps

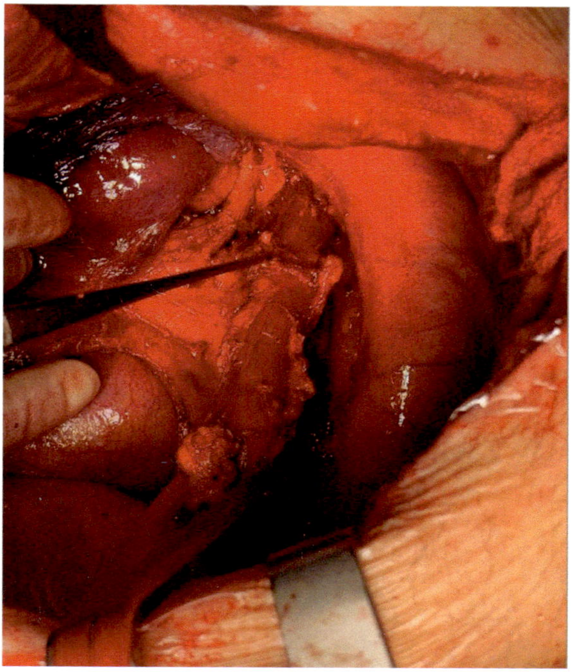

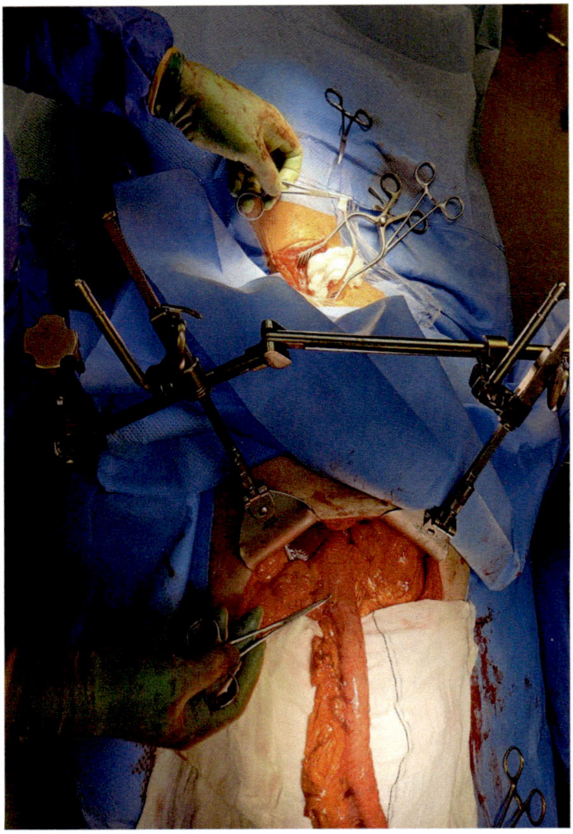

Fig. 7.14 View of the cervical and abdominal field showing the gastric tube ready for transposition

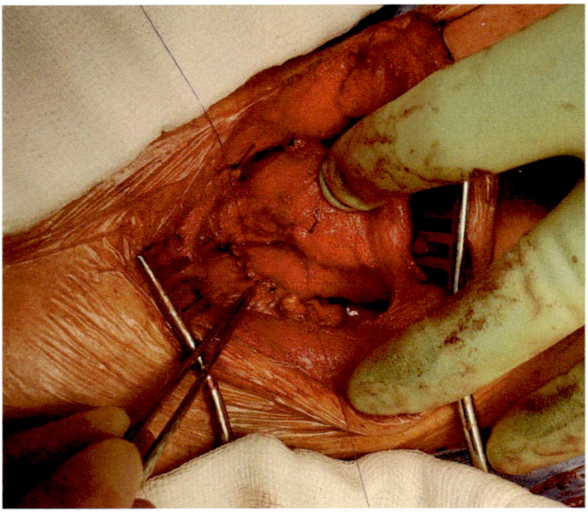

Fig. 7.15 Completed anastomosis in the neck indicated by forceps with the mobilised left lobe of the thyroid reflected anteriorly

7.3.2 Learning Points

Access into the thoracic cavity can prove difficult or impossible in some situations, as in this case. However, it is well to remember that the oesophagus can easily be approached through the left chest. The aortic arch makes it difficult to perform a high intrathoracic anastomosis, although this can be achieved by flipping the oesophagus from under the arch to above it. Even then, space is quite restricted through the left chest and it is easier to perform the anastomosis in the neck, as in this case.

7.4 Thoracic Incisional Hernia

7.4.1 Case Summary

A man in his 50s who had undergone an Ivor-Lewis oesophagectomy for a T3 N1 M0 adenocarcinoma of the GOJ three years previously complained of pain and swelling in his thoracotomy scar.

On examination, the scar was well healed, but there was a wide gap between the sixth and seventh ribs, and an incisional hernia was easily demonstrable as a bulge when he exhaled or coughed. There was indrawing of the skin over the rib space on inspiration. It was initially managed expectantly, but the hernia continued to enlarge. Repeat imaging showed no evidence of recurrent tumour or metastatic disease but quite a large gap between the sixth and seventh ribs on the right with prolapsing lung (Fig. 7.16). This is also well shown in the reconstructed images (Fig.7.17).

The patient was offered a repair. He was positioned for a right thoracotomy, the thinned-out scar was excised, and the lung carefully separated from the underlying atrophic intercostal muscles and the ribs. Careful dissection was required to separate the lung which was stuck to the thoracic wall above and below the level of the original thoracotomy. The sixth and seventh ribs were strong, and there was no evidence of a fracture associated with the original thoracotomy. After fully mobilising the right lung and inserting a chest drain, the rib space was closed with five #5 Ethibond figure-of-eight sutures, apposing the ribs and almost obliterating the rib space (Fig. 7.18).

The patient made an uneventful post-operative recovery with no hernia recurrence two years later. He continued to have some pain in the region, which was eventually treated with intercostal nerve cryotherapy.

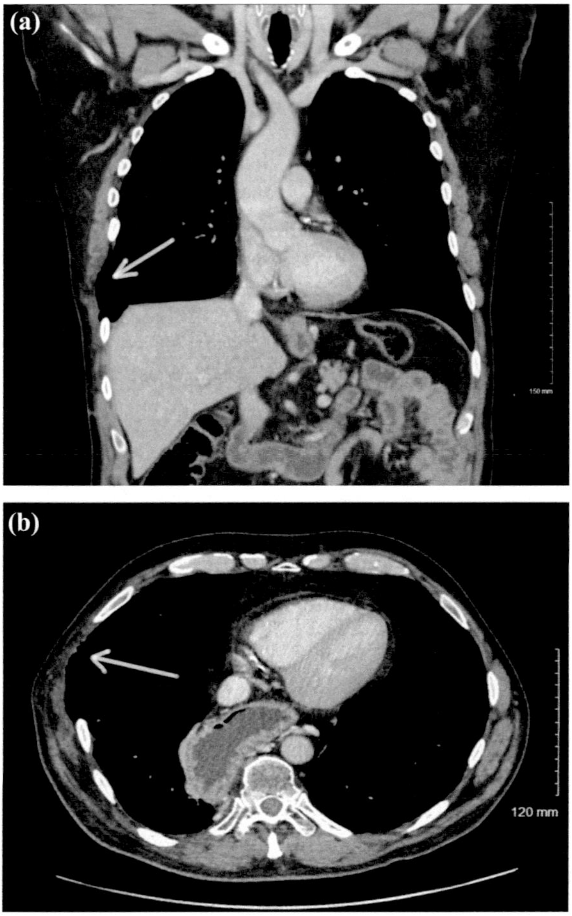

Fig. 7.16 Coronal (a) and axial (b) views with arrows showing right lung hernia

7.4.2 Learning Points

Lung hernias are uncommon, and the aetiology includes congenital, traumatic and postsurgical causes. The majority are a result of penetrating or blunt trauma.[2] Post thoracotomy hernias are uncommon, and the same aetiological factors apply as with abdominal wall hernias, i.e., technical factors, early wound dehiscence, immunosuppression, steroid treatment and chronic cough. In our patient, the hernia must have occurred as a result of technical factors, although the thoracotomy wound had healed without infection or early dehiscence. The patient had been reviewed and scanned every six months for the first two years during which no hernia was apparent.

[2] Scelfo et al. [2].

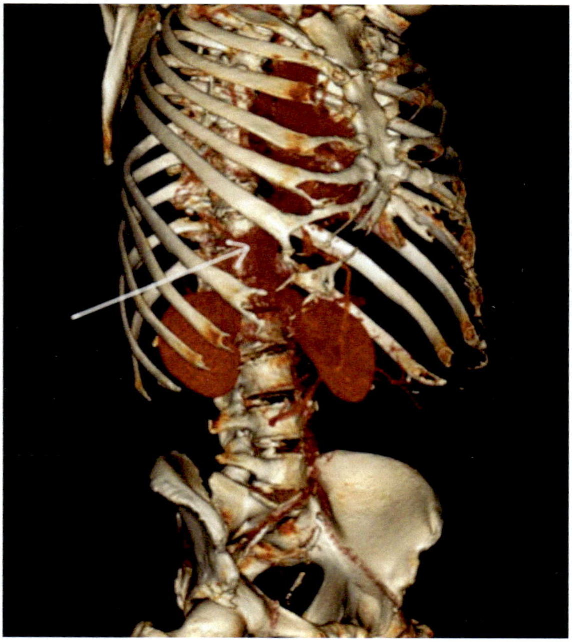

Fig. 7.17 Reconstructed image with arrow showing the gap between intact right sixth and seventh ribs

Before contemplating repair, it was important to carry out up-to-date imaging to ensure that there was no evidence of tumour recurrence or metastatic disease that might have changed the treatment plan. CT scan with 3-D reconstruction showed a clear the gap between the ribs. Imaging also showed that the ribs above and below were intact and normal without fractures, and therefore amenable to suture approximation. Just as with an abdominal wall hernia and the likelihood of bowel adherent to the sac, we found a similar adherence of the lung, which had to be carefully separated. This was performed using diathermy with a spatula point that was bent at an angle to enable the dissection to be kept close to the chest wall without damaging lung parenchyma.

In this case, we did not have to use mesh to augment the repair.

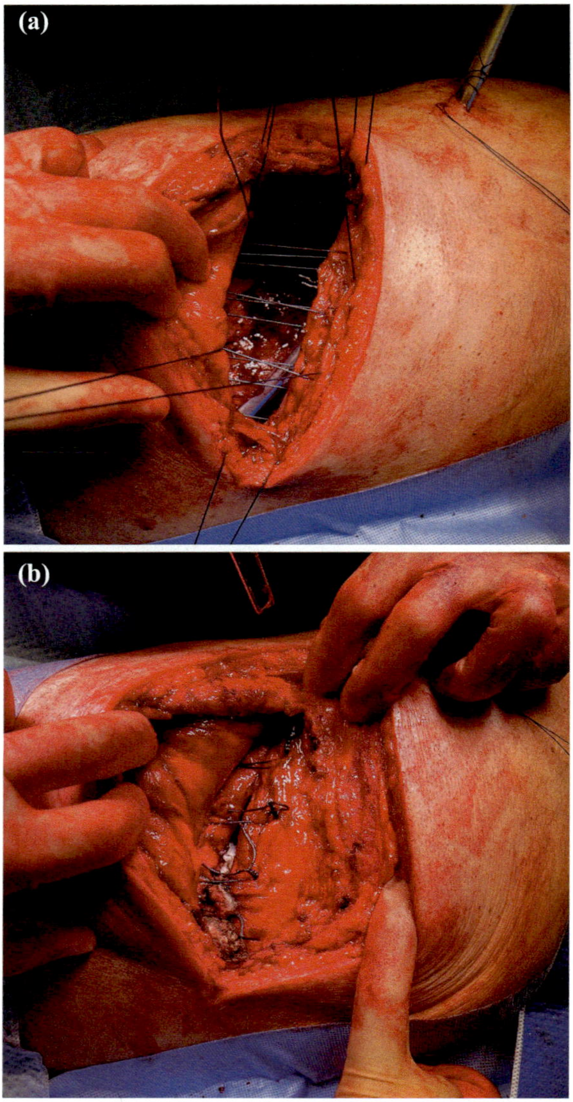

Fig. 7.18 Chest closure sutures placed (a) and tied (b)

7.5 Unusual Anatomy

7.5.1 Case Summary

A woman in her 40s was diagnosed with a T2 N0 M0 adenocarcinoma of the GOJ. Staging CT also showed left-sided isomerism/heterotaxy syndrome. This was made up of the following abnormalities: azygous continuation of the IVC (in essence, the azygous vein was the IVC) malposition of the stomach, which was situated to the right, malrotation of the bowel with the caecum lying in the left upper quadrant of the abdomen, polysplenia and a truncated pancreas.

The main difficulty anticipated was in the dissection of the oesophagus at the level of the carina where it was completely surrounded by vital structures (Fig. 7.19). Starting with the spine at the 6 o'clock position working clockwise, next is the IVC replaced by the azygous, at 9 o'clock the left main bronchus, at 2 o'clock the right main bronchus and at 4 o'clock the descending aorta.

The operation commenced with a laparotomy. Although the stomach was on the right, it had a conventional arterial supply, and it was possible to mobilise it in the usual way based on the gastroepiploic arch. After performing a lymphadenectomy and placing a feeding jejunostomy the abdomen was closed, and the patient was

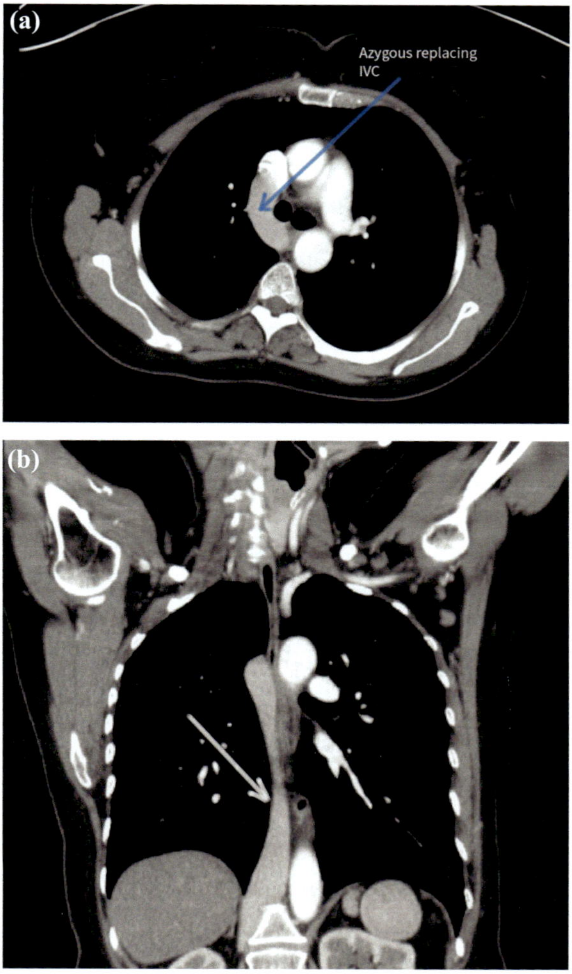

Fig. 7.19 CT sections with arrows showing replacement of inferior vena cava with the azygous vein

Fig. 7.20 Diagram depicting pre-operative anatomy

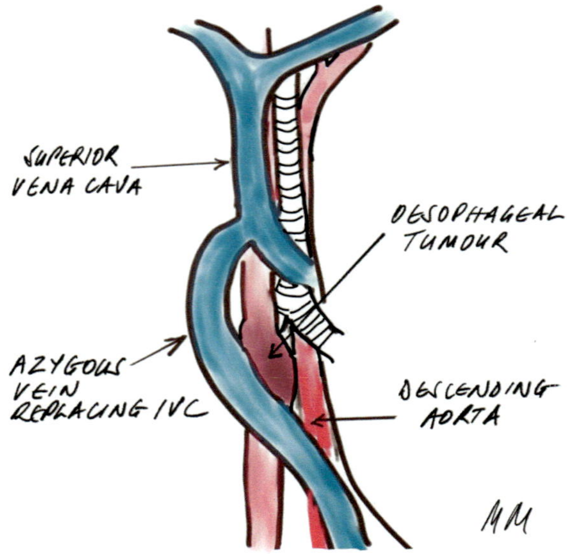

repositioned. A right thoracotomy was carried out which revealed the abnormality as depicted in Fig. 7.20.

The oesophagus was dissected from behind the arching azygous vein and after transection at the level of the carina, it was brought in front of the azygous and anastomosed to the gastric conduit (Figs. 7.21 and 7.22).

The patient made an uneventful post-operative recovery.

7.5.2 *Learning Points*

Heterotaxy syndrome and interrupted inferior vena cava (IVC) with azygos continuation is rare.[3] It is estimated to affect 1 in 10,000 people in the Western World. We had never encountered it previously.

In this case, the anatomy had to be carefully considered both in terms of the usability of the stomach for a conventional gastric conduit and the ability to safely dissect out the oesophagus and carry out an anastomosis in the chest. Luckily, the tumour was at the GOJ, below the difficult dissection in the chest, where, essentially, it was a normal oesophagus that had to be carefully separated from crowded vital structures.

We spent a long time going through the images with radiologists to understand the anatomy and discuss our surgical strategy, which worked out as planned.

---

[3] Dolatkhah et al. [3].

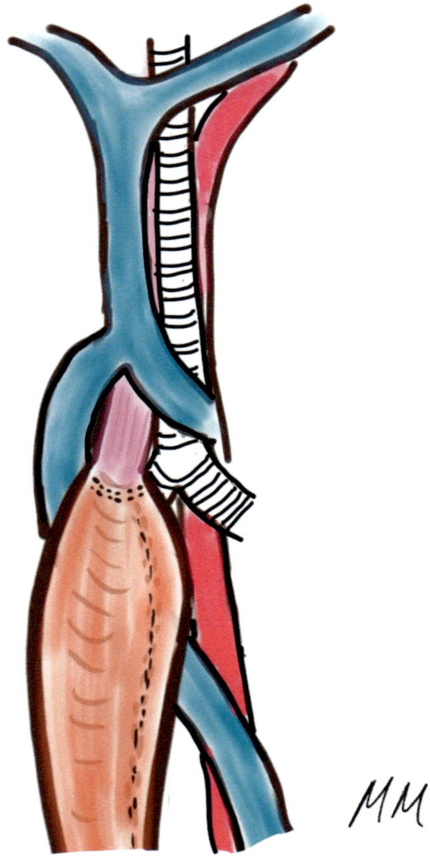

Fig. 7.21 Resection and reconstruction showing the conduit lying anterior to the azygous vein

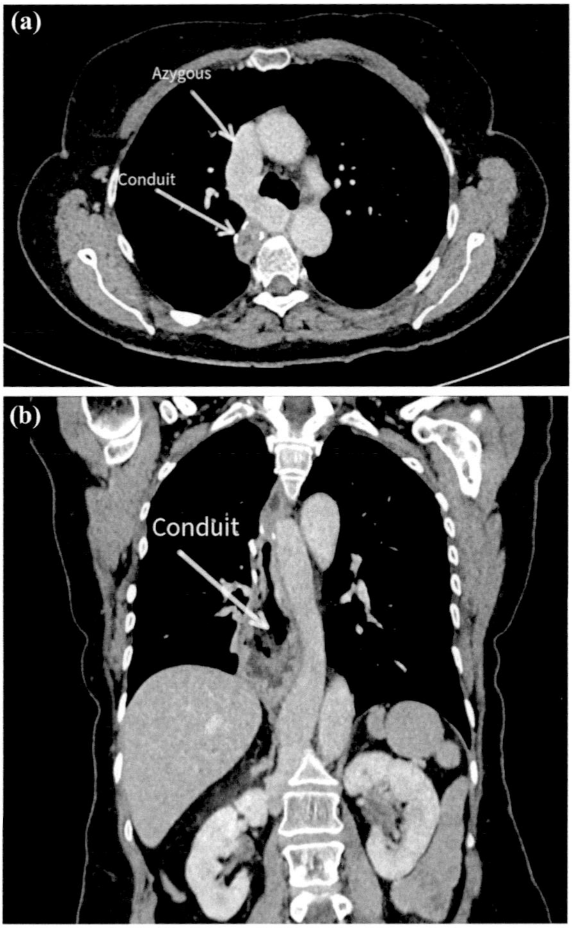

Fig. 7.22 Axial (a) and coronal (b) CT sections showing the position of the conduit relative to the azygos vein

7.6 Abdomen

Access to the abdomen can be gained by a variety of incisions. The long midline incision is adequate for most cases and has the advantage of providing exposure to the entire abdominal viscera, which is particularly useful if a colonic interposition is contemplated. However, if optimum exposure is required mainly in the supracolic compartment, the alternative incisions are a rooftop or an L-shaped incision. Both of these lend themselves to optimal application of table-mounted retractors to lift up the costal margin to open up the subdiaphragmatic field of dissection (Figs. 7.23, 7.24 and 7.25).

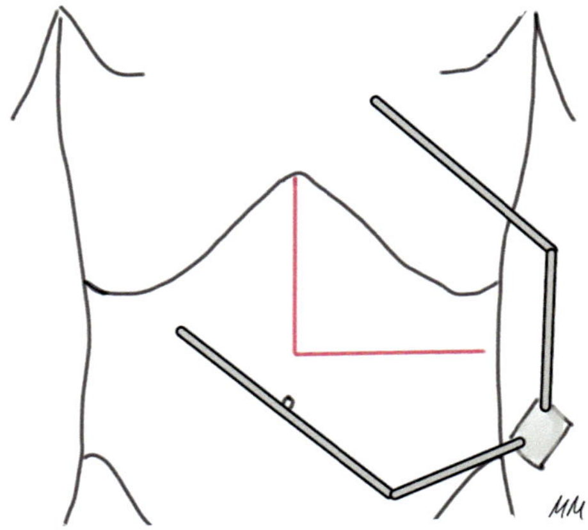

Fig. 7.23 L-shaped incision and positioning of table-mounted retractor

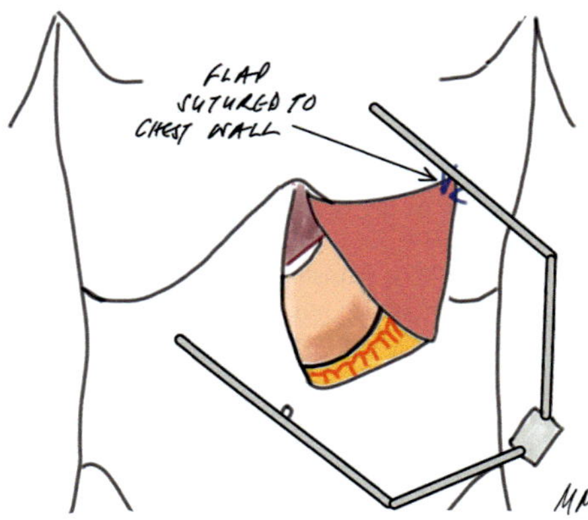

Fig. 7.24 Resulting triangular myocutaneous flap folded and sutured above the left costal margin

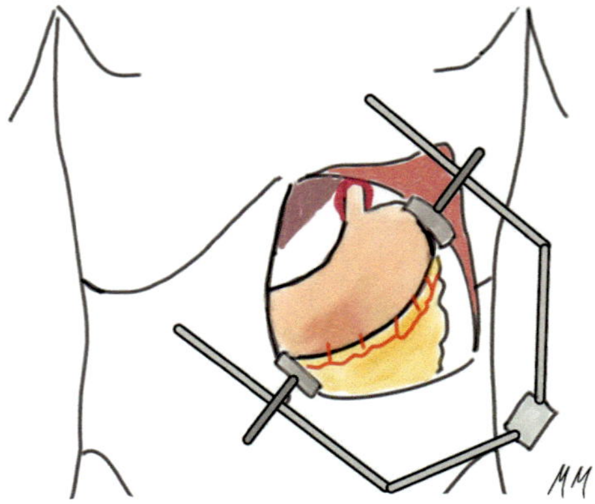

Fig. 7.25 Table-mounted retractor in place

References

1. Manabu H, Taro O. This link will open in a new window Link to external site, Gosuke T, Naoki U, Hasegawa H, Masashi Y et al. Laparoscopic creation of a retrosternal route for gastric conduit reconstruction. Surg Endoscopy **36**(4), 2680–87. https://doi.org/10.1007/s00464-021-08745-y
2. Scelfo C, Longo C, Aiello M, Bertorelli G, Crisafulli E, Chetta A. Pulmonary Hernia: case report and review of the literature. Respirology Case Reports. 2018;6(8): e00354. https://doi.org/10.1002/rcr2.354.
3. Dolatkhah MA, Farashah MSG, Hesam N. Heterotaxy syndrome and interrupted inferior vena cava (IVC) with azygos continuation. 2020;27(2).

Chapter 8
Bridging Strategies and 'Toolbox' of Reconstruction

Abstract This chapter explores oesophageal exclusion as a method of diverting contaminants like saliva, fluids, and gastric contents, particularly in cases of large perforations or fistulas. The goal is to control mediastinal and chest sepsis while awaiting definitive treatment. Various exclusion techniques are discussed, including loop oesophagostomy, lateral oesophagostomy, and end oesophagostomy, each with its benefits and considerations for future reconstruction. Additionally, the chapter covers the use of intercostal muscle flaps for bolstering repairs, gastric exclusion to prevent reflux, and techniques for feeding jejunostomy. It also delves into the management of thoracic collections and sepsis, highlighting the importance of choosing the right intervention at the right time. Endoscopic vacuum therapy, including the EsoSponge and VAC-Stent, are presented as effective options for managing oesophagogastric perforations and leaks, with emphasis on proper placement and regular monitoring for optimal outcomes. Overall, the chapter provides a comprehensive overview of bridging strategies and reconstruction techniques essential for managing complex oesophageal conditions.

Keywords Oesophageal exclusion · Bridging strategies · Reconstruction · Oesophagostomy · Gastric exclusion · Intercostal muscle flaps · Thoracic drainage · Feeding jejunostomy · Endoscopic vacuum therapy · EsoSponge · VacStent

8.1 Oesophageal Exclusion

Oesophageal exclusion is used to keep it free of saliva, ingested fluids and food, and from reflux of gastric contents. It is most often considered when there is a large perforation of the oesophagus or in cases of fistulation to the airways. It is a useful bridging strategy to minimise or control mediastinal and chest sepsis in the hope that the underlying pathology can eventually be dealt with and continuity of the oesophagus restored. When considering oesophageal exclusion, it is important to consider the likelihood of eventual reconstruction because that dictates how the exclusion is carried out.

M. Mughal, *Reconstructive Surgery of the Oesophagus and Stomach*,
https://doi.org/10.1007/978-3-031-66846-3_8

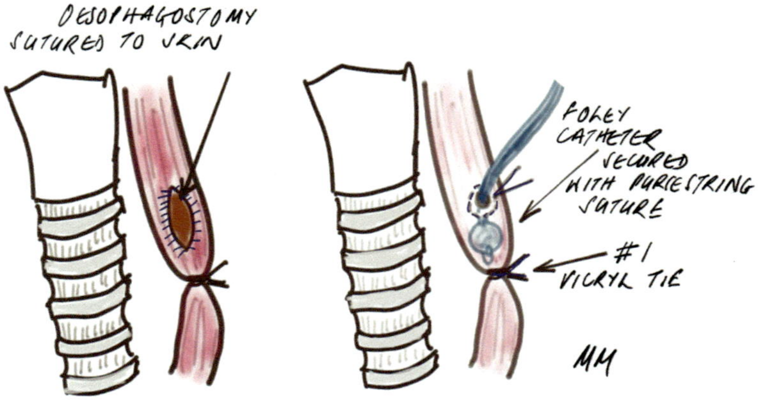

Fig. 8.1 On the left is the technique described by Urschel and on the right is my technique, which does not require bringing the oesophagus to the skin

In principle, to exclude the oesophagus from all fluids and food, an oesophagostomy is required proximally, and the oesophagus needs to be either closed off temporarily at the gastro-oesophageal junction or some other strategy is adopted to prevent gastro-oesophageal reflux. Examples of different strategies are described in some of the cases presented in this book.

Forming an oesophagostomy is not simple. The cervical oesophagus is deeply buried in the neck, with important structures surrounding it. Also, a normal oesophagus is essentially a straight tube tethered proximally at the hypopharynx and distally at the hiatus. Therefore, unless a substantial part of the oesophagus is fully mobilised and the gastro-oesophageal junction released, it is impossible to easily perform a loop oesophagostomy. In my experience, there is not enough give in the oesophagus for this, even if 10 to 15 cm can be freed up in the neck. Having said that, a form of loop or side oesophagostomy has been described, mobilising the cervical oesophagus and then carrying out a longitudinal oesophagotomy, the edges of which are then sutured to the skin.[1] This results in a lateral oesophagostomy leaving the oesophagus in continuity. The authors do not explain how the technique can divert saliva and oral fluids since the oesophagus remains in continuity. They also describe a technique of the temporary closure of the distal oesophagus with a Teflon band tied with nylon tape below an oesophageal perforation with a gastrostomy to drain the stomach.

Another group has described a variation to this by tying the oesophagus with a heavy absorbable suture below a lateral oesophagostomy, ensuring that no secretions reach oesophagostomy the distal oesophagus.[2] The beauty of this technique is that the absorbable suture dissolves after a few weeks, and oesophageal continuity is restored naturally. I have used this technique on several occasions and can attest to its success (Fig. 8.1).

---

[1] Urschel et al. [1].

[2] Koniaris et al. [2].

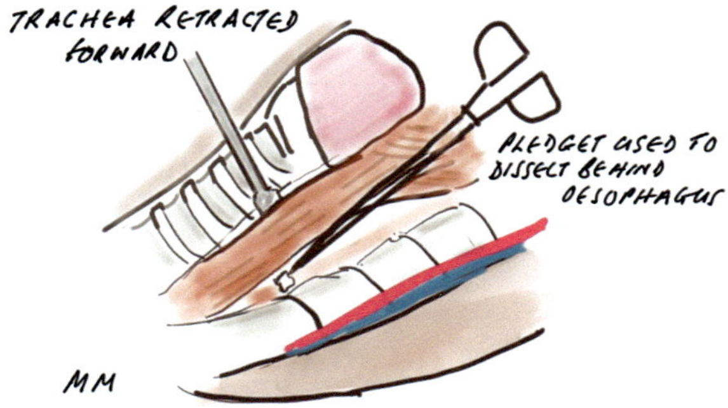

Fig. 8.2 Separating the oesophagus from the spine, posteriorly with a pledget

Raymond and Watson have described a more conventional end oesophagostomy resulting in complete exclusion of the oesophagus from the oropharynx. It involves mobilising a length of the cervical oesophagus, transecting it, closing off the distal end and bringing out the proximal end as a stoma in the neck.[3] The gastro-oesophageal junction is closed off with a non-cutting stapler. They have found that the staple line lasts about two weeks before it opens up. Therefore, this is an ideal technique, if exclusion is only required for a short time. In many cases, this may be all that is needed and has the great advantage of avoiding the need for further, potentially challenging, surgery to re-establishing continuity between the oesophagus and the stomach.

To create an end oesophagostomy, it is important to dissect the oesophagus well down into the superior mediastinum before transection. Otherwise, there may be insufficient length for a tension-free free oesophagostomy and, also, reconstruction is made more difficult by a short stump. After encircling the cervical oesophagus, as described in the previous section, a nylon tape is passed around the oesophagus to provide traction, and the trachea is gently retracted medially, safeguarding the recurrent laryngeal nerve. The oesophagus can be easily freed posteriorly by blunt dissection with a pledget. Anteriorly, it is separated from the trachea using bipolar diathermy. At least 6–8 cm of the oesophagus is freed up in this way and then transected using a stapler or by suture-ligation (Figs. 8.2 and 8.3).

I have described diagrammatically the three types of oesophageal exclusion I have used.

Figure 8.4 shows a formal end cervical oesophagostomy. A drainage gastrostomy is performed along with a feeding jejunostomy. This completely diverts oral fluids from the oesophagus, but even with the drainage gastrostomy, gastric juices can reflux into the oesophagus. It therefore works well with a perforation in the proximal oesophagus, but not one near the gastro-oesophageal junction.

A different technique is illustrated in Fig. 8.5. The cervical procedure is the same as the configuration illustrated in Fig. 8.4, but the stomach is transected in the same way as it would be in creating a gastric conduit, but leaving the lesser curve attached to the oesophagus. I call this the gastric partioning procedure. The lesser curve of

[3] Raymond and Watson [3].

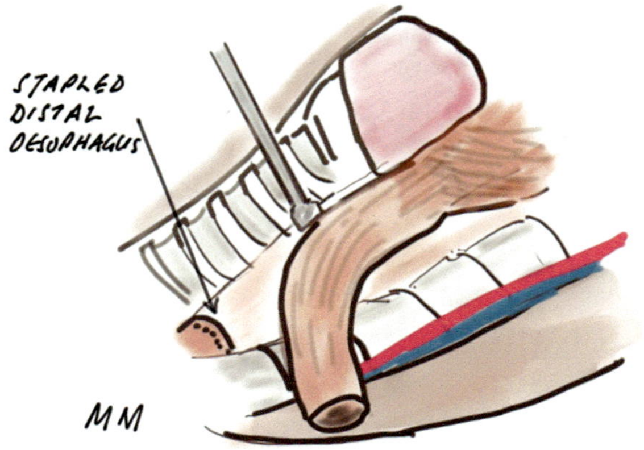

Fig. 8.3 The oesophagus transected low down in the superior mediastinum, providing a good length for the oesophagostomy

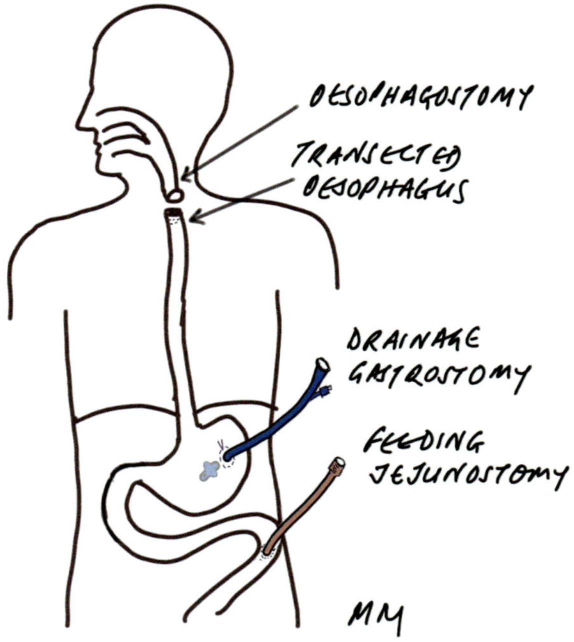

Fig. 8.4 Transection of cervical oesophagus with end oesophagostomy, drainage gastrostomy and feeding jejunostomy

the stomach is drained with a Foley catheter (Fig. 8.6). This completely excludes the oesophagus whilst retaining access to the oesophagus which may be useful in certain circumstances, as will be illustrated in some of the cases described later. The partitioned greater curve side of the stomach can be used as a conduit for oesophageal replacement or bypass at the same operation or later as required. I have not seen this procedure described before.

Figure 8.7 shows a way of achieving temporary oesophageal exclusion without the need for a later reconstruction. The cervical oesophagus is closed with a 0 or 1

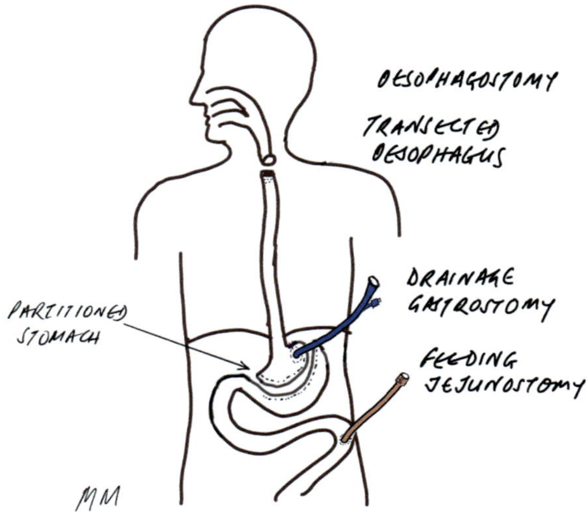

Fig. 8.5 Transection of cervical with end oesophagostomy, partitioning of stomach and drainage of oesophagus through the attached lesser curve

Vicryl suture and a Foley catheter is placed in the oesophagus above it and secured with a purse string suture. The gastro-oesophageal junction is closed with a non-cutting stapler. The oesophagus between the Vicryl suture above, and the staple line below is thereby excluded. A drainage gastrostomy and feeding jejunostomy are also placed. Oesophageal continuity is restored naturally by the suture reabsorbing and the staple line opening up in 2 to 6 weeks, although both areas of temporary closure may need dilatation to achieve full patency. This configuration obviates the need for a reconstruction, provided this is only required for a short period of time. It is also only suitable for treating a perforation, as closing the intact oesophagus would create a closed tube resulting in the accumulation of mucus.

I have used a similar strategy for temporarily isolating a large leak from the proximal staple line following a sleeve gastrectomy.

An end oesophagostomy usually requires the creation of a conduit to restore continuity, even if the excluded oesophagus were to become technically usable by complete healing of a perforation or leak. Even when the oesophagostomy has been performed by simply transecting the oesophagus, the transected end becomes fibrotic, and the excluded oesophagus shortens over time. In any case, the distal end of the oesophagus is difficult to free up, and a tension-free end-to-end anastomosis would not be achievable. It is important to emphasise that an end oesophagostomy almost always requires a conduit to restore continuity. Therefore, the technique for oesophageal exclusion must be chosen with care with future implications in mind.

There is an interesting case report describing the transection of the oesophagus in the neck with a stapler for oesophageal exclusion with the proximal end intubated rather than being brought out as a formal oesophagostomy.[4] However, eventually, there was a leak from the transected proximal end, which 'broke' into the stapled

[4] Ryohei [4].

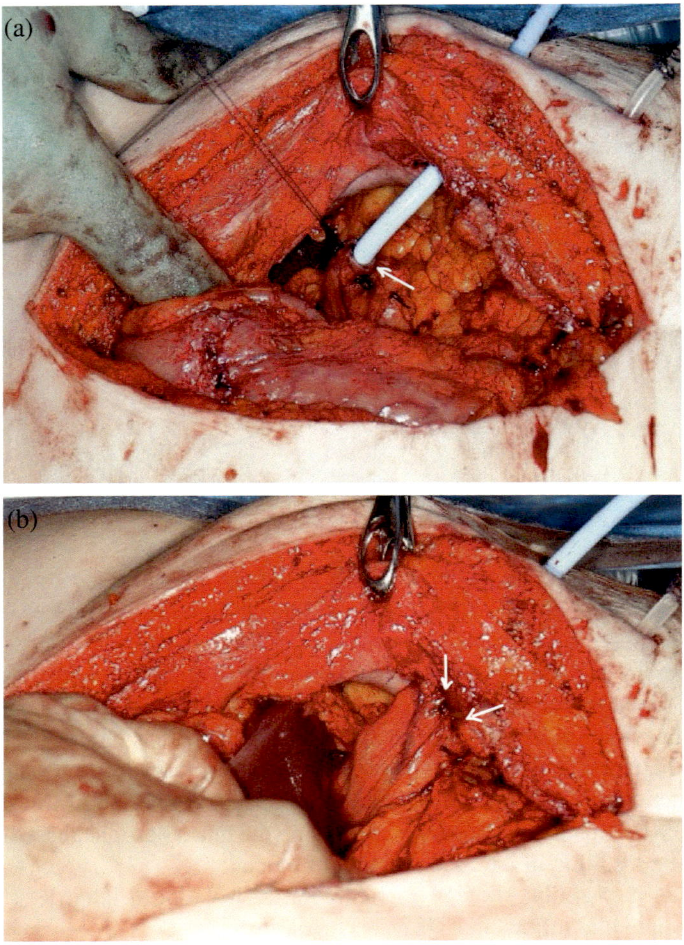

Fig. 8.6 Foley catheter placed in the partitioned lesser curve of the stomach (a) and brought up to the anterior abdominal wall (b) shown by arrows

distal end, resulting in spontaneous re-establishment of continuity! This is plausible, considering that the two ends would have been close to each other (Fig. 8.8). But my technique of achieving temporary closure of the cervical oesophagus by tying it with absorbable suture with a tube oesophagostomy above is a simple and reliable technique obviating the need for reconstruction once the oesophageal perforation has healed.

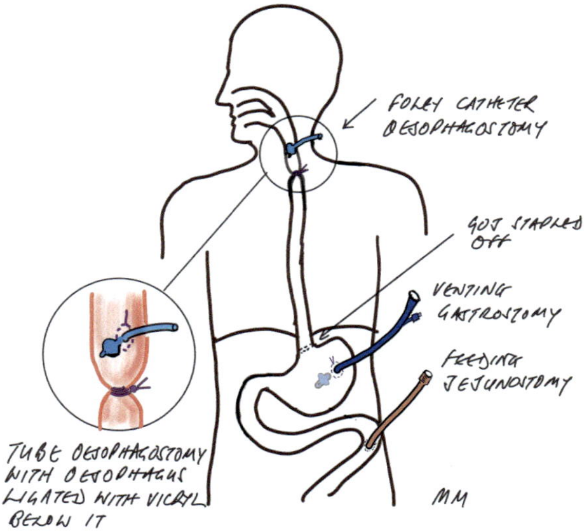

Fig. 8.7 T-Tube oesophagostomy with ligation of cervical oesophagus and stapling of GOJ to provide temporary exclusion without the need for interventions to re-establish patency

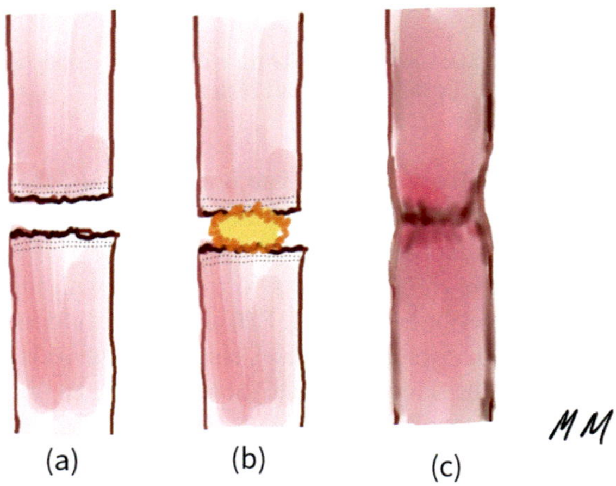

Fig. 8.8 Oesophagus divided with a stapler with ends lying close together (a), complicated by disruption of staple line with abscess formation between the ends (b) resulting in re-establishment of continuity with stricture formation (c)

8.2 Intercostal Muscle Flap

Intercostal muscle flaps are useful for bolstering repairs of the airways and the oesophagus. Although technically the flap can be raised from any of the rib spaces apart from the first and second, the lower rib spaces provide a longer flap. However, selection of the space to harvest the flap depends on the exact requirement. Basically, the level of the flap is chosen for its proximity to the area of the repair and to obtain as long length as possible.

Once the need for an intercostal flap has been established, the rib retractors are removed and re-appled to the chest wall exposing several intercostal spaced. The

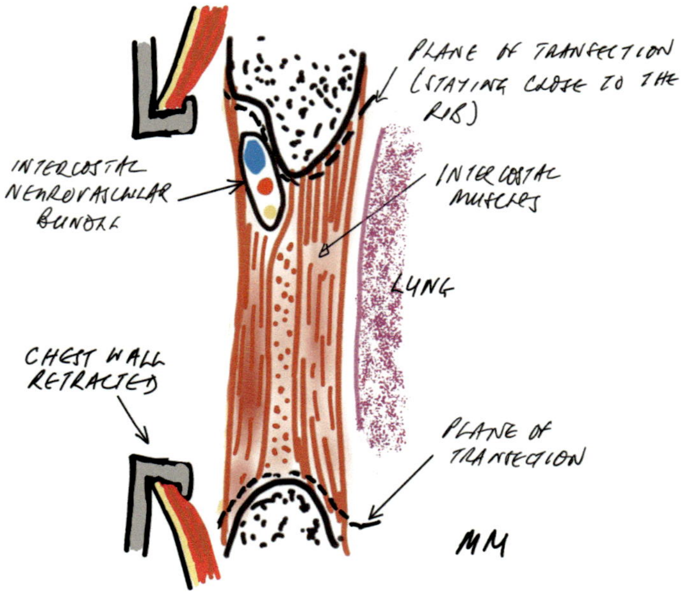

Fig. 8.9 Diagram showing the neurovascular bundle closely applied to the under surface of the rib, and the plane to be followed for safe separation

interspace for harvesting the flap is identified and the flap can be raised in two ways. It can be raised by keeping the associated rib in situ or excising it subperiosteally. I prefer not to excise the rib.

I score the rib above the selected space with the diathermy a few millimetres above its inferior border (Fig. 8.9) and along its length as far back as possible to the level of the paraspinal muscles. Using a periosteal elevator, the periosteum is scraped down from the scored edge and then, hugging the rib, and keeping subperiosteally, a plane is developed on the inside of the superior rib, detaching the intercostal muscle with the neurovascular bundle (Fig. 8.10). Once the correct plane has been entered, and the vascular bundle becomes visible the dissection is relatively easy, keeping the neurovascular bundle in view whilst separating it gradually from the rib as far back as possible. The flap is detached as anteriorly as possible and mobilised as posteriorly as possible to give a longer length. Once any bleeding has been stopped, the flap is wrapped in a warm, damp swab and kept carefully out of the way until needed (Fig. 8.11). The rib retractors should be replaced with care so as not to damage the intercostal flap.

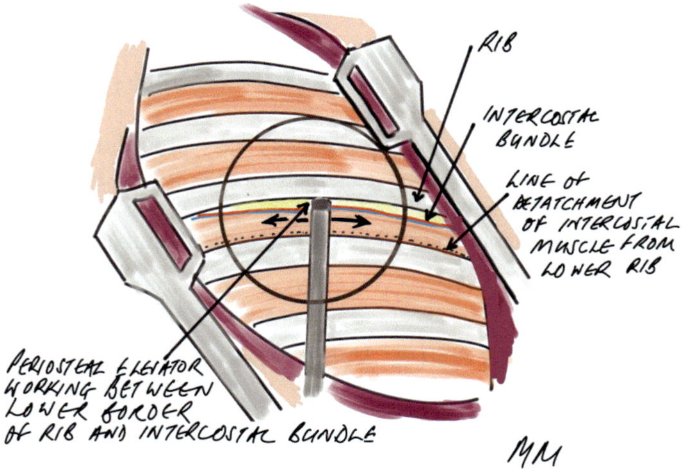

Fig. 8.10 Diagram showing separation of the neuromuscular bundle and intercostal muscle from the rib using a periosteal elevator

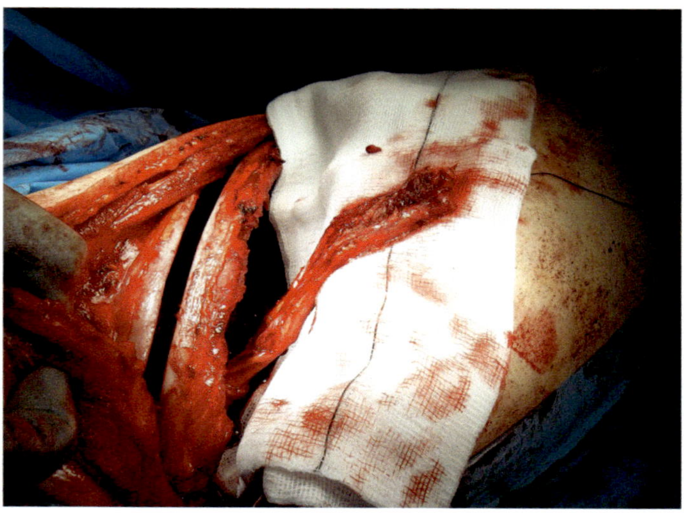

Fig. 8.11 Intercostal muscle flap, fully harvested and ready for use. Note that it has been taken from the space above the level of the thoracotomy

8.3 Indications for and Techniques for Gastric Exclusion

Gastric exclusion can be used as part of oesophageal exclusion to stop the reflux of gastric contents into the oesophagus or for gastric perforations. For instance, I have used it as a bridging strategy in a large chronic perforation from a gastric sleeve to isolate the stomach from the adjacent cavity. It is also helpful, again as a bridging strategy, for large and complex gastroduodenal perforations. I have used it for traumatic rupture of the duodeno-pancreatic complex and large iatrogenic perforations of the duodenum associated with a chronic cavity when the patient is not fit for definitive treatment.

Applying a non-cutting stapler is a relatively easy procedure, often requiring minimal dissection, simply to be able to get around the full width of the stomach. However, the exclusion is temporary and can only be relied on to be effective for two to six weeks. It does not require surgery to re-establish the lumen of the stomach.

8.3.1 Techniques for Feeding Jejunostomy

A large variety of commercially available tubes is available to establish a feeding jejunostomy. My preference is to use the MIC because it is secure and durable. It has two wings near the inner tip of the tube, which are used to secure the tube into a Witzel tunnel as well as a Dacron cuff in the extra-abdominal portion, which becomes incorporated in the subcurtaneous tissues over time (Fig. 8.12). This obviates the need for permanent retaining sutures needed to secure tubes without cuffs and which can damage the tube. In my experience and practice, MIC tubes have lasted up to two years, provided they are well cared for. Also, the external part of the tube, particularly the connector, can be replaced using a repair kit, further increasing the tube's lifespan.

The tube is inserted into the jejunum, usually 25 to 30 cm distal to the DJ flexure, with one wing just inside the bowel. A Witzel tunnel is then created between the two wings. The tube is then brought through the selected exit site using the extroducer, and secured to the parietal peritoneum and posterior sheath with sutures passed through the eyelets of the external wing. It is important to ensure some laxity in the bowel

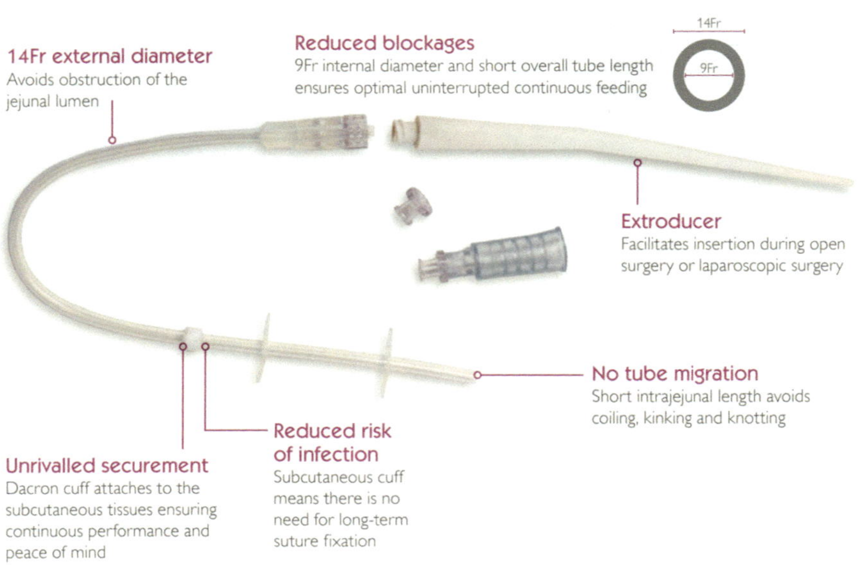

Fig. 8.12 MIC Feeding jejunostomy kit

loop at this point to allow for postoperative distension of the abdomen, which would otherwise cause kinking of the bowel and potentially an obstruction. The bowel is attached to the posterior sheath with two further sutures one centimetre away from the exit point on each side to prevent twisting of the bowel.

8.4 Indications and Techniques of Thoracic and Oesophageal Drainage

Perforations of the intrathoracic oesophagus, anastomotic leaks and extension of sub-diaphragmatic sepsis into the chest require effective drainage.

Many different interventions are now available, including radiologically guided placement of pigtail stents and video-assisted surgery. It is important to select the most appropriate intervention for the circumstances and at the right time. Fluid can be easily drained through pigtail stents, but they are ineffective when there is debris or loculated collections. Like other aspects of managing perforations of the oesophagus, the management of thoracic collections and sepsis should also be discussed in a multidisciplinary context. Poor choice of initial interventions can result in unnecessarily prolonged sepsis and empyema that could have been avoided by a more appropriate initial intervention.

VATS can be carried out as a separate procedure or combined with the deployment of a stent or VAC-stent and placement of a drainage gastrostomy and feeding jejunostomy.

With the increased use and demonstrated benefit of stents for oesophageal perforation, it is not often that surgical drainage of the perforation is required. However, if appropriate stents or the expertise to deploy them is not available, a T-tube can be placed into the oesophagus to control the leak (Figs. 8.13 and 8.14). My experience and that of others who have used this technique is that there is always leakage

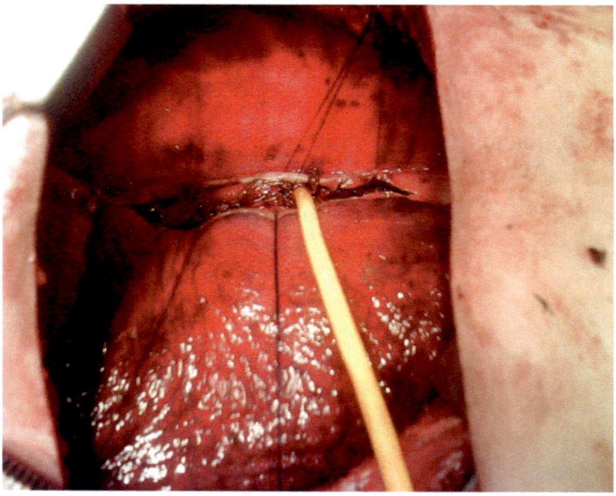

Fig. 8.13 T-tube placed in an oesophageal perforation

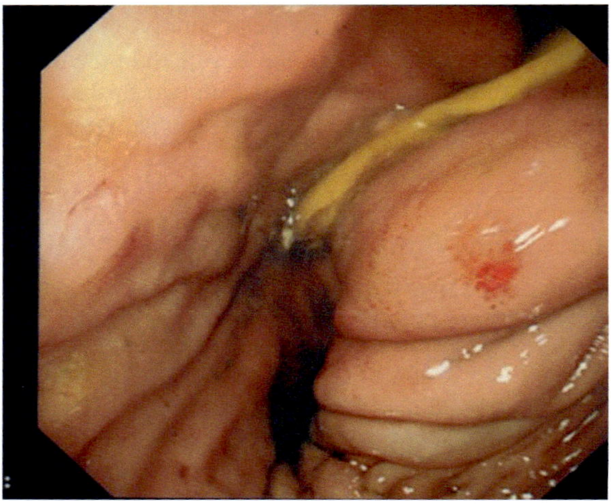

Fig. 8.14 T-tube viewed endoscopically

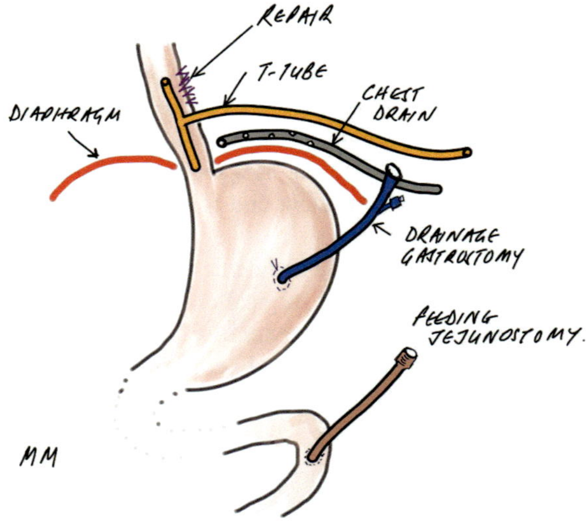

Fig. 8.15 Repair of oesophageal perforation around a T-tube

around the stent, so placing a drain alongside a T-tube is important (Fig. 8.15). It is not a technique I would use now, preferring instead a thoracoscopic washout and appropriately positioned chest drains to drain the perforation effectively.

8.5 Endoluminal Vacuum Therapy in the Management of Oesophagogastric Perforations and Leaks

The EsoSponge is a specialised endoscopic vacuum-assisted closure (EVAC) system, designed specifically for managing esophagogastric perforations (Fig. 8.16). The VAC-Stent is a fully covered, self-expanding metal stent, measuring 70 mm in length and 14 mm in width. Its central part is covered by a macroporous polyurethane sponge, which is connected to a tube that can be attached to a negative pressure source. This unique design combines the benefits of intraluminal EVT while preserving the patency of the gastrointestinal tract (Fig. 8.17).

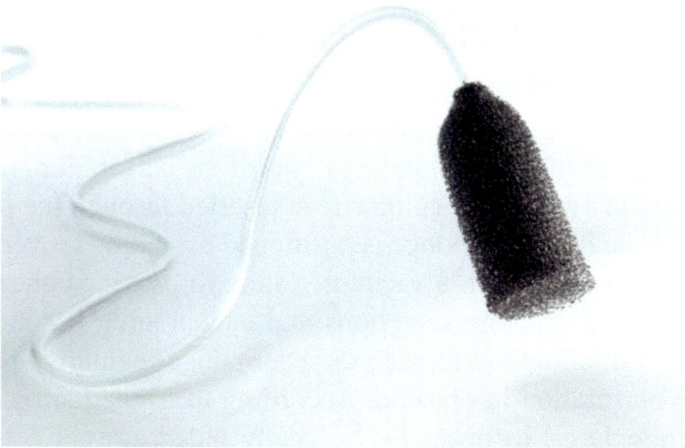

Fig. 8.16 EsoSponge

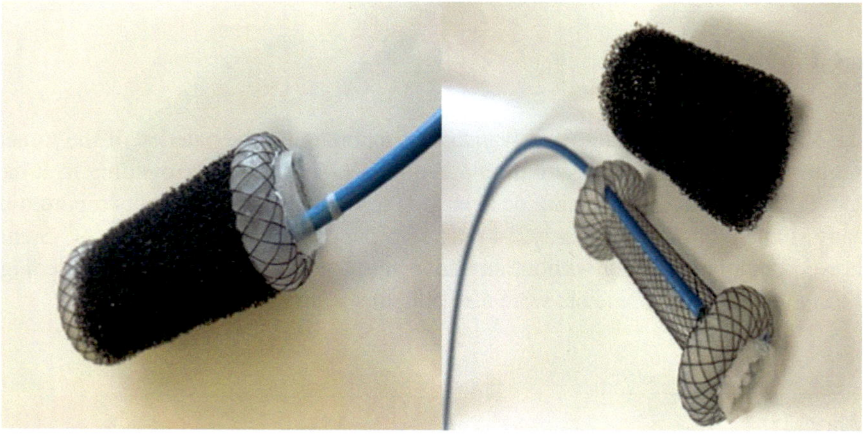

Fig. 8.17 Vac-Stent

8.5.1 Indications for EsoSponge Use

The EsoSponge is indicated for managing esophagogastric perforations, including those resulting from iatrogenic injury, spontaneous rupture, or anastomotic leakage after oesophageal surgery. EVT can be used in nearly every area of the oesophagus, stomach, and duodenum. Studies have reported success rates of over 80%, with minimal morbidity and mortality. However, like any technique, it is important to know when and how to use EVT.

EVT is best avoided in early leaks where a cavity has not yet formed and in complete anastomotic dehiscence with tissue necrosis. Several studies have shown 87 to 90% success rate in using EVT for leaks from sleeve gastrectomy.[5]

8.5.2 Technique for EsoSponge Placement

The initial step involves conducting an endoscopic evaluation to determine the location, size, and condition of the surrounding tissue of the perforation. If the evaluation confirms the feasibility of EVT, a guidewire is inserted through the perforation into the adjacent cavity, and the EsoSponge is positioned by sliding it over the guidewire. The sponge is then connected to a vacuum system to provide continuous negative pressure. This helps in draining secretions and encouraging tissue granulation. It is recommended to monitor and replace the EsoSponge regularly, usually every 3–5 days, until the perforation has healed. According to Kouladouros, it is crucial to place the device into the cavity instead of luminally and ensure correct placement and sizing of the sponge to prevent cavity segmentation.[6] Monitoring the cavity through CT scans is necessary to confirm proper drainage and avoid partitioning of the cavity.

8.5.3 VAC-Stent

The VAC-Stent has the unique advantage of maintaining the patency of the lumen and providing negative pressure drainage through the sponge surrounding it. It has been effectively used in treating oesophageal leaks with positive results reported in many studies. In one such study, 14 out of 15 patients treated with the VAC-Stent, showed complete healing without any adverse effects such as erosion or bleeding. During the treatment, patients were also able to consume liquids orally.[7]

---

[5] Ahrens [5].
Josselyn Mariana Vera [6].

[6] Konstantinos [7].

[7] Lange [8].

Endoscopic Vacuum Therapy (EVT) plays a vital role in managing anastomotic leaks and perforations of the upper gastrointestinal tract. With advancements in technology and endoluminal interventions, cases of oesophageal perforation that were previously treated surgically with either repair or drainage are now considered suitable for EVT. However, a robust decision-making framework is essential to optimise outcomes and select the best treatment option based on the patient's condition.

Although VAC-Stent is a useful option, it may not be suitable for all cases, such as a large cavity adjacent to a small perforation in the oesophagus. In such cases, it would be better to enlarge the perforation and insert the EsoSponge directly into the cavity. Therefore, regular assessment of the leak and associated cavities by both endoscopy and CT scans is crucial. This assessment should be done in a multidisciplinary setting, considering all available treatment options, such as interventional endoscopy, radiology, VATS and surgery.

References

1. Urschel HC, et al. Improved management of esophageal perforation: exclusion and diversion in continuity. Ann Surg. 1974;179(5):587–91. https://doi.org/10.1097/00000658-197405000-00010.
2. Koniaris LG, Spector SA, Staveley-O'Carroll KF. Complete esophageal diversion: a simplified, easily reversible technique. J Am Coll Surg. 2004;199(6):991–3. https://doi.org/10.1016/j.jamcollsurg.2004.07.024.
3. Raymond DP, Watson TJ. Esophageal diversion. Oper Tech Thorac Cardiovasc Surg. 2008;13(2):138–46. https://doi.org/10.1053/j.optechstcvs.2008.05.001.
4. Matsui R, et al. Iatrogenic esophageal perforation that could be treated indirectly by cervical esophagostomy and laparoscopic surgery. Int J Surg Case Rep. 2019;60:4–7. https://doi.org/10.1016/j.ijscr.2019.05.053.
5. Markus A et al. Endoscopic Vacuum therapy in salvage and standalone treatment of gastric leaks after bariatric surgery. Langenbeck's Archives of Surgery 2022;407(3): 1039–46. https://doi.org/10.1007/s00423-021-02365-9
6. Intriago JMV et al. Endoscopic vacuum therapy (EVT) for the treatment of post-bariatric surgery leaks and fistulas: a systematic review and meta-analysis. Obesity Surgery 2022;32(10):3435–51. https://doi.org/10.1007/s11695-022-06228-0
7. Konstantinos K. Applications of endoscopic vacuum therapy in the upper gastrointestinal tract. World J Gastrointestinal Endoscopy 2023;15(6):420–33. https://doi.org/10.4253/wjge.v15.i6.420
8. Lange J et al. The VACStent trial: combined treatment of esophageal leaks by covered stent and endoscopic vacuum therapy. Surgical Endoscopy 2023;37(5):3657–68. https://doi.org/10.1007/s00464-023-09861-7

Chapter 9
Oesophageal Replacement

Abstract This chapter discusses the necessity of surgical reconstruction in situations where the oesophagus is damaged or needs removal due to various reasons. It highlights the use of different conduits, including the stomach, colon, and jejunum, for replacing part or the entire oesophagus. Factors such as conduit availability, blood supply, and functional outcomes are crucial considerations in choosing the appropriate conduit. Surgical techniques for preparing and transposing conduits, as well as managing complications like leaks, are detailed. Additionally, advancements in creating artificial oesophagi and the use of neck muscles and biological patches for repair are explored. The chapter emphasizes the importance of careful planning and expertise in achieving successful oesophageal reconstruction outcomes.

Keywords Oesophageal replacement · Surgical reconstruction · Conduit selection · Gastric conduits · Colonic conduits · Jejunal conduits · Functional outcomes · Surgical techniques · Surgical complications · Flaps using neck muscles · Biological patches · Oesophagoplasty

In situations where the oesophagus is damaged or requires removal due to disease or trauma, surgical reconstruction is necessary to restore the continuity of the gastrointestinal tract. Various types of conduits can be used to replace the oesophagus.

The stomach, colon and jejunum can be used to replace the entire or part of the oesophagus. In choosing a conduit, the first consideration is what is available, followed by the distance that needs to be spanned by the conduit, mainly dictated by its blood supply. The functional outcome from the conduit is also important, but tends to be a secondary consideration. However, I think it should also be considered in the planning stages. This is particularly important in surgery for benign conditions in young patients where the long-term outcome of the particular conduit is very important. As patients are living longer, in my experience, it is not uncommon to have to revise a conduit created many years ago that no longer works well. This is a particular issue with colonic conduits.

The stomach, if available, tends to be the most common part of the gastrointestinal tract used in substituting the oesophagus. It has the advantage of a generally rich and

M. Mughal, *Reconstructive Surgery of the Oesophagus and Stomach*,
https://doi.org/10.1007/978-3-031-66846-3_9

fairly constant blood supply. It is usually mobilised, preserving the gastroepiploeic arch carrying the arterial blood supply from the right side of the stomach. By tubularising the stomach, the full length of the greater curvature can be utilised and by full mobilisation of the duodenum, the tip of the tube will usually reach the base of the skull in most cases.

The colon is also suitable for use as a conduit as long as it is not diseased and there is no significant deviation from the usual blood supply.[1] It requires more expertise in choosing the appropriate part of the colon and preparing its blood supply. Also, the nature of the colon is such that it is prone to redundancy and other complications depending on which part is used and this can impact its function. Surgeons with experience of using colonic conduits usually have a personal preference as to which side of the colon to use. That being so, those specialising in oesophageal reconstruction must be able to use any part of the colon, depending on availability and blood supply. If the right colon is used in an isoperistaltic fashion, the caecum can be too bulky to bring up to the neck through the restricted space at the thoracic inlet. There are ways of addressing this, including retaining the last 10–15 cm of terminal ileum on its blood supply and using that for the proximal anastomosis.[2] Necrosis and loss of the conduit are more common with the colon than the stomach.[3] Although many patients will achieve good long-term functional results, some will have problems requiring further surgery.[4]

The jejunum can be used on a vascular pedicle to replace the distal oesophagus either as a pedicled conduit to bridge a gap between the oesophagus and the stomach or as a conventional Roux-en-Y to replace the stomach as well. With careful preparation and selection of the appropriate loop, it is possible to take the jejunum quite high into the chest. However, replacing the entire oesophagus with jejunum is difficult because of the disposition of its vascular arcades making it difficult to maintain a blood supply to a long segment based on one proximal pedicle. However, this obstacle can be overcome by using a free graft transfer with microvascular anastomosis or supercharging a pedicled jejunal loop by augmenting its proximal blood supply using neck vessels.[5]

In some cases, only part of the oesophageal wall needs to be replaced. In such cases, a patch may be sufficient and different techniques are described to deal with this situation.[6] In my experience, this situation is rare and usually arises in the cervical oesophagus.

Lastly, there has been progress in creating an artificial oesophagus from seeding scaffolds with the appropriate cells and developing a muscle tube with an inner

[1] Greene et al. [1].
[2] Matsumoto et al. [2].
[3] Larson et al. [3].
[4] Greene et al. [1].
[5] Baker et al. [5].
[6] Nieponice et al. [6].

lining of mucosa.[7] However, there remain challenges in developing vasculature and innervation to mimic the oesophagus.

9.1 Reconstruction with Stomach

If the stomach is available and has a normal blood supply, it is the ideal conduit for replacing the oesophagus. With proper preparation, a gastric tube can be fashioned to reach the pharynx. The critical elements of fashioning a long conduit are ensuring a good blood supply, mobilisation of the duodenal loop and creating a new lesser curve which is as long as the greater curve. The gastroepiploic arch is preserved right up to the short gastric vessels which are divided well away from the fundus. If the duodenum is Kocherised fully, in my experience, dividing the right gastric artery does not help to achieve a greater length of conduit. Transecting the stomach 4 to 5 cm parallel to the greater curvature provides sufficient length in most cases to reach the pharynx. To ensure that the resection line is kept parallel to the greater curvature, it is important to carry out the transection using multiple firings of 40 or 50 mm stapler, from the incisura to the angle of His (Fig. 9.1).

In cases where there has been previous surgery involving the stomach, for instance fundoplication or the creation of a gastrostomy, the length of the gastric conduit may be limited. Depending on the gastrostomy site, it may not be possible to transect the stomach optimally. Although it may be possible to recruit the fundus of the stomach after dismantling a previous fundoplication, that part of the stomach may not be suitable for the conduit because of compromised blood supply.

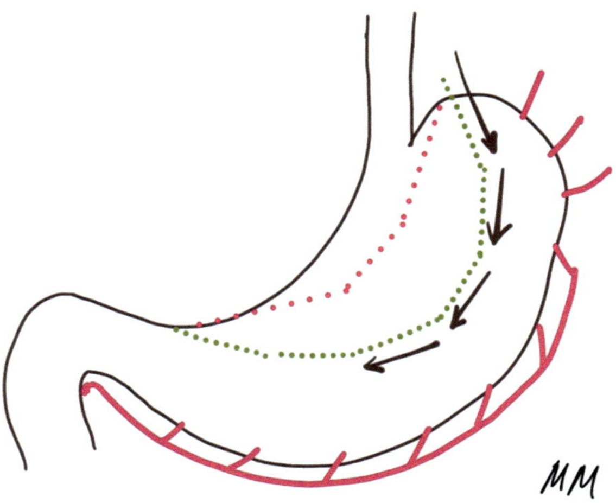

Fig. 9.1 Arrows showing the correct path of transection to obtain the maximum length of gastric conduit. In red is the incorrect transection line resulting in a shorter, wider conduit

[7] Nieponice et al. [6].

9.2 Reconstruction Using Colon

Provided that the colon is not diseased and has a good blood supply, different segments can be used as a pedicled conduit depending on the length required. Most of the literature on the subject reports using the left colon based on the left colic artery which is more constant than the other feeding vessels. The resulting conduit is also said to be of a more appropriate diameter and less prone to dilatation than, say, the right colon. Most published series of colonic interposition have reported using the left colon[8] with a graft necrosis rate of 0 to 9.4% and an anastomotic leak rate of 0 to 12.5%.

9.2.1 *Selecting and Preparing the Conduit*

I prefer using the right colon as I have usually found the middle colic vessels and the marginal artery of the ascending colon to be suitable for a pedicled conduit (Fig. 9.2). Also, provided there is a good ileal branch of the ileocaecal artery, it is often possible to obtain a 15–20 cm length of the ileum for the conduit (Fig. 9.3).[9] This has several advantages for a conduit to the neck. It provides extra length, the ileum matches the diameter of the cervical oesophagus, and the ileum is not constricted by the limited space in the thoracic inlet, as the caecum sits lower in the mediastinum or the retrosternal tunnel, where there is more space. The final decision as to which part of the colon to use is made during the laparotomy.

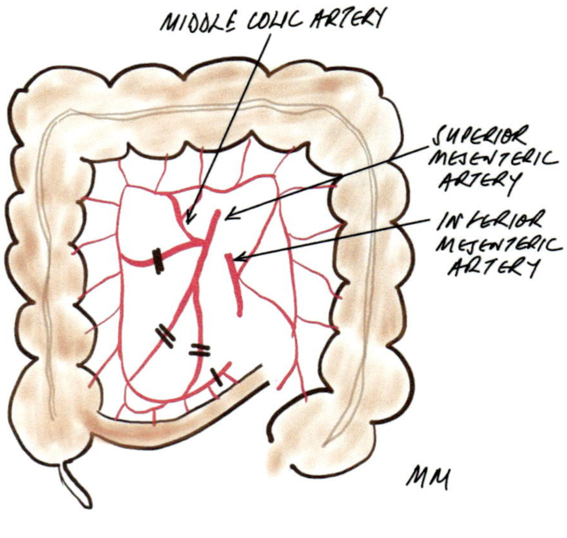

Fig. 9.2 Diagram showing the blood vessels which need to be typically divided to prepare a right colon conduit, including the terminal ileum

---

[8] Klink et al. [8].

[9] Matsumoto et al. [2].

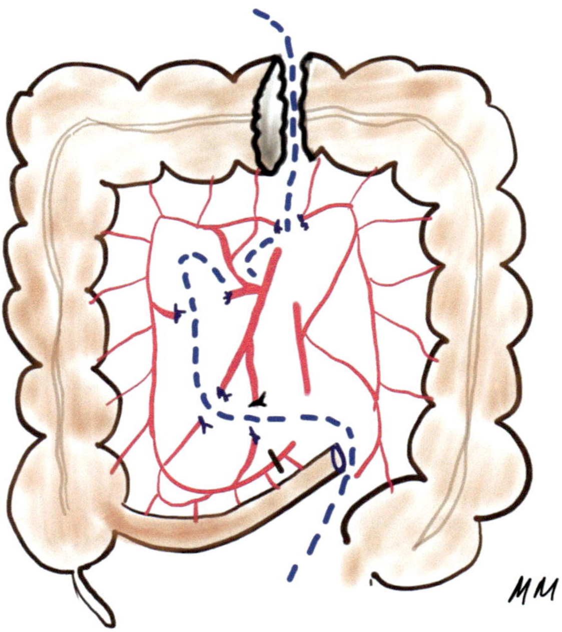

Fig. 9.3 Diagram showing vessel division for use of the right colon as a conduit

I have also used the transverse and left colon. The principles of preparing the conduit loop are the same as for right colon, starting with a careful inspection of the bowel to ensure that it does not harbour unexpected pathology and then studying the vasculature to select the pedicle which will support a conduit of the required length. Preparation of transverse or left colon colon conduits is illustrated in Figs. 9.4 and 9.5. I have never used an antiperistaltic colonic conduit, but this has been reported in cases where it has been possible to harvest a longer loop than would have been possible with an isoperistaltic conduit.[10] Surgeons who have performed this procedure report that the incidence of regurgitation is no higher with an antiperistaltic conduit than isoperistaltic conduits.[11] This is worth knowing in case one encounters a situation where the vascular supply and the anatomy of the conduit appear best suited to an isoperistaltic conduit.

Previous colonic resection and significant colonic pathology (inflammatory bowel disease, severe diverticular disease, polyposis coli) may make the colon unsuitable. At the planning stage, imaging with a CT scan of the neck, chest and abdomen is carefully reviewed for any obvious abnormalities of the colon and its blood supply. However, I do not routinely request a CT angiogram unless indicated by a standard contrast-enhanced CT.

I do not routinely perform bowel preparation. At laparotomy, the colon is carefully examined and after detaching the greater omentum from the transverse colon, I

[10] Pai and Kumar [10].

[11] Klink et al. [8].

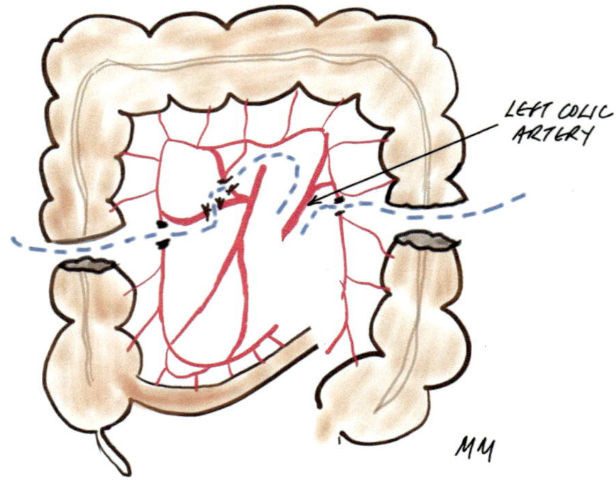

Fig. 9.4 Diagram showing a transverse colon conduit based on the left colic artery

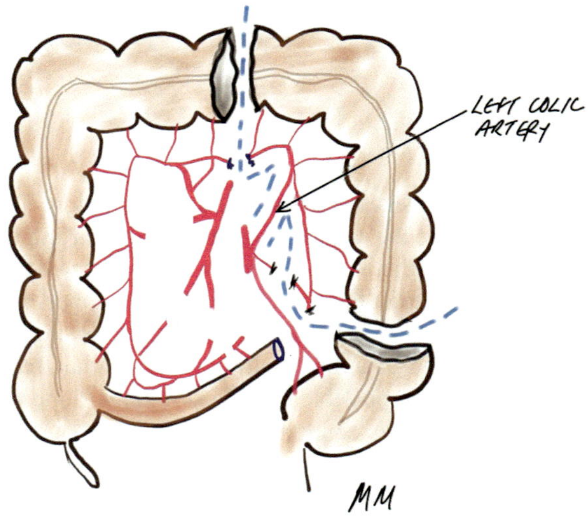

Fig. 9.5 Diagram showing a left colon conduit based on the left colic artery

mobilise the right colon with the ileocaecal junction as well as the transverse colon and the splenic flexure. I then examine the vasculature by transillumination and select the part of the colon to be used based on the vasculature and the length needed, although my preference is to use the right colon and ileum. Once I have determined that there is a good marginal artery and middle colic vessels, I create windows in the mesocolon and occlude the right colic and ileocolic vessels with small bulldog clamps (Figs. 9.6 and 9.7).

I then look for the ileal branch of the ileocaecal artery, following it along the terminal ileum to see if it joins the last ileal branch. If that proves to be the case, it is possible to harvest a good length of vascularised ileum that can be used as part of the conduit. Before the bulldog clamps are applied, I ensure the patient is normotensive

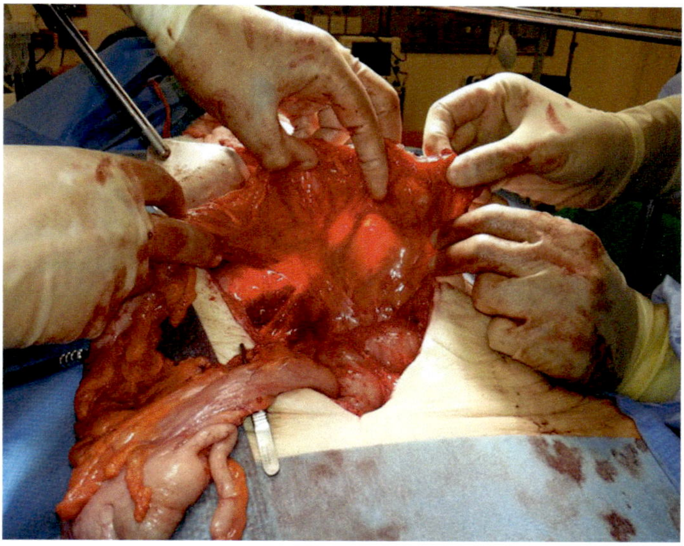

Fig. 9.6 Inspecting the vascular supply with mesenteric windows created

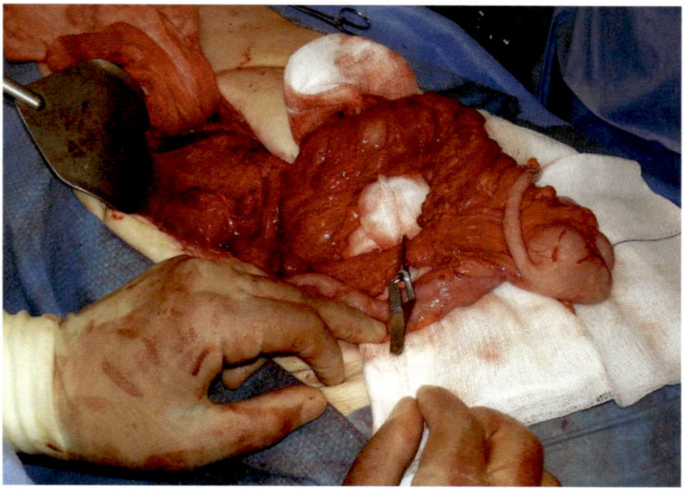

Fig. 9.7 Isolating and temporarily occluding the blood vessels with bulldog clamps

and not on vasopressors. It is also important to divide the mesentery to origin of the middle colic vessels to obtain as long a pedicle as possible. Furthermore, to gain as much length of the ascending colon as possible, the mesentery needs to be divided close to the marginal artery.

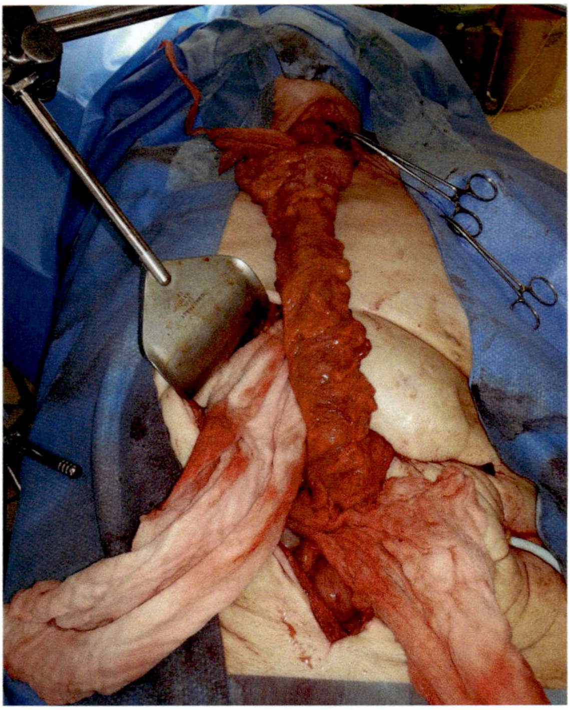

Fig. 9.8 Colonic conduit laid on chest, ready for transposition

After milking distally any faeces out of the loop to be harvested, the bowel is divided with a stapler at the appropriate level proximally and distally. The conduit can then be prepared to be routed through the mediastinum or the retrosternal space. The sequencing of conduit preparation and preparing the route depends on several factors, including whether the operation is being carried out as a primary procedure combined with a resection, or as a secondary procedure where an oesophagostomy has been previously constructed. In the latter situation, I prepare the conduit first (Fig. 9.8) so that I can be certain that it will be possible to obtain a long enough length before carrying out the neck dissection, taking down the oesophagostomy.

9.2.2 *Transposing the Conduit*

Transposing the conduit must be carried out with care to avoid damaging the blood supply and ensuring that the bowel is not twisted. After trying different techniques, I have developed one that I have found to be consistently reliable for a smooth and safe transposition. I use a sterile plastic camera sleeve to protect the conduit as it is conveyed to the neck. A nylon tape is sutured to the proximal end of the conduit at three points to distribute tension, and the conduit is drawn up through a length of the

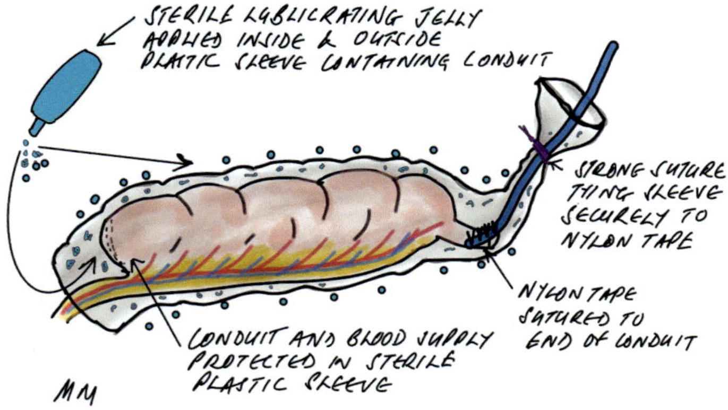

Fig. 9.9 Diagram showing the conduit enclosed in a plastic sleeve ready to be pulled to the right (cranial direction). Note that the nylon tape is sutured to the conduit, but the tape is also secured with a strong transfixion stitch to the sleeve

sleeve, which is 10–20 cm longer than the length of the conduit. It is important to lubricate both the inside and outside of the sleeve with sterile gel. With the conduit completely enclosed within the sleeve, the nylon tape is secured firmly to the sleeve using a strong transfixion suture tied around the top of the sleeve. Thus traction of the nylon tape is applied to the sleeve rather than the contained bowel (Fig. 9.9).

I recommend a surgical pause before transposing the conduit. At this point, it is important to check that the blood supply is not compromised, that the space within the tunnel is adequate, and the conduit is correctly orientated without a twist. Once the conduit has been transposed and unsheathed, correcting a twist or any other problem can become very difficult, and repeated manipulations of the conduit can endanger its vascularity (Fig. 9.10).

After coating the outside of the plastic sleeve liberally with sterile gel, the conduit is passed through the tunnel using a combination of gentle traction on the tape and ‘feeding’ it from the abdomen, the push–pull technique. Once the top of the conduit is comfortably in the neck, it is unsheathed by gently pulling on the sleeve. After checking that the conduit is still well vascularised, the nylon tape is detached from the conduit and it is ready for the anastomosis.

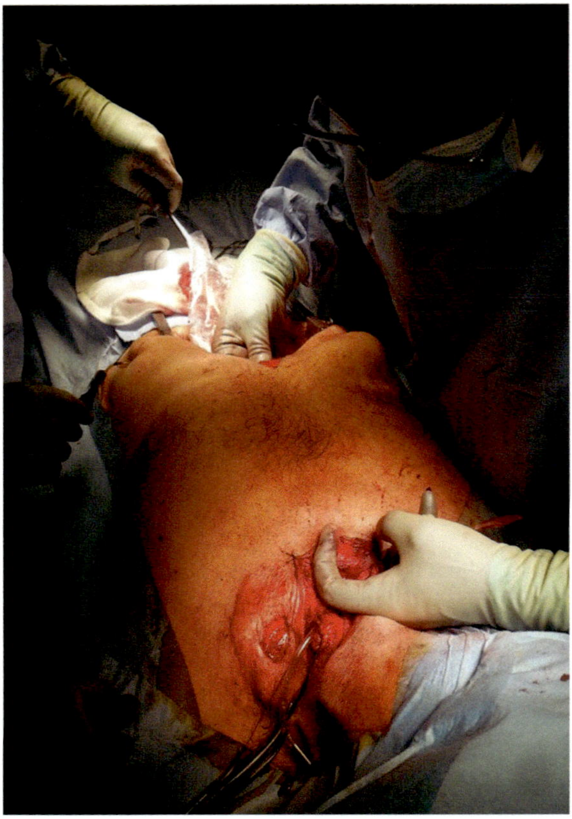

Fig. 9.10 Checking the lie of the conduit and space within the tunnel before removing the sheath

9.2.3 *Mobilising the Oesophagostomy and Cervical Anastomosis*

If there has been a previous oesophagostomy, it is taken down with great care to avoid damage and maximise the available length of the residual oesophagus. I start by placing a series of sutures around the circumference of the mucocutaneous junction (Fig. 9.11). These are kept long and used to provide traction whilst mobilising the stoma. I have found this to be better and safer than applying instruments to the stoma, which inevitably leads to sacrificing a few millimetres of the oesophagus due to damage by the instruments (Figs. 9.11, 9.12 and 9.13). The top of the conduit is anastomosed to the oesophageal stump and the bottom to proximal jejunum or stomach depending on the circumstances of the reconstruction (Figs. 9.14 and 9.15).

I routinely place a Penrose train in the neck in case of a leak and insert a feeding jejunostomy (Fig. 9.16).

In my personal series of 32 reconstructions with a colonic conduit, leak rate from the cervical anastomosis is 16% (5 cases). However, 18 cases were reoperations with

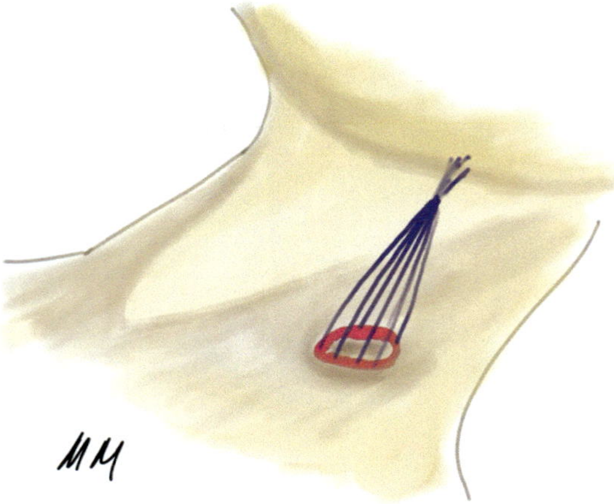

Fig. 9.11 Traction sutures placed around the stoma

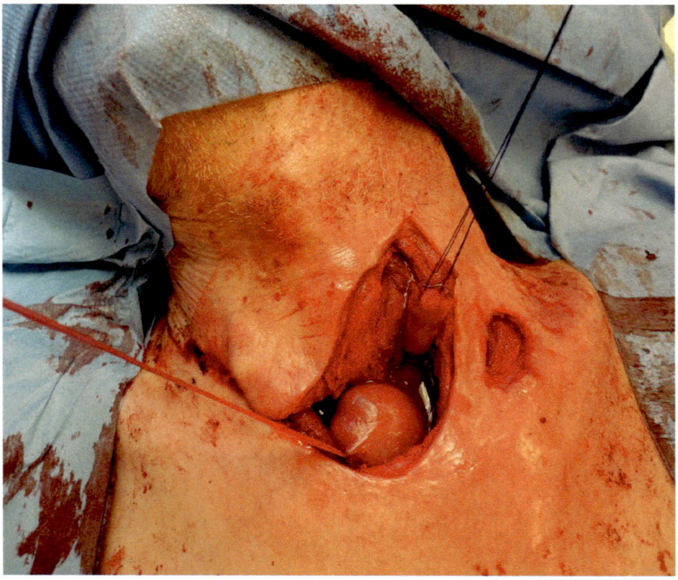

Fig. 9.12 View of neck showing stoma trephine and oesophageal stump held by traction sutures and top of retrosternal colonic conduit ready for anastomosis

a second or third operation on the neck, and in three cases the anastomosis was to the pharynx rather than the oesophagus. A leak from the neck usually manifests with saliva in the drain bag. In some cases the leak tracks into the chest along the plane of dissection, rather than appearing at the neck. I request a contrast swallow to assess its size and, more importantly, to see if contrast is flowing through the anastomosis

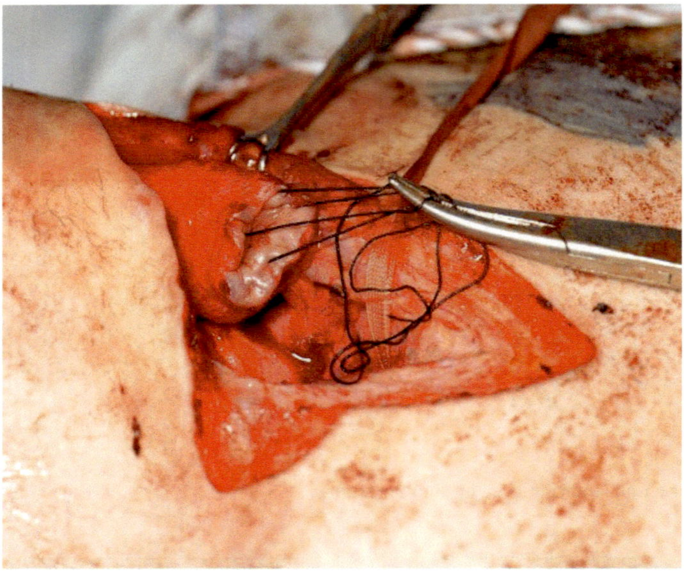

Fig. 9.13 Stoma detached from the skin with the traction sutures attached

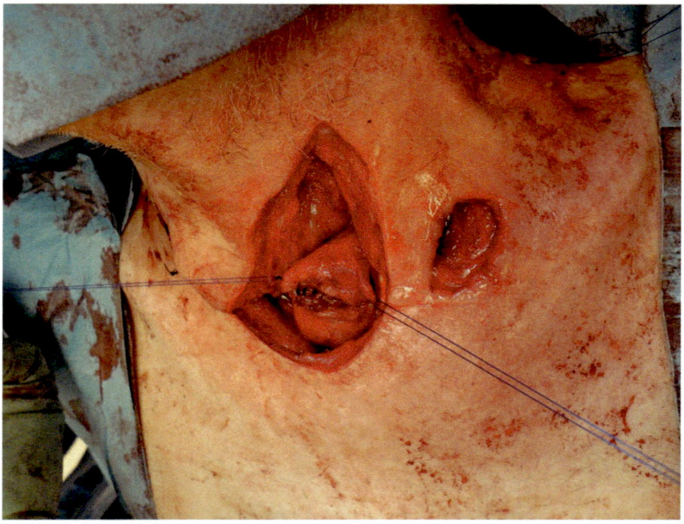

Fig. 9.14 Cervical anastomosis

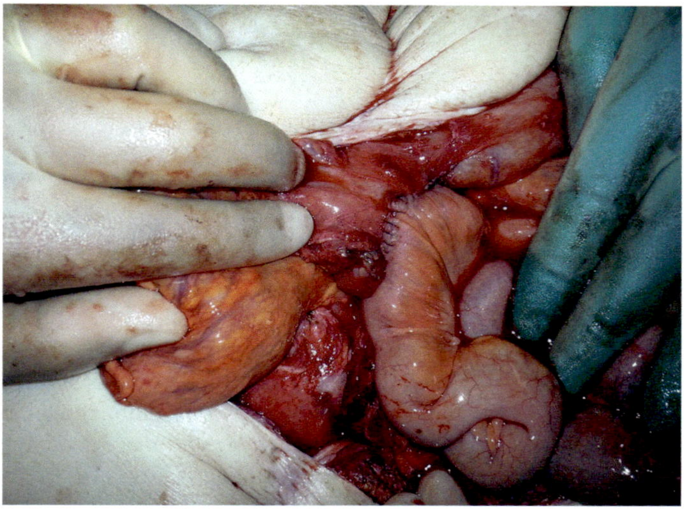

Fig. 9.15 Distal anastomosis of the colonic conduit to the jejunum

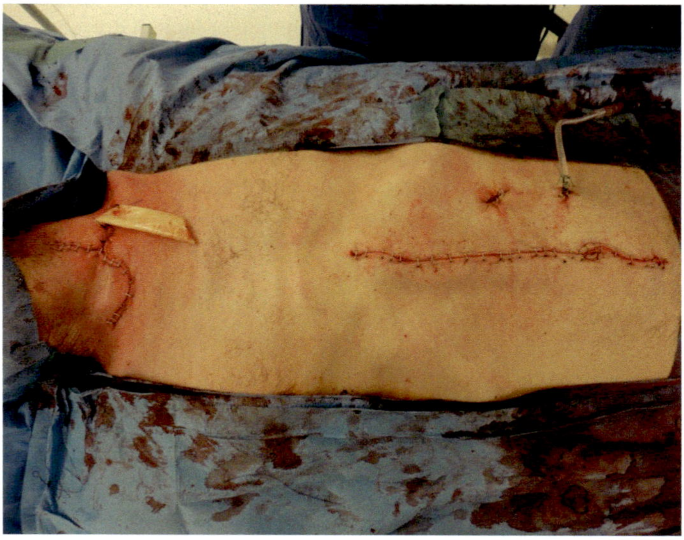

Fig. 9.16 Completed operation showing Penrose drain in the neck and feeding jejunostomy

into the conduit. Healing is likely with conservative treatment if the leak is small and there is free flow of contrast into the conduit. Management includes stopping oral intake, antibiotics and continuing with jejunostomy feeding. The drain is kept in place until the leak has healed.

9.2.4 Jejunal Conduits

The jejunum can be used as a pedicled graft or a free graft. A free graft can be transferred to wherever it is needed and requires a microvascular anastomosis to establish a blood supply. To understand the utility and limitations of using jejunum as a pedicled conduit, it is important to appreciate its blood supply. The superior mesenteric artery gives off around 12 to 15 branches that supply the jejunum. These branches further lead to secondary arcades, which ultimately form a marginal branch located near the border of the bowel. The proximal jejunum, characterized by longer and straighter branches, is more suitable for a longer conduit.

In order to prepare a long jejunal loop, the ideal point for the proximal transection is 20 to 30 cm distal to the DJ flexure. This is marked, but transection is not performed until the supply of the jejunum has been examined by transillumination. Depending on the length of the loop required, the seventh or eighth branch from the superior mesenteric artery is chosen as the vascular pedicle (Fig. 9.17).

Windows are then carefully created in the jejunal mesentery, close to the superior mesenteric artery to enable the application of bulldog clamps to the selected jejunal branches. It is important to occlude the branches close to their origins from the superior mesenteric artery to maintain the arcades. If the bowel loop remains well vascularised during the test occlusion. the jejunal branches are carefully ligated and divided and the bowel loop is detached on its pedicled and prepared for the transposition.

A long enough loop of jejunum to reach the neck can be obtained by maintaining the marginal branches but the most proximal part of the bowel is likely to become ischaemic. In this case, supercharging the loop by augmenting its blood supply to a

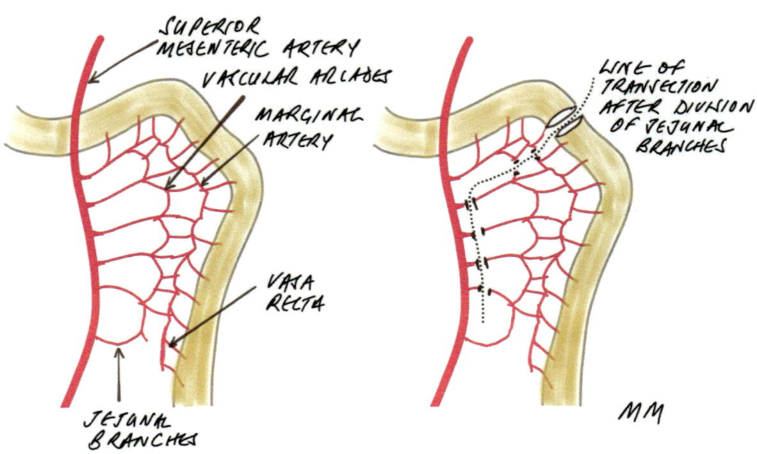

Fig. 9.17 The diagram on the left shows the typical blood supply to the proximal jejunum with the typical arrangement of the vascular arcades. On the right is shown the transection line to obtain a proximal jejunal conduit

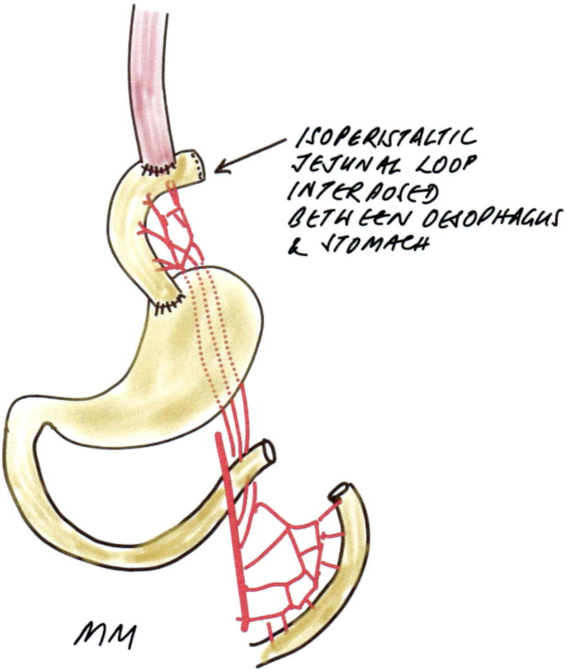

Fig. 9.18 The Merendino procedure

proximal pedicle from the neck is an option.[12] This, however, needs the assistance and expertise of a plastic surgeon.

Short lengths of the jejunum have been used as free grafts to replace small segments of the cervical oesophagus.

The Merendino operation is a particular type of jejunal transposition which can be useful for replacing relatively small segments of the distal oesophagus and the gastro-oesophageal junction. It has the advantage of retaining the stomach in its normal position by using a short length of pedicled jejunum to bridge the gap between the stomach and the oesophagus (Fig. 9.18).[13]

It is not widely used, but its proponents report good outcomes. It may be the most appropriate reconstruction after a limited gastro-oesophageal junction, e.g., for a large GIST or a leiomyoma. In their original description of the procedure, Merendino and colleagues suggested that the isoperistaltic jejunal interposition would minimise gastro-oesophageal reflux and therefore the procedure has also been used to treat failure of both Heller's operation for achalasia and antireflux surgery. However, a study of its use after failed antireflux surgery has reported poor outcomes.[14]

---

[12] Baker et al. [5].

[13] Alvin and Dillard [8].

[14] Analatos et al. [9].

9.3 Use of Neck Muscles for Repairing the Cervical Oesophagus

If the oesophageal defect is not circumferential, it may be feasible to repair and patch it with muscle. The choice of muscle depends on the site and size of the defect. There are several choices in the neck, including sternomastoid, trapezius and pectoralis major flaps. These do not need microvascular anastomoses, but it is important to understand the blood supply in order to obtain a well-vascularised length and width of muscle.

The inferior part of the sternomastoid is broad and has a segmental blood supply such that the flap can be based superiorly on the occipital artery or inferiorly on the thyroid cervical trunk. The whole muscle can be used or just the anterior portion.

My personal experience is limited to the use of the strap muscles and the omohyoid. The superior belly of the omohyoid muscle is ideal for small defects in the cervical oesophagus.[15] The strap muscles can also be used by detaching them from their superior attachments as they have a segmental blood supply from branches of the superior and inferior thyroid arteries with anastomoses within and around the muscles. By carefully mobilising and maintaining the inferior blood supply, it is possible to divide the muscles superiorly and obtain a well vascularised flap of a reasonable size for interposition or bolstering a repair (Figs. 9.19 and 9.20).

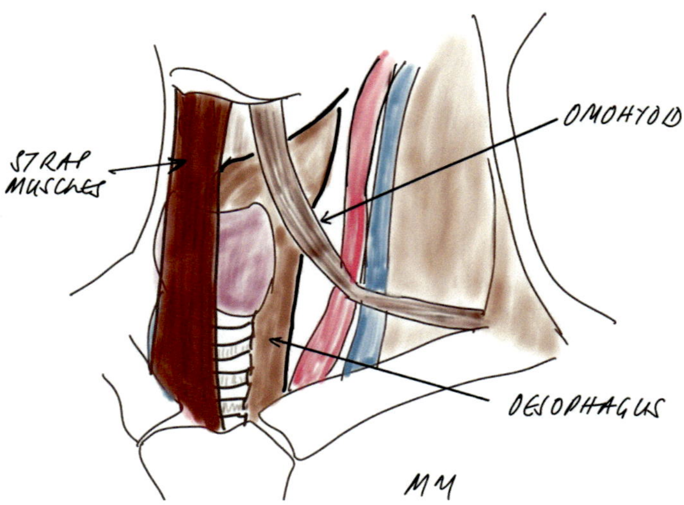

Fig. 9.19 Right strap muscles and left omohyoid shown with attachments and proximity to cervical oesophagus

[15] . Surek [10].

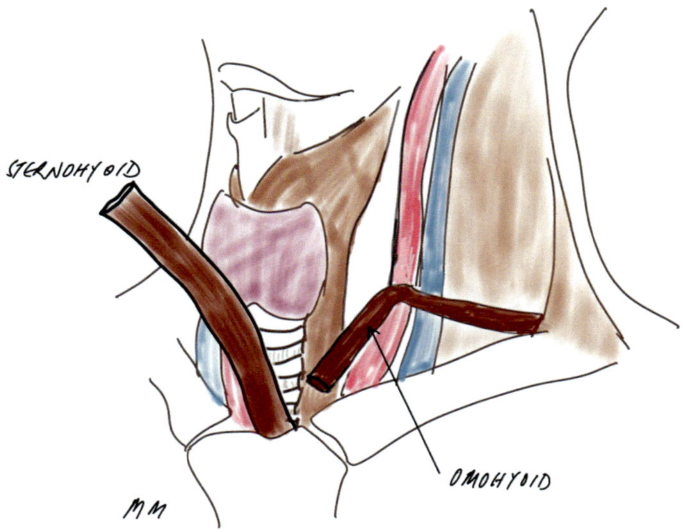

Fig. 9.20 Strap muscles and omohyoid detached from their superior attachments

9.4 Biological Patches

Successful use of patch oesophagoplasty using biological scaffolds has also been reported.[16] Nieponice and colleagues used an extracellular matrix bioscaffold made of porcine urinary bladder to patch oesophageal defects. Gastroscopy showed the formation of mucosa over the patch at two months, with the defect indistinguishable from surrounding healthy tissue. Biopsy from the patch showed normal squamous epithelium. The group have used patches in different parts of the oesophagus with up to a 5 cm diameter defect without the need for muscle or skin flaps.

References

1. Greene CL, DeMeester SR, Augustin F, Worrell SG, Oh DS, Hagen JA, DeMeester TR. Long-term quality of life and alimentary satisfaction after esophagectomy with colon interposition. The Annals of Thoracic Surgery 2014;98(5):1713–20. https://doi.org/10.1016/j.athoracsur.2014.06.088
2. Matsumoto H, Hirai T, Kubota H, Murakami H, Higashida M, Hirabayashi Y. Safe esophageal reconstruction by ileocolic interposition: ileocolic esophageal reconstruction. Dis Esophagus. 2012;25(3):195–200. https://doi.org/10.1111/j.1442-2050.2011.01232.x.
3. Larson III, Theodore C, Shuman LS, Libshitz HI, McMurtrey MJ. Complications of colonic interposition. Cancer 1985;56(3):681–90. https://doi.org/10.1002/1097-0142(19850801)56:3<681::AID-CNCR2820560341>3.0.CO;2-U

[16] Nieponice et al. [6].

4. Baker CR, Forshaw MJ, Gossage JA, Ng R, Mason RC. Long-Term outcome and quality of life after supercharged jejunal interposition for oesophageal replacement. The Surgeon 2015;13(4):187–93. https://doi.org/10.1016/j.surge.2014.01.004
5. Nieponice A, Ciotola FF, Nachman F, Jobe BA, Hoppo T, Londono R, Badylak S, Badaloni AE. Patch esophagoplasty: esophageal reconstruction using biologic scaffolds. Ann Thorac Surg. 2014;97(1):283–8. https://doi.org/10.1016/j.athoracsur.2013.08.011.
6. Klink CD, Binnebösel M, Schneider M, Ophoff K, Schumpelick V, Jansen M. Operative outcome of colon interposition in the treatment of esophageal cancer: a 20-year experience. Surgery 2010;147(4):491–96. https://doi.org/10.1016/j.surg.2009.10.045
7. Pai E, Kumar T. Technique of antiperistaltic left colonic conduit. Indian J Surgery. 2020;82(5):959–62. https://doi.org/10.1007/s12262-020-02117-x.
8. Alvin MK, Dillard. DH. The concept of sphincter substitition by an interposed jejunal segment for anatomic and physiologic abnormalities at the esophagogastric junction. Annals of Surgery 1955;142(3):486–506.
9. Apostolos A, Lindblad M, Rouvelas I, Elbe P, Lundell L, Nilsson M, Tsekrekos A, Tsai JA. Evaluation of resection of the gastroesophageal junction and jejunal interposition (Merendino Procedure) as a rescue procedure in patients with a failed redo antireflux procedure. a single-center experience. BMC Surgery 2018;18(1). https://doi.org/10.1186/s12893-018-0401-8
10. Surek CC, Girod DA. Superior omohyoid muscle flap repair of cervical esophageal perforation induced by spinal hardware. Ear, Nose and Throat J 2014;93(12): E38–42. https://doi.org/10.1177/014556131409301203

Chapter 10
Anastomotic Techniques

Abstract This chapter discusses various methods for creating anastomoses in different regions of the gastrointestinal tract, focusing on neck, chest, and oesophago-jejunal anastomoses. In neck anastomoses, hand-sewn techniques are favoured over staplers due to limited space. Techniques involve careful preparation of the oesophageal stump and the conduit, followed by meticulous suturing in two layers. In chest anastomoses, both stapled and hand-sewn methods are detailed, emphasising technical nuances to ensure proper alignment and integrity of the anastomosis. For oesophago-jejunal anastomoses, hand-sewn techniques are discussed, particularly in situations with limited space, with detailed steps outlined to achieve optimal outcomes. The chapter provides valuable insights into the surgical principles and techniques essential for successful anastomotic procedures in various clinical scenarios.

Keywords Anastomotic techniques · Neck anastomosis · Chest anastomosis · Oesophago-jejunal anastomosis · Hand-sewn · Stapled · Surgical principles · Conduit preparation · Surgical procedures

10.1 Neck Anastomoses

There are many techniques for anastomosing a conduit to the cervical oesophagus. I have never used staplers and prefer to do a hand anastomosis. I find this works well in the limited space available in the neck.

Once mobilised, the oesophageal stump is prepared by cutting the oesophageal muscle circumferentially with point diathermy on a low coagulation setting. Care is taken not to damage the underlying mucosa. By applying gentle traction to the end of the oesophageal stump, as the muscle is cut, a mucosal cylinder appears, which is then cut 5 mm distal to the muscle edge (Fig. 10.1). I then make a transverse enterotomy about 1 cm below the top of the conduit, ensuring that the length matches the diameter of the oesophagus. Gentle traction on stay-sutures at the 3 and 9 o'clock

M. Mughal, *Reconstructive Surgery of the Oesophagus and Stomach*,
https://doi.org/10.1007/978-3-031-66846-3_10

positions on the oesophageal stump helps to estimate the diameter and the subsequent performance of the anastomosis.

Interrupted 4/0 PDS sutures are used for the anastomosis in two layers. The posterior part of the anastomosis is started with interrupted sutures, taking the full thickness on the stomach side and the mucosa on the oesophagus (Fig. 10.2). Once this latter is completed, a nasogastric tube is passed across the anastomosis and sited appropriately. The anterior layer is completed similarly. Sutures at the 3 and 9 o'clock positions are tied but left long (Fig. 10.3). The second layer of anterior interrupted sutures is placed through the seromuscular layer of the stomach and the muscle of the oesophagus. The stay sutures help twist the anastomosis to complete the second layer posteriorly (Figs. 10.4 and 10.5).

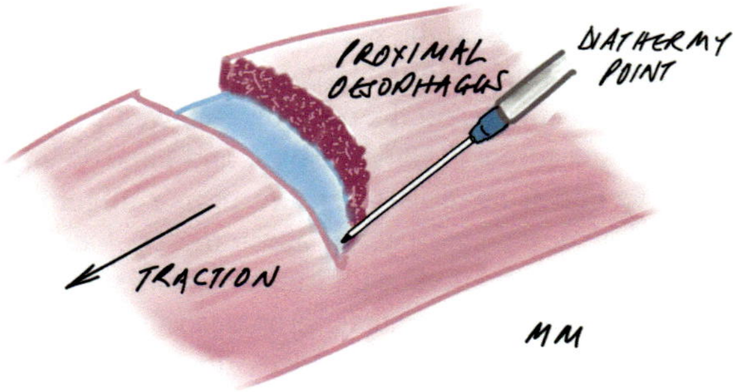

Fig. 10.1 Dividing the muscle layer of the oesophagus to create a mucosal cylinder

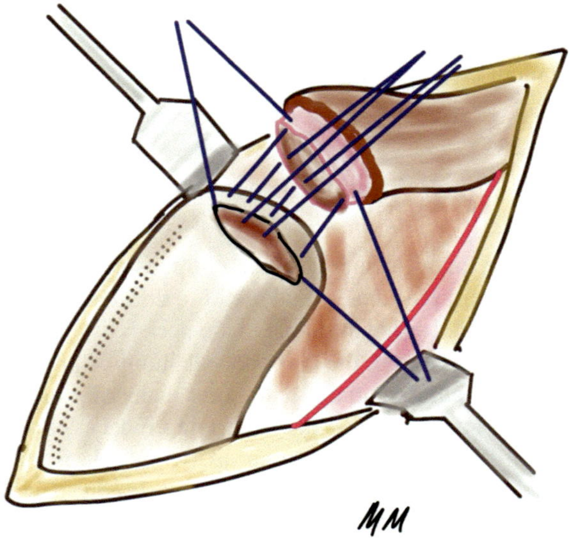

Fig. 10.2 Interrupted sutures taking full-thickness bites of the stomach and bites through the oesophageal mucosal cylinder

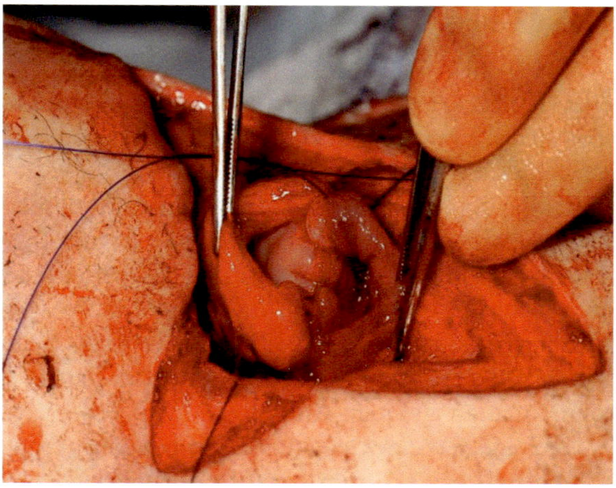

Fig. 10.3 Completed posterior layer of sutures

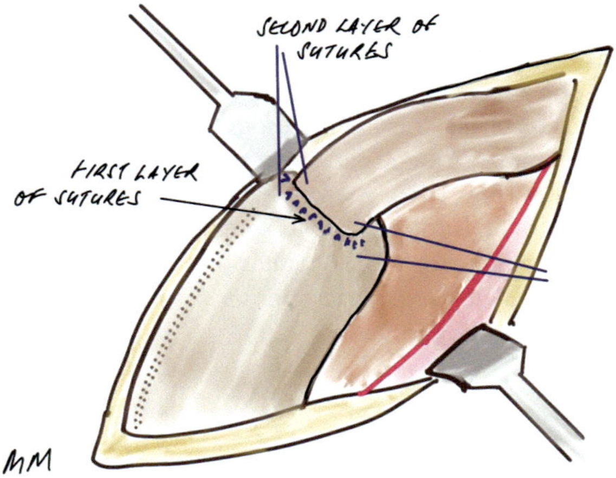

Fig. 10.4 Second layer of anterior sutures being placed

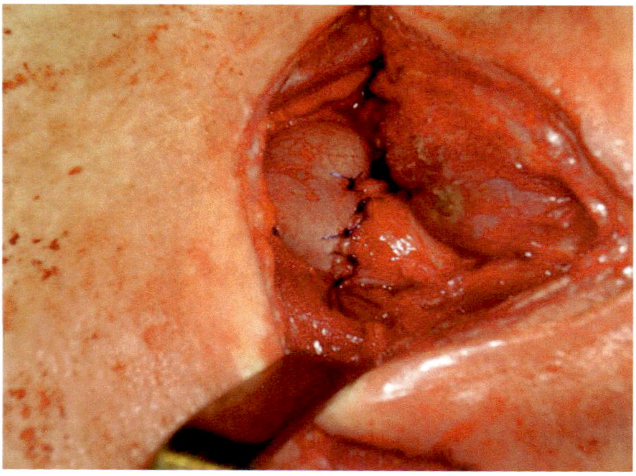

Fig. 10.5 Second layer of sutures through the seromuscular layer of the stomach and the oesophageal muscle

10.2 Chest Anastomosis

There are many techniques for carrying out anastomosis of the conduit to the oesophagus in the chest. I will describe my preferred techniques for stapled and hand anastomoses.

For the stapled anastomosis, I use a circular stapler. The most important technical detail for this anastomosis is to use the largest diameter anvil in the oesophagus ensuring that the purse string closes the oesophagus snugly around the spindle without gaps or undue bunching. On transection, the oesophagus always shrinks both in length and width. Using the widest anvil ensures that any bunched tissue around the spindle is as far away as possible from the staples and the knife, ensuring proper approximation and join. After dividing the oesophagus, I place four stay sutures at 9, 12, 3 and 6 o'clock positions for traction to keep the oesophagus open. I avoid placing Babcock's forceps or other instruments on the oesophagus to avoid trauma. Also, I insert the anvil into the oesophagus before placing the purse string suture. In my experience, placing the purse-string first, results in compromising the width of the oesophageal opening and therefore the size of the anvil that can be used.

The spindle of the anvil is held with a long clip and moved from side to side to expose each quadrant of the oesophageal circumference to enable accurate placement of the purse-string. Gentle traction on the stay sutures aids the accurate spacing of the bites (Fig. 10.6). After tying the purse-string, the staple gun is inserted through an anterior gastrotomy, and its spindle is brought out through the opposite wall about 2 cm from the top of the conduit. The gastrotomy is closed after firing the gun and ensuring a satisfactory anastomosis. A nasogastric tube placed across the anastomosis into the gastric conduit.

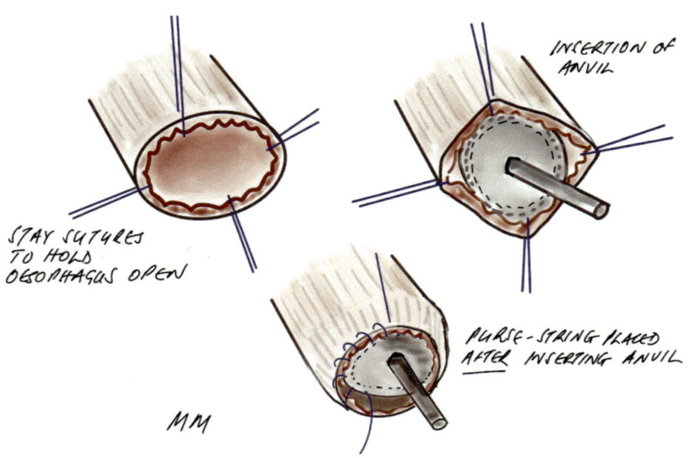

Fig. 10.6 Technique of securing the circular stapler anvil in the oesophagus

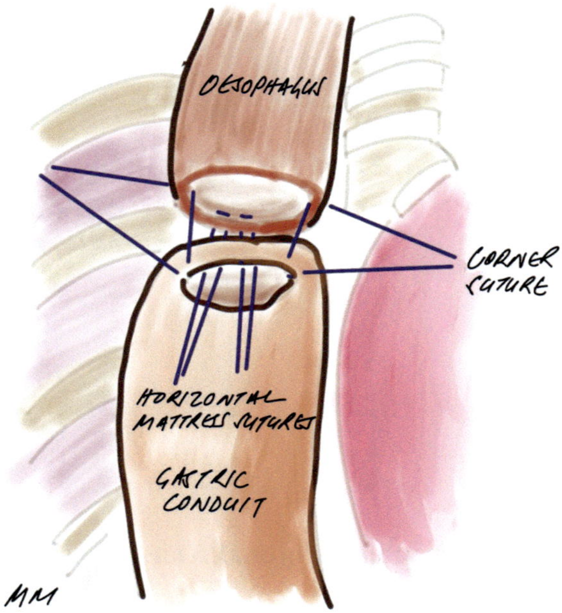

Fig. 10.7 Hand-sewn anastomosis of the oesophagus to the gastric conduit in the chest showing posterior mattress sutures being placed

For a hand anastomosis, a gastrotomy is made in the appropriate part of the conduit to match the diameter of the oesophagus and two full-thickness stay sutures are placed at either end between the oesophagus and the conduit (Fig. 10.7). A posterior layer of interrupted full-thickness horizontal mattress sutures is placed. Each suture passes through the inside of the stomach 5 mm from the edge of the gastrotomy, then through the posterior wall of the oesophagus, and back the other way into the stomach. Four or five such sutures usually suffice and are carefully tied after all the sutures have been placed, ensuring that any slack is taken and the knots are seated on the gastric mucosa. This is followed by a full-thickness continuous suture of the back wall working around to the front. Interrupted, horizontal mattress sutures are finally placed anteriorly between the stomach and the oesophagus to complete the anastomosis (Fig. 10.8).

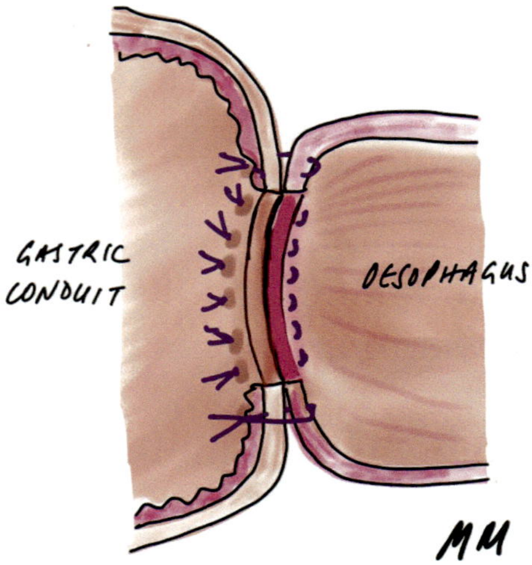

Fig. 10.8 'Cut-away' diagram showing posterior layer of full-thickness mattress sutures tied on the stomach side

10.3 Oesophago-Jejunal Anastomosis

Numerous techniques have been described for anastomosing the jejunum to the oesophagus at the hiatus. When space is limited, particularly when performing a high anastomosis in the mediastinum, I have found hand anastomosis to be a dependable technique.

After preparing the Roux loop, full-thickness sutures are placed at 3 and 9 o'clock positions from outside-in on the oesophageal side and inside-out on the jejunum side. The jejunal loop is kept well out of the field whilst a series of interrupted full-thickness sutures are placed in the front wall of the oesophagus from the outside in keeping the needles attached (Fig. 10.9). When using a table-mounted retractor, it is convenient arrange these sutures held by mosquito forceps along the bar. It is important to keep them in order, so they do not become tangled. Next, the posterior wall sutures are inserted. These are placed from inside-out on the oesophagus and outside-in on the jejunum, with each held with mosquito forceps sequentially threaded on a Roberts clamp. The jejunum is held away from the oesophagus during the placement of these sutures. Once all the sutures are in place, the jejunum is parachuted down to the oesophagus. The end sutures are tied first, followed by the posterior layer of sutures, ensuring that each suture is 'run' before being tied to take up any slack. Once all the sutures have been tied, they can be held up, which brings up the posterior wall. The suture line is inspected for any undue gaps that can easily be closed with extra sutures. Only then are the sutures cut. Next, the needles on the previously inserted anterior wall oesophageal sutures, are used to pick up the anterior wall of the jejunum. Again, all the sutures are placed before being tied. As with the posterior layer, all the sutures are held up before being tied, revealing any gaps requiring extra sutures.

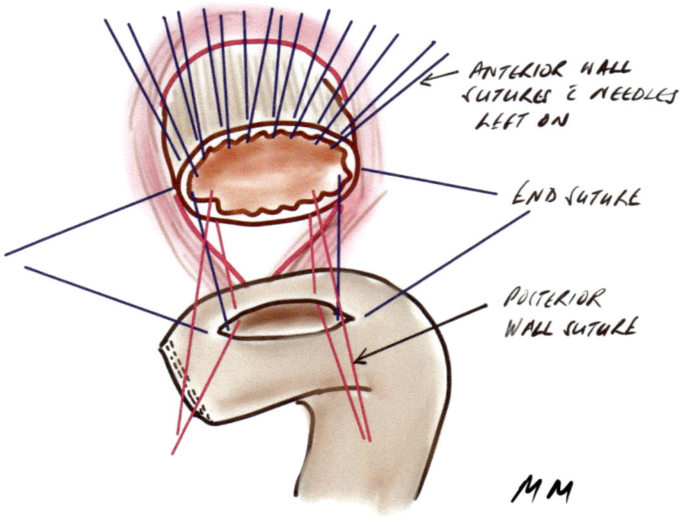

Fig. 10.9 Diagram showing sutures in the anterior part of the stomach in place and commencement of the posterior layer

Chapter 11
Perioperative Care

Abstract This chapter underscores the critical importance of comprehensive patient management alongside surgical expertise. Recognising that many patients may require preoperative optimisation due to illness-related deconditioning; the text emphasies early involvement of multidisciplinary teams including dieticians, physiotherapists, and anaesthetists to address nutritional and respiratory needs. Specialized counseling by dieticians and speech therapists is highlighted, particularly regarding adjustments post-procedure, such as modifying diets for patients with gastric or colonic conduits. Clear post-operative care pathways, including pain management and respiratory support guidelines, are stressed, along with the necessity for 24/7 access to interventional resources for managing complications. Lastly, the chapter underscores the significance of promptly identifying and addressing post-operative complications, emphasizing the principle of "failure to rescue" in optimizing patient outcomes.

Keywords Perioperative care · Preoperative optimization · Multidisciplinary teams · Nutritional assessment · Respiratory function · Post-operative care pathways · Pain management · Interventional resources · Complications management

Needless to say, perioperative care is as important as choosing the right operation and doing it well. Some patients may have been deconditioned by the illness or complication that ultimately required reconstruction. Their nutritional state and respiratory function must often be addressed before they can be considered for a complex operation. In addition to carrying out the appropriate assessments and investigations, patients benefit from seeing dieticians, physiotherapists and anaesthetists as early as possible so that they can be given a plan on how to make the necessary improvements before surgery.

Specialist dieticians working in the reconstruction team can explain to patients the implications of having a gastric or colonic conduit and how their swallowing will be affected and advise them on how to accommodate the changes by modifying their diets and lifestyles. Speech therapists should also be involved in the counselling,

M. Mughal, *Reconstructive Surgery of the Oesophagus and Stomach*,
https://doi.org/10.1007/978-3-031-66846-3_11

particularly when a neck dissection is likely to be performed with the potential for injury to the recurrent laryngeal nerve and its implications.

It is important to have clear pathways for post-operative care so that everybody involved in the patient's care understands what is expected regarding oral intake, management of chest drains, pain management, mobilisation, enteral feeding etc. The HDU or ITU team also need a clear idea of what they can and cannot do if the patient requires respiratory support. For instance, CPAP (continuous positive airway pressure) is probably best avoided, particularly with a high oesophageal anastomosis, because of the risk of anastomotic disruption. Education of the entire team includes highlighting the fact that a patient who develops unexplained atrial fibrillation a few days after surgery could have an anastomotic leak, a known presenting feature.

It is also important to have interventional facilities and expertise available 24/7. This includes endoscopic expertise, for instance, to clip or stent a leak if appropriate. Access to urgent imaging with urgent reporting is also essential.

Complications are expected after major surgery, and this will have been discussed with patients. It is important to have a low threshold for investigating a patient who isn't progressing as expected and deal with any complications expeditiously. It is well-known that "failure to rescue" often explains the difference between the outcomes of different units undertaking the same case mix of complex surgery. The complication rate may be the same, but the speed with which complications are detected and treated may explain the variation in outcomes.

Part I
Case Studies

Chapter 12
Emergencies

Abstract This chapter covers the management of emergencies such as oesophageal perforation, acute gastric volvulus, aorto-oesophageal fistula and atrio-oesophageal fistula illustrated by cases. The management of Boerhaave syndrome is considered, which is influenced by factors like clinical condition, comorbidities, and the extent of mediastinal and systemic sepsis. Historically, mortality rates ranged from 20 to 40%, with various treatment options from supportive care to radical surgery. With the advent of minimally invasive techniques, there is a shift towards endoscopic interventions like endoscopic vacuum therapy and VAC-Stent, showing promising outcomes in recent case series. However, the choice of intervention relies more on available expertise than evidence-based algorithms. Multidisciplinary collaboration, resuscitative measures, and timely referrals to specialist centres play pivotal roles in optimising patient outcomes. The management of gastric volvulus with and without ischaemia is discussed as well as the aetiology, presentation and management of the rare and catastrophic complications of aorto-oesophageal and atrio-oesophageal fistula. The early recognition of these complications is emphasised with rapid assessment and treatment by teams with appropriate expertise.

Keywords Oesophagogastric emergencies · Boerhaave syndrome · Iatrogenic oesophageal perforation · Gastric volvulus · Minimally invasive surgery · Endoscopic interventions · Damage limitation surgery · Aorto-oesophageal fistula · Atrio-oesophageal fistula · Thoracoscopic approaches · Laparoscopic approaches · Multidisciplinary approach

12.1 Boerhaave Syndrome

The management of a patient with Boerhaave syndrome depends on several factors, including the clinical condition and comorbidity, the duration of the perforation and the extent of mediastinal and systemic sepsis. Most publications up to the early

M. Mughal, *Reconstructive Surgery of the Oesophagus and Stomach*,
https://doi.org/10.1007/978-3-031-66846-3_12

2000s report a mortality of 20 to 40% with a high morbidity. Because of this variation, it is not surprising that the literature on the subject describes different management options ranging from supportive treatment with minimal intervention to radical surgery.

Before the evolution of minimally invasive surgery and endoscopic procedures such as clipping and suturing, the aim of treatment of a substantial oesophageal tear with mediastinitis and/or soiling of the thoracic cavity was to repair the oesophageal tear if possible, or create a fistula by placing a T-tube into the tear. This was supported by adjunctive measures of nil by mouth, antibiotics and enteral or parenteral nutrition. However, it was common for leakage to continue around a T-tube, and repairs often gave way. Oesophagostomy was sometimes carried out to defunction the oesophagus. However, this did not necessarily speed up healing of the tear and usually required transection of the oesophagus, necessitating a complex reconstruction eventually. Small, contained leaks without systemic sepsis have been successfully treated without attempts to close the perforation, other than draining an associated collection and supportive measures.

Minimally invasive approaches are increasingly being used with good outcomes, but exactly what combination of interventions to use in each patient is not so much defined by evidence-based algorithms but by the availability of expertise. So that the best intervention can be considered for a particular patient, treatment should be carried out at a centre capable of offering all interventions, including radical surgery. As the diagnosis is likely to be made in a variety of healthcare settings, it is important that beyond immediate resuscitative measures such as IV fluids, antibiotics and addressing respiratory problems, further interventions are carried out by discussing the case with the nearest specialist centre. This may include advice to place a chest drain if there is a large hydropneumothorax, but complex interventions are best left to the specialist centre.

A recent case series with a systematic review [1] reported mortality rates of 2%, 13% and 33% for thoracoscopic, endoscopic, and laparoscopic approaches, with successful outcomes in 98%, 38% and 67% of patients, respectively. This included four patients with free perforation treated with left-sided thoracoscopic irrigation, placement of apical and basal drains and endoscopic placement of two gastrostomies, one for drainage of the stomach and the other to facilitate the placement of a jejunal extension for enteral nutrition. No attempt was made to either intubate or repair the oesophageal tear. In this small series, there was no mortality and all the leaks healed without requiring subsequent surgical intervention.

There is increasing use of endoscopic interventions for selected cases of Boerhaave syndrome, such as the use of EVLT [2] and VAC-Stent [3].

Despite the trend for effective minimally invasive and endoscopic interventions for Boerhaave syndrome, some patients cannot be managed without surgical intervention.

12.2 Boerhaave's Requiring Colonic Interposition

12.2.1 Case Summary

A man in his 40s presented with severe chest pain after prolonged vomiting. He had a history of chronic alcoholic pancreatitis with known oesophageal varices. He was on insulin and Creon due to pancreatic insufficiency and also suffered from chronic schizophrenia.

A CT scan with oral contrast showed a right hydropneumothorax and extravasation of contrast into the right chest (Fig. 12.1).

After resuscitation and treatment, including commencement of antibiotics, he was taken to theatre, and a gastroscopy was performed, which showed an oesophageal perforation at 41 to 42 cm with dusky mucosa around it. A laparotomy was carried

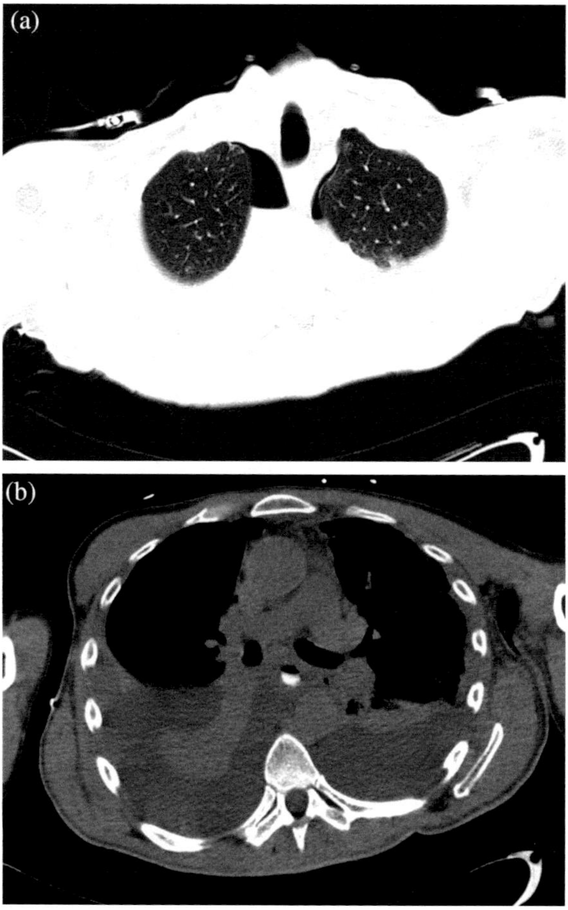

Fig. 12.1 CT sections showing a large hydropneumothorax

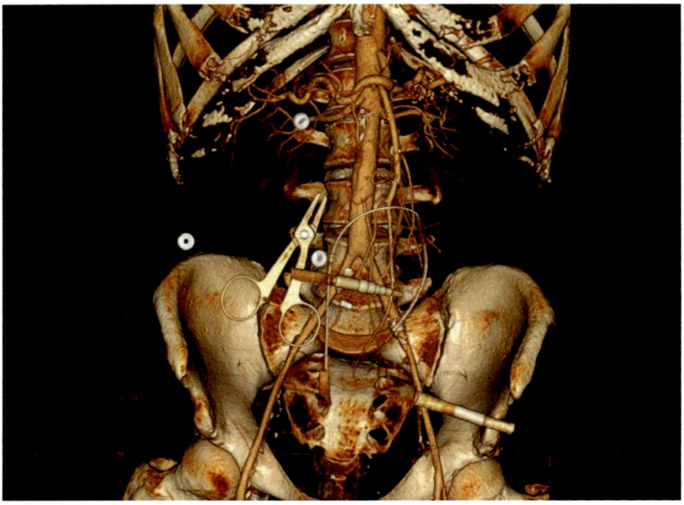

Fig. 12.2 CT reconstruction to show arterial supply to the GI tract

out to repair the perforation, but extensive varices prevented transhiatal dissection. A venting gastrostomy and feeding jejunostomy were carried out, as well as a right thoracoscopic washout and placement of a chest drain. He continued to deteriorate, and a gastroscopy ten days later showed a necrotic distal oesophagus with a much-enlarged perforation. A cervical oesophagostomy was performed, dividing the oesophagus in the superior mediastinum through a neck approach. A right thoracotomy was also carried out for debridement of the necrosed oesophagus below the azygous arch. The patient recovered and was discharged from hospital four weeks later and was readmitted for reconstruction after four months. As he was a heavy smoker, a CT angioram was carried out to assess the mesenteric vessels (Fig. 12.2).

At laparotomy, multiple varices were again noted in the upper abdomen around the stomach and the splenic flexure (Fig. 12.3). The decision was therefore made to use the right colon for reconstruction. This was routed through a substernal tunnel, anastomosed to the cervical oesophagus (Fig. 12.4), and distally to the stomach. The patient made an uneventful post-operative recovery with a normal contrast swallow at day 5 (Fig. 12.5).

12.2.2 Learning Points

This was a particularly challenging case of spontaneous oesophagus rupture associated with oesophageal necrosis in a patient with varices. Although the perforation was distal and could have been approached through the abdomen, a hiatal dissection could not be performed safely in view of extensive varices. Ultimately, a cervical oesophagostomy was required to control the mediastinal sepsis and reconstruction

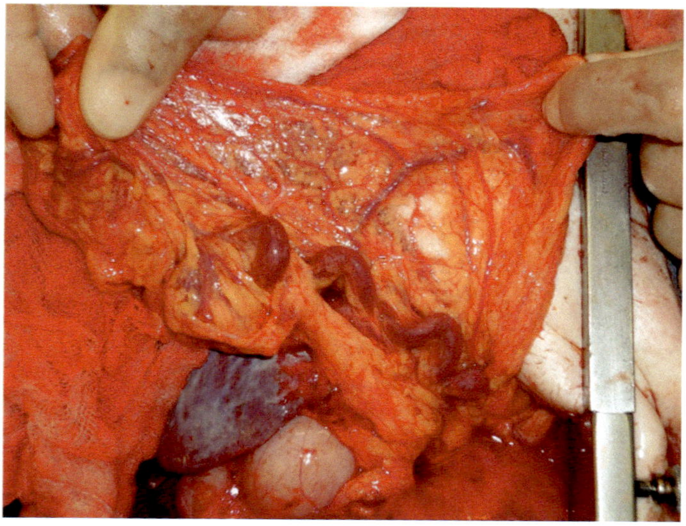

Fig. 12.3 Varices around the stomach and splenic flexure

Fig. 12.4 Colo-oesophageal anastomosis in the neck

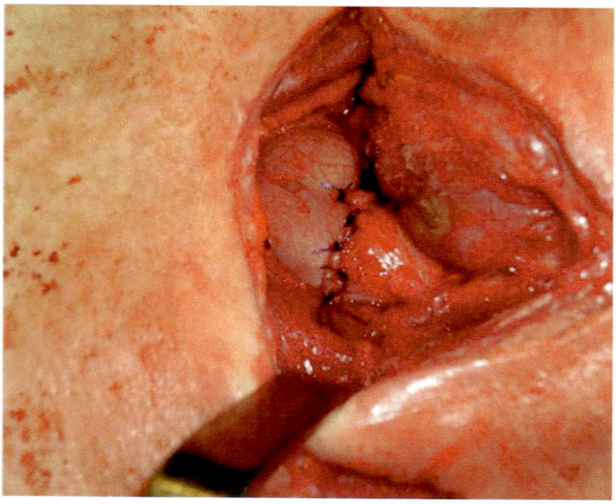

was only possible with a colonic loop. Although the stomach was intact it was unusable due to varices.

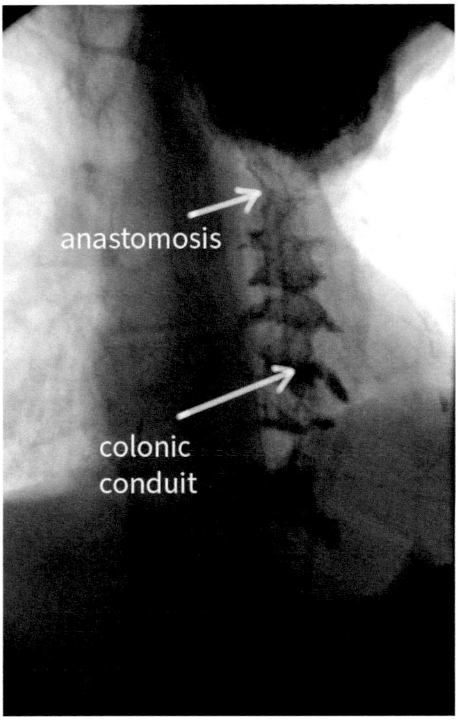

Fig. 12.5 Contrast swallow 5 days post-op showing no leak

12.3 Iatrogenic Perforations of the Oesophagus

Iatrogenic causes account for almost half of oesophageal perforations, with the most common cause being endoscopic interventions [4]. Presentation depends on the site and size of the perforation and the time elapsed since the perforation occurred. Because perforation is a risk of endoscopic interventions, patients should be observed for signs and symptoms of perforation and undergo appropriate investigations if there is any suspicion to exclude perforation before discharge. However, in some cases, the signs and symptoms of a perforation only arise after discharge, delaying the diagnosis and treatment.

If a perforation is suspected a CT scan of the neck, chest and abdomen with intravenous and oral contrast should be performed. This will not only show a perforation but also provide essential information about the site and possibly the size of the perforation, as well as the degree of extravasation of oral contrast. Although all patients with a perforation, however small, should initially be treated with intravenous antibiotics and nil by mouth, the information obtained from the CT scan helps to decide further management. In general terms, a contained perforation (i.e., ingested contrast does not diffuse out widely, with the majority of contrast passing on beyond the perforation into the stomach) can be treated conservatively in the absence of systemic sepsis. Larger perforations will require some form of intervention, which depends on the level of the perforation, associated collections, general condition of the patient and associated comorbidity.

Because of the expertise and experience required, significant oesophageal perforation should be dealt with in a specialist centre. There is evidence that this is already happening in the UK and is associated with improving outcomes [5]. Large or complex perforations are best managed by a multidisciplinary approach to decide on the best method or, more commonly, a combination of interventions for optimum outcomes. Minimally invasive techniques, including stents [6], endoscopic vacuum therapy [7] and VAC-stents [8] are increasingly being shown to be effective tools in the armamentarium of treatments for oesophageal perforation. There is, however, still a place for surgery in some circumstances and when minimally invasive and endoscopic treatment has failed [9].

Perforations of the cervical oesophagus are generally easier to treat than those in the thoracic oesophagus. In the neck, the tissue planes often contain the perforation, resulting in local rather than systemic sepsis. Many cases can be treated conservatively, but some require surgery, as in the example below.

12.4 Perforation During Trans-oesophageal Echocardiography

12.4.1 Case Summary

A man in his 50s underwent left atrial ablation for persistent AF guided by transoesophageal echography (TOE). There were no apparent technical issues in placing the TOE probe. The ablation was successful, and protamine was administered intravenously at the end of the procedure with instructions to continue with warfarin.

After the procedure, he developed surgical emphysema in the neck associated with difficulty in swallowing. The treating team placed a nasogastric tube and requested a CT scan of the neck, before obtaining a specialist opinion. The scan showed the nasogastric tube had traversed the oesophagus through the perforation and extravasation of the swallowed contrast (Figs. 12.6, 12.7 and 12.8).

Because of the misplaced nasogastric tube and extent of mediastinal soiling, it was decided to treat the perforation surgically. The perforation level meant that an approach through the neck would be at the extreme limit of accessibility. On the other hand, access from the chest would have been equally challenging. Furthermore, as the perforation was in the midline posteriorly, the question was which side of the neck to choose for the approach. After positioning the patient with the neck extended, it was decided to approach the neck through an anterior collar incision 2 cm above the sternal notch as for a total thyroidectomy. The strap muscles were divided to allow approach to both sides of the neck, and the left paratracheal space was opened. There was a posterior tear starting in the retropharyngeal area and extending 8–10 cm to the thoracic inlet.

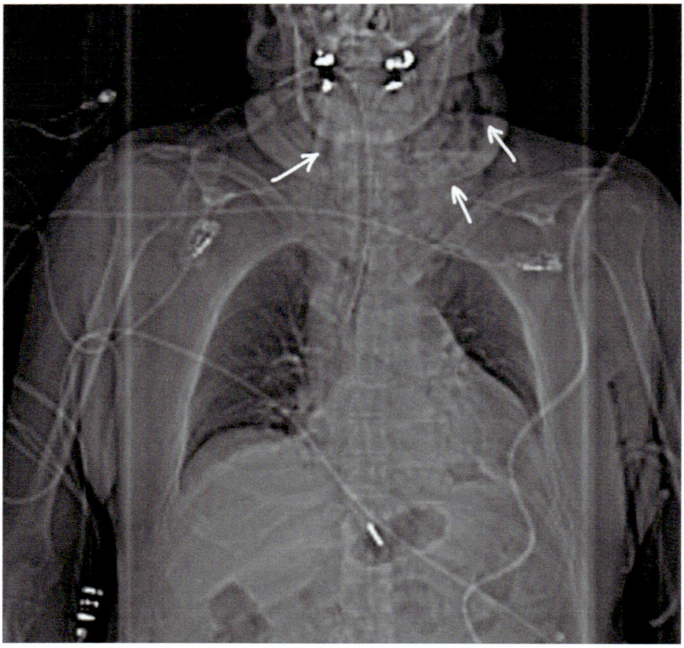

Fig. 12.6 CT scout film with arrows showing extensive surgical emphysema

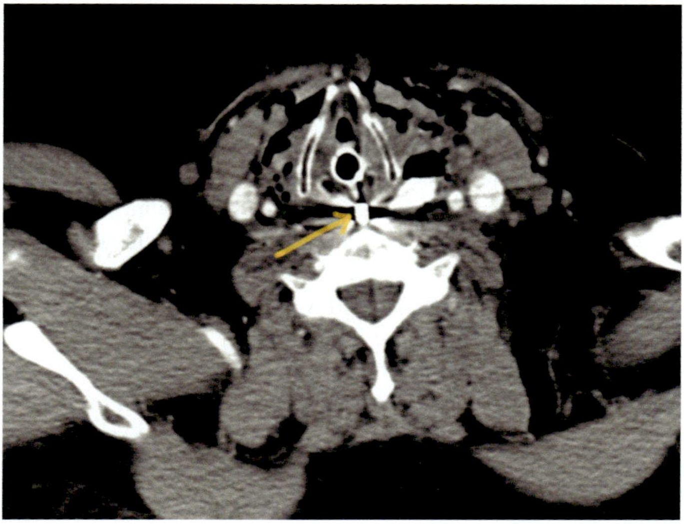

Fig. 12.7 CT showing the tip of the nasogastric tube lying outside the oesophagus posteriorly

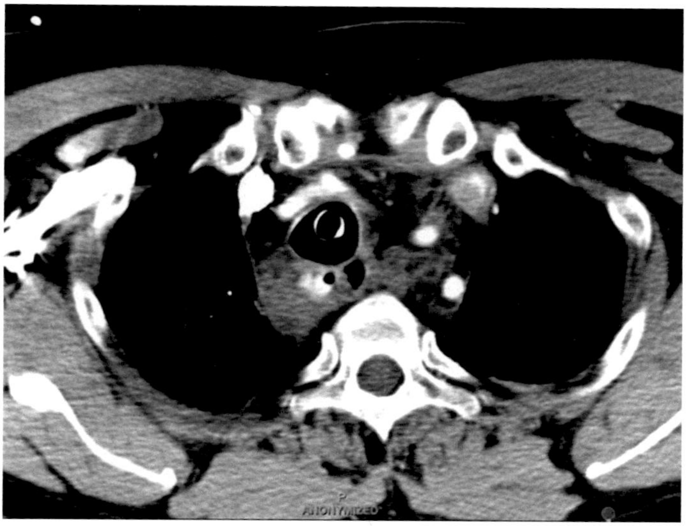

Fig. 12.8 CT showing extravasation of swallowed contrast in the upper mediastinum as well as a large amount of mediastinal air

The left recurrent laryngeal nerve was identified and safeguarded. The oesophagus was dissected as distally as possible. By placing a stay-suture at the proximal and distal limit of the tear and applying gentle traction to these, it was possible to twist the oesophagus to make the tear accessible for suturing. As the tear was somewhat ragged, it was felt that a primary repair was not appropriate, and therefore, it was closed with interrupted 3/0 PDS sutures around a 16 Fr T-tube. The T-tube was fashioned so that the proximal limb was short, measuring 2 cm, and the distal limb measuring 4 cm. The T-tube was placed in the distal end of the tear to keep the proximal limb of the T-tube from extending to and irritating the cricopharyngeus. The operation was completed by placing two drains in the neck, and a feeding jejunostomy was also placed.

As is common with a T-tube placed in the oesophagus, some leakage of oral contrast was noted when imaging was carried out five days after the procedure. However, the leak exited through the paraoesophageal neck drains. The leak dried up in two weeks, the neck drains were removed, and the patient was discharged with the T-tube in place (Figs. 12.9, 12.10 and 12.11). The T-tube was removed six weeks after a satisfactory contrast swallow (Fig. 12.12).

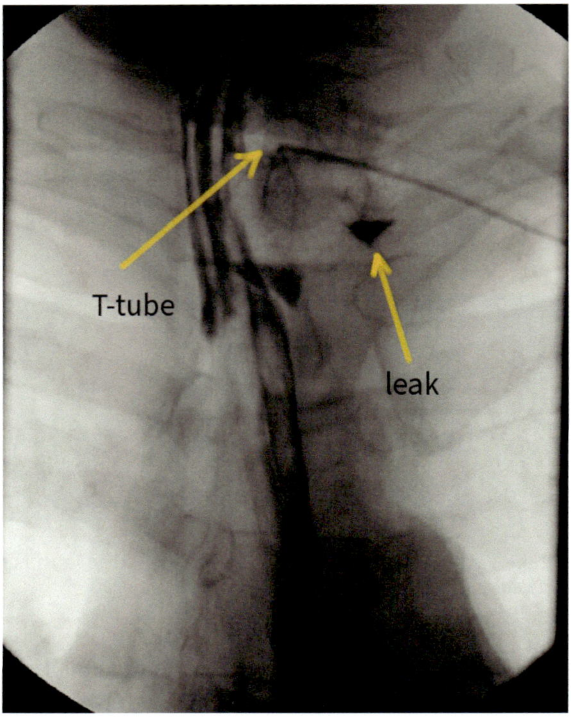

Fig. 12.9 Gastrografin swallow 10 days post-op showing T-tube in position with a small leak around it

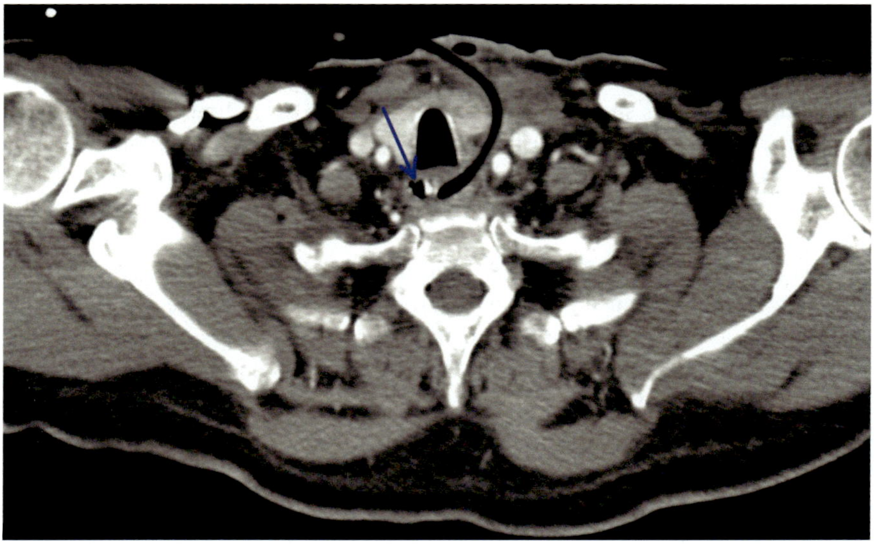

Fig. 12.10 CT showing the T-tube (arrowed) in position

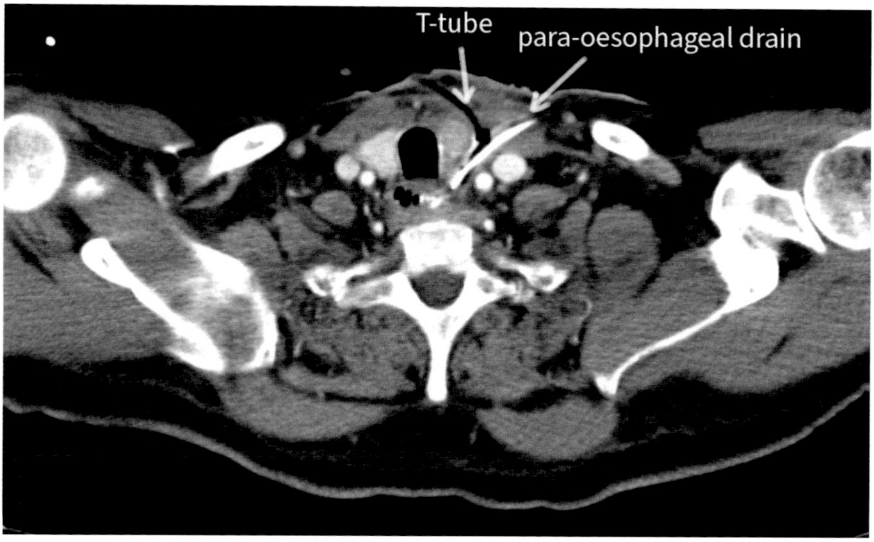

Fig. 12.11 CT showing swallowed contrast leak passing through the para-oesophageal drain

Fig. 12.12 Contrast swallow at 6 weeks, showing no leak

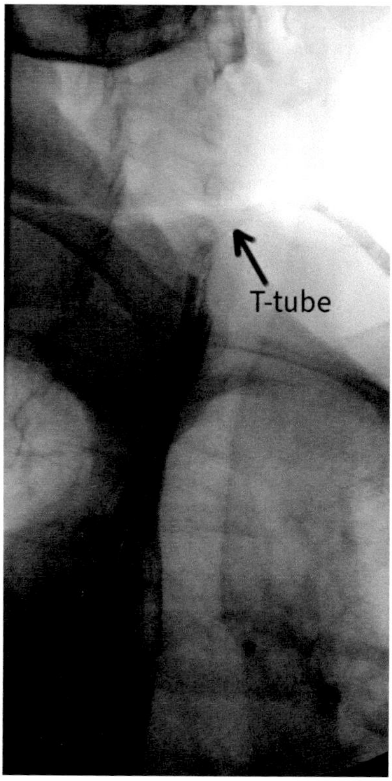

12.4.2 *Learning Points*

Perforations of the cervical oesophagus can often be treated conservatively with antibiotics, nil by mouth and either enteral or parenteral feeding. In this case, the imaging suggested a large perforation with extravasation of swallowed contrast into the mediastinum. A nasogastric tube had also been placed by the treating team, the tip of which was seen to be lying outside the oesophagus. This would have to be removed, but we were concerned about what would happen if we decided to do that and pursue conservative treatment. We opted for a surgical approach, leaving the nasogastric tube in place to assess its position and any secondary damage it might have caused.

This case posed a particular difficulty for the surgical approach as the tear was situated posteriorly and also in the "no man's territory", being very deep from a neck approach and very high if we had chosen a thoracic approach. We decided to approach this through a collar incision in the neck and, after dividing the omohyoid and the strap muscles and dividing the middle thyroid veins and inferior thyroid arteries to mobilise the left lobe of the thyroid, it was possible to mobilise the laryngo-pharyngeal complex and gain good exposure of the oesophagus in the superior mediastinum. Once the nasogastric tube had been removed, stay sutures were replaced at the upper and lower extent of the tear in the oesophagus posteriorly and used to "corkscrew" or rotate the oesophagus to permit the placement of the repair stitches and the T-tube. It was important to sculpt the T-tube appropriately so that its superior limb was kept short and did not emerge at the cricopharyngeus.

12.5 Acute Gastric Volvulus

Gastric volvulus can present with acute or chronic symptoms. It arises from the rotation of the stomach along its horizontal or vertical axis.

Gastric volvulus can be classified as primary or secondary. Primary gastric volvulus is believed to occur due to weakened gastric ligaments, which can be further exacerbated by skeletal deformities like kyphoscoliosis. This typically affects older patients. On the other hand, secondary gastric volvulus is associated with other anatomical abnormalities, of which a hiatal hernia is the most common.

There are two types of primary gastric volvulus, the more common organoaxial volvulus and the less common mesenteroaxial volvulus. In organoaxial volvulus, the stomach rotates along its long axis, causing the antrum to rotate anteriorly lying above the fundus, while the fundus rotates posteriorly and lies below the antrum. In contrast, mesenteroaxial volvulus occurs when the stomach rotates around its middle, leading to the antrum ending up above the gastro-oesophageal junction.

Symptoms depend on the degree of rotation, and often there are none, with the diagnosis being made incidentally during radiological imaging for some other indication. However, if the stomach rotates more than 180°, it can lead to complete gastric outlet obstruction. When the volvulus is associated with a hiatus hernia, the stomach can become incarcerated resulting in ischaemia and necrosis, presenting as a medical emergency. The symptoms of a volvulus depend on whether the presentation is acute or chronic [10]. Borchardt's triad [11], which is usually indicative of acute volvulus, comprises three symptoms. These are a sudden onset of severe epigastric pain, retching without producing much vomitus, and the inability to pass a nasogastric tube into the stomach.

Management of acute gastric volvulus depends on the presentation, age and comorbidity, as illustrated in the following two cases.

12.6 Gastric Volvulus with Perforation of the Stomach

12.6.1 Case Summary

A woman in her 70s was transferred from another hospital where she had been admitted with a 48-hours history of vomiting and chest pain. A CT scan showed aspiration pneumonia secondary to gastric volvulus. She was septic, ventilated and on high doses of noradrenaline when transferred. Her white cell count was 24 and albumin was 23.

An emergency laparoscopy showed the stomach incarcerated in a large hiatus hernia. Partial reduction of the stomach revealed ischaemic perforation of the body with food contents in the mediastinum. It was decided to convert to a laparotomy, and a subtotal gastrectomy was performed, removing the antrum and body of the stomach. The proximal stomach was viable and was stapled off and a venting gastrostomy was placed. Immediate reconstruction was not carried out because of the mediastinal sepsis, treatment with inotropes and low albumin. A feeding jejunostomy was placed and enteral nutrition commenced.

After a good recovery, three months later, the patient was reassessed for reconstruction. Gastroscopy showed a healthy stomach remnant with a hiatus hernia. In order to determine if reconstruction could be carried out without opening the chest, a CT scan was performed to determine the position of the stomach remnant in relationship to the oesophageal hiatus (Fig. 12.13).

The stomach was distended with fluid instilled through the gastrostomy prior to the CT scan. This showed a hiatus hernia but a good capacity stomach remnant, with a reasonable portion below the diaphragm. Reconstruction was carried out with a Roux-en-Y jejunal loop anastomosed to the stomach. As most of the stomach remnant was within a hiatus hernia and was firmly adherent to the surroundings, no attempt was made to reduce the stomach remnant into the abdomen.

The patient made an uneventful recovery and was able to resume oral feeding and remained well on follow-up three years later.

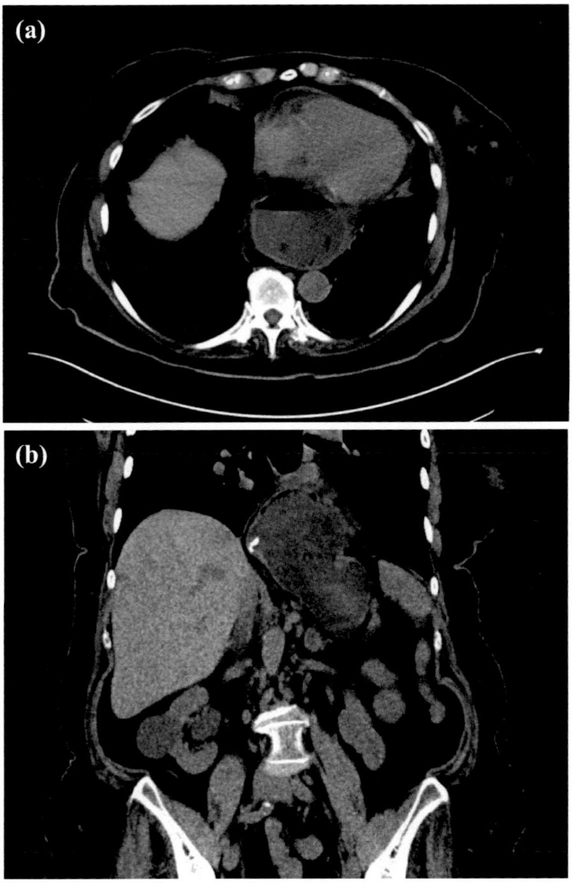

Fig. 12.13 Axial (a) and coronal (b) CT sections three months following initial surgery, prior to reconstruction

12.6.2 Learning Points

At the initial presentation of a perforated, partially necrotic stomach involved in a paraoesophageal hiatus hernia, the procedure was limited to dealing with the sepsis and excising the necrotic stomach. Reconstruction was carried after the patient had recovered fully and an assessment of the stomach remnant had been carried out endoscopically and by CT. No attempt was made to reduce the stomach remnant from a hiatus hernia because of dense adhesions. It was felt that a difficult reduction and repair of the hiatus would add to the morbidity without significant benefit.

12.7 Gastric Volvulus

12.7.1 Case Summary

A woman in her 90s presented with a six-month history of intermittent severe upper abdominal and chest pain associated with episodic dysphagia. Her general health was reasonable for her age but there was a history of hypertension and ischaemic heart disease.

A CT scan showed a large hiatus hernia with an air-fluid level, and a configuration in keeping with a chronic organoaxial gastric volvulus (Fig. 12.14).

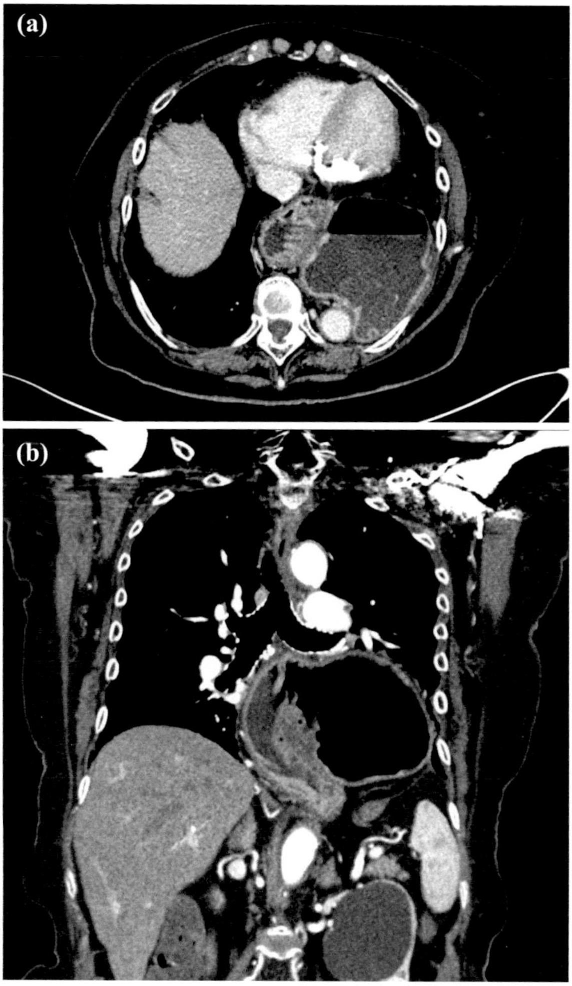

Fig. 12.14 Axial (a) and coronal (b) CT scans at presentation

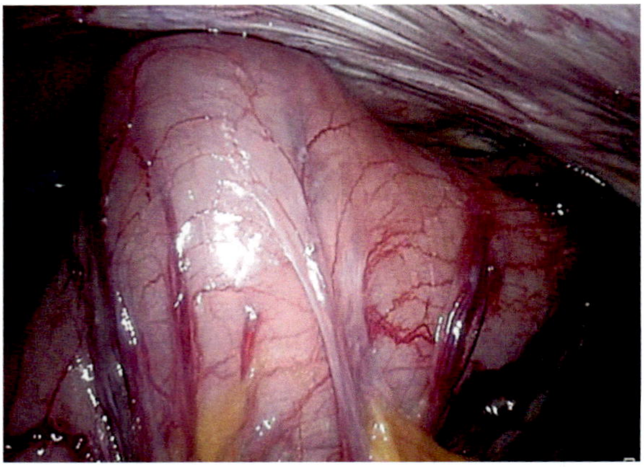

Fig. 12.15 Laparoscopic view showing fixation of stomach with PEG tubes

In view of her age and comorbidity, after a detailed discussion with the patient, it was decided to opt for a reduction of the hiatus hernia and gastropexy rather than a formal repair. A laparoscopy was performed, and as much of the stomach as possible was reduced without a formal dissection through the hiatus. The reduction was assisted with a simultaneous gastroscopy which was then also used for the placement of two PEG tubes to fix the antrum to the abdominal wall (Fig. 12.15). The tubes were removed six weeks later.

The patient recovered well but suffered from symptoms of gastro-oesophageal reflux which were managed with a combination of lifestyle advice and PPIs. She underwent a CT scan for the investigation of lower abdominal pain two years later. This showed a large left-sided hiatus hernia. The stomach had come away from the anterior abdominal wall at the site of the previous gastropexy. There was new herniation of the splenic flexure of the colon (Fig. 12.16).

12.7.2 Learning Points

Because of the patient's age and comorbidity it was decided to manage the volvulus with a gastropexy rather than a formal repair. It is accepted that this is a temporary measure to deal with an acute problem, and it is often not resilient. Despite fixation of the antrum to the abdominal wall by two PEG tubes for 6 weeks, the stomach became detached in due course. This is not uncommon with any form of gastropexy. A CT scan two years later showed a recurrence of the hiatus hernia but without a volvulus. In addition, the splenic flexure of the colon had also herniated. Despite that, the patient remained free of attacks of dysphagia and chest pain until four years later. This highlights the fact that symptoms do not always correlate with findings on radiological imaging, and it is important to have a pragmatic approach to managing large hiatus hernias in elderly patients and those with significant comorbidity.

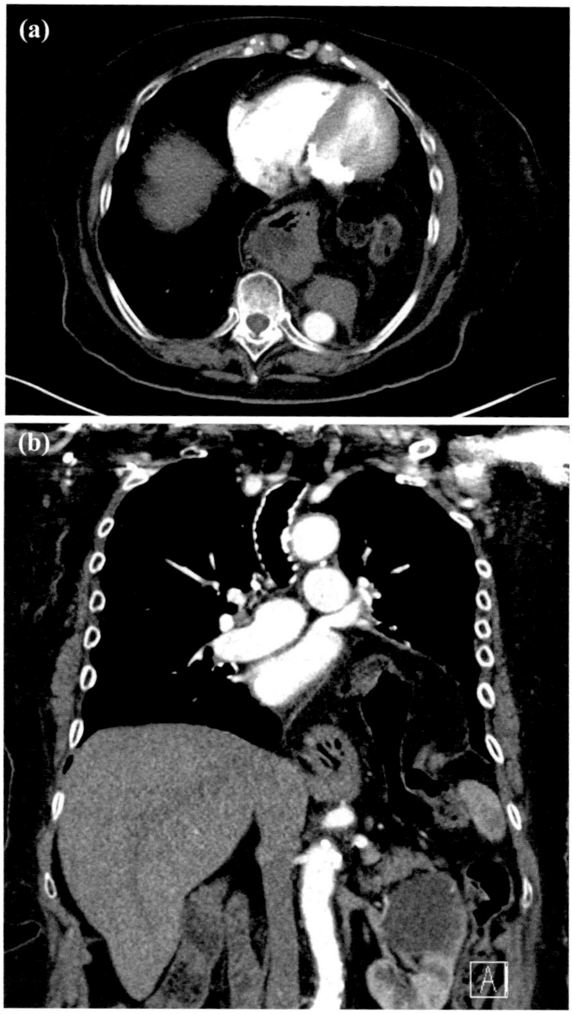

Fig. 12.16 Axial (a) and coronal (b) CT sections two years following gastropexy

12.8 Aorto-oesophageal Fistula

Aorto-oesophageal fistula (AOF) is an extremely rare condition. According to a study by Lee et al., the incidence of primary aorto-oesophageal fistula is low, with only 500 cases reported in the literature between 1928 and 1991 [12]. It has been reported as a rare but lethal complication after thoracic endovascular aortic repair [13] and other aortic interventions [14]. However, it can also complicate chemoradiotherapy for thoracic cancer, oesophagectomy and oesophageal stenting, resulting in catastrophic haemorrhage [15].

AOF is a serious complication that can cause severe gastrointestinal bleeding but may present with small bleeds commonly known as "herald bleeding." In addition to this, patients may experience chest pain, dysphagia, and sepsis. Diagnosing AOF can be challenging and often requires a high level of suspicion, particularly in patients with a history of aortic surgery or oesophageal pathology. CT angiography and endoscopy is useful to diagnose the condition.

The management of AOF can be challenging and is associated with a high mortality. The most durable and successful approaches include radical oesophagectomy and extensive aortic reconstruction [16]. Although endovascular management may be an initial treatment option, it is often complicated by recurrent sepsis, which necessitates long-term clinical and radiological surveillance. Treatment with a combination of antibiotics, graft replacement and oesophagectomy have the best outcomes with a survival of 50% at 60 months.

I have included two different examples AOF and how they were managed. One of these was a mycotic aneurysm of the thoracic aorta [17]. AOFs fistulae present in a wide variety of different ways and degree of urgency. Management is therefore dictated by many factors, including the primary pathology, urgency of presentation, as well as the patient's general condition and comorbidity. However, the principles are the same, which are to stop the bleeding and carry out an oesophageal exclusion, diversion followed by addressing the primary cause which usually requires an oesophagectomy and reconstruction as staged procedures.

AOF is a rare but life-threatening condition that requires prompt diagnosis and aggressive surgical management. Due to its rarity and high mortality rate, a multidisciplinary approach involving vascular surgeons, gastroenterologists, and radiologists is essential for optimal patient outcomes.

12.9 Aorto-oesophageal Fistula from a Mycotic Aneurysm

12.9.1 Case Summary

woman in her 50s presented a few weeks history of fever, with weakness and lethargy. Her history included a 2.5 cm abdominal aortic aneurysm and retroperitoneal fibrosis which had been treated with tamoxifen. A CT scan showed thoracic and abdominal aortic aneurysms as well as an aneurysm at the origin of the right subclavian artery. A PET scan (Fig. 12.17) showed features of an inflammatory or mycotic aetiology as well as discitis affecting the lower lumbar spine. She was managed by a MDT comprising of rheumatologists, vascular surgeons, and specialists in infectious diseases. Treatment was commenced with intravenous antibiotics and steroids, although blood cultures were negative.

A repeat CT scan one week later showed that the aneurysms had enlarged and therefore endovascular repair was carried out. Before that, she required a bilateral

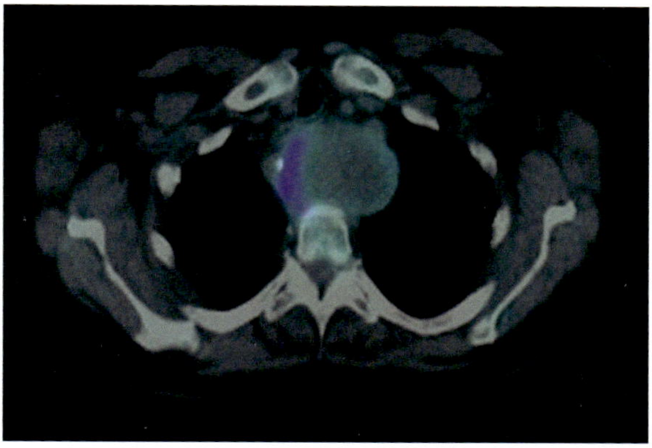

Fig. 12.17 PET scan at presentation showing mycotic aneurysm

carotid to subclavian bypass to ensure perfusion to the upper limbs, followed by bilateral subclavian artery and thoracic stent grafts. This was followed by a fenestrated stent graft for an enlarging abdominal aneurysm. One month after discharge, she was readmitted with systemic infection and back pain. CT and oral contrast showed a fistula between the oesophagus and the sac of the thoracic aneurysm.

She was commenced on antibiotics and antifungals and was transferred to our unit. An OGD was performed under general anaesthetic, which showed two well-established fistulae between the oesophagus and the sac of the thoracic aneurysm. The stent graft was visible through the larger, more proximal fistula (Fig. 12.18). The decision was taken to carry out oesophageal exclusion to minimise infection of the stent graft.

The cervical oesophagus was approached through a left neck incision, but access was limited by a very narrow window due to the carotid to subclavian graft.

The oesophagus was transected as low down as possible in the superior mediastinum, and the proximal end was brought out as an oesophagostomy. The fistula and related anatomy is illustrated in Fig. 12.19. A laparotomy was performed, and the stomach was portioned using a stapler, leaving a narrow part attached to the oesophagus and the remaining part left for future reconstruction. A venting gastrostomy was placed in the part attached to the oesophagus to provide drainage and access to the excluded oesophagus (Figs. 12.20 and 12.21) feeding jejunostomy was placed and enteral nutrition commenced. The patient made a good recovery and was discharged on long-term antibiotics.

Against expectations she remained well for the next three months, hence a decision was made to offer her a reconstruction. The previously partitioned stomach with the tube gastrostomy was left undisturbed. The thoracic oesophagus and the gastro-oesophageal junction were not disturbed as excision would have been extremely hazardous and jeopardised the previous stent repair. The previously created gastric conduit was brought up into the neck via a retrosternal tunnel and anastomosed to the oesophageal stump (Figs. 12.22, 12.23, 12.24, 12.25 and 12.26). Post-operative imaging showed satisfactory appearances (Figs. 12.27 and 12.28). The patient made

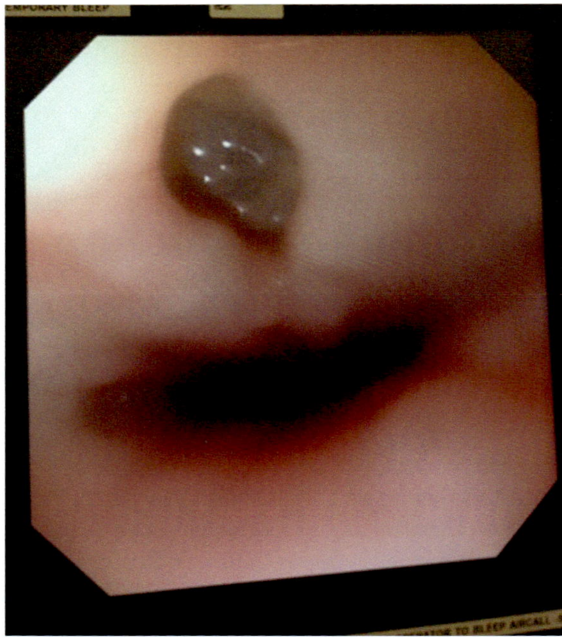

Fig. 12.18 Endoscopy showing a fistula between the oesophagus and the aneurysm sac, through which can be seen the stent graft

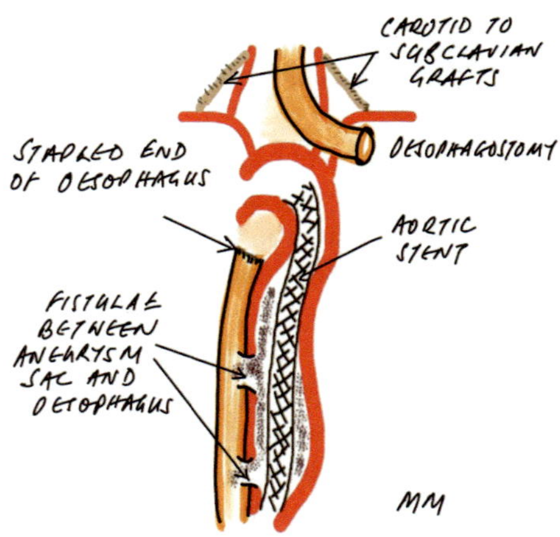

Fig. 12.19 Diagrammatic depiction of the aortoesophageal fistula

an uneventful recovery and was discharged on oral feeding and long-term antibiotics. She survived for four years, eventually succumbing to spinal sepsis (Fig. 12.29).

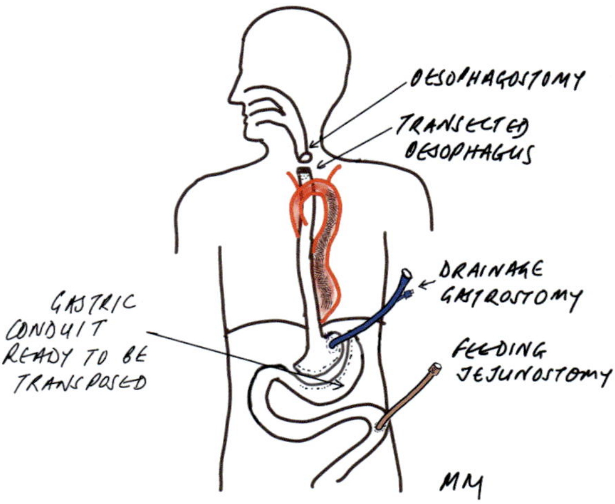

Fig. 12.20 Excluded oesophagus, venting gastrostomy and feeding jejunostomy

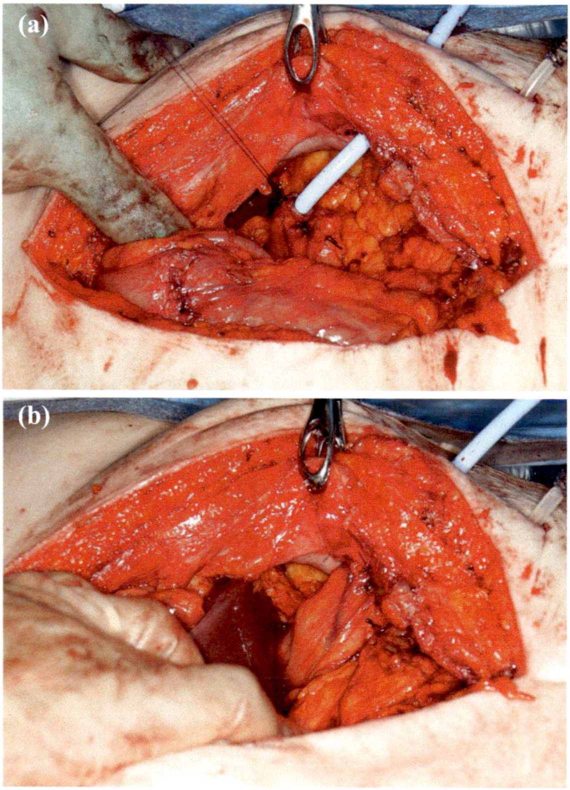

Fig. 12.21 Foley catheter at the tip of the partitioned lesser curve of the stomach secured with a purse-string suture (a). The second picture (b) shows the lesser curve hitched up to and sutured to the anterior abdominal wall

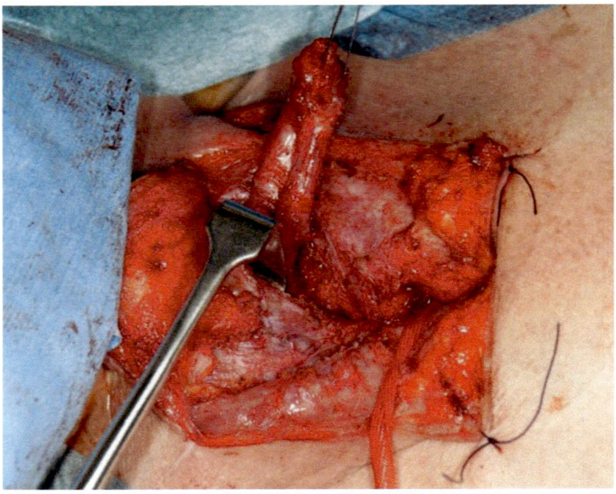

Fig. 12.22 Oesophagostomy taken down and oesophageal stump mobilised for the anastomosis. Note traction sutures placed around the liberated mucocutaneous junction

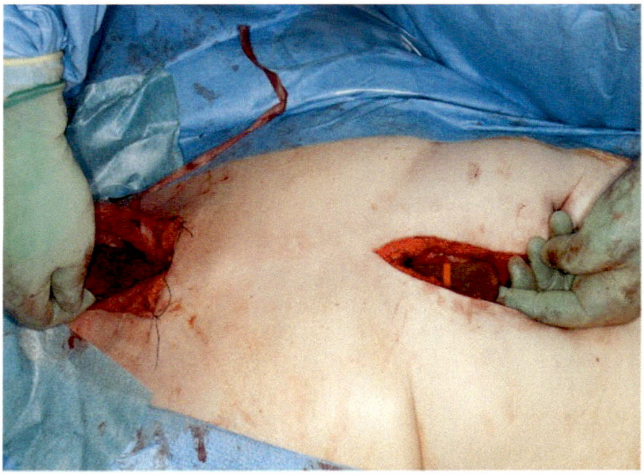

Fig. 12.23 Retrosternal tunnel created with malleable retractor

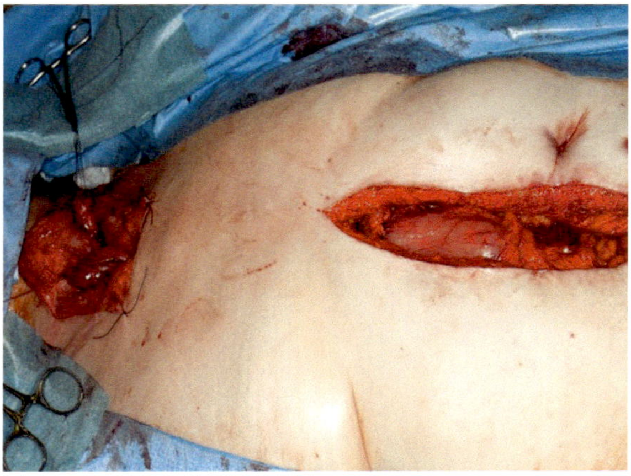

Fig. 12.24 Gastric conduit routed through the retrosternal tunnel to the neck

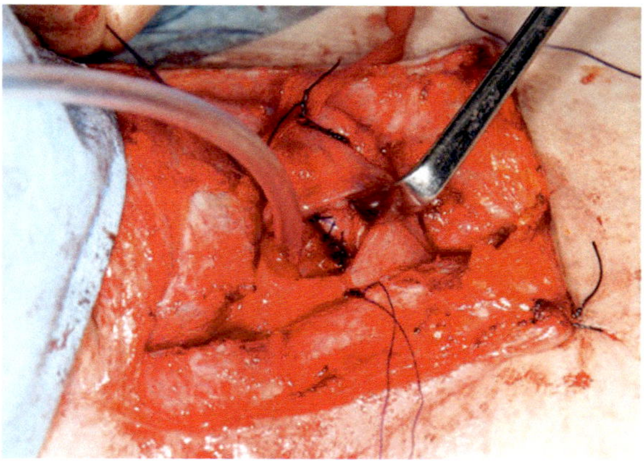

Fig. 12.25 Completed posterior layer of the anastomosis with the NGT about to be placed into the conduit before suturing the anterior layer

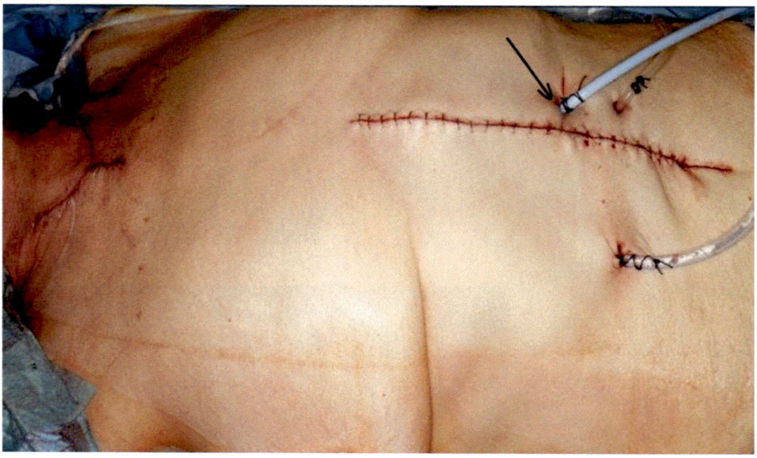

Fig. 12.26 Completed operation with feeding jejunostomy and Foley catheter (arrowed) to the left of the incision and an abdominal drain to the right

12.9.2 Learning Points

This was an extremely complex case. The decision to exclude the oesophagus was taken to minimise infection of the aortic stent graft. The fistula was between the oesophagus and the stent without an endoleak. So, the immediate concern was sepsis rather than aortic bleeding. We did not expect that the sepsis could be controlled and that the patient would survive long enough or remain well enough to have a reconstruction, but she did. Reconstruction was carried out using the stomach to bypass the excluded oesophagus, as it would have been too hazardous to remove the oesophagus. The lesser curve of the stomach was retained after construction of the gastric conduit, and a Foley catheter was placed into it to both drain the provide

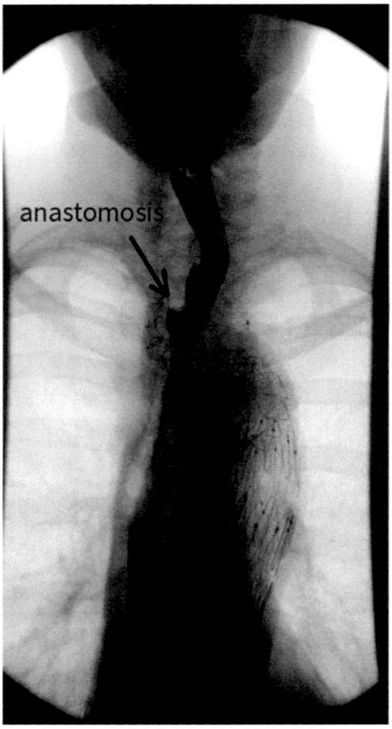

Fig. 12.27 Contrast swallow 7 days after surgery

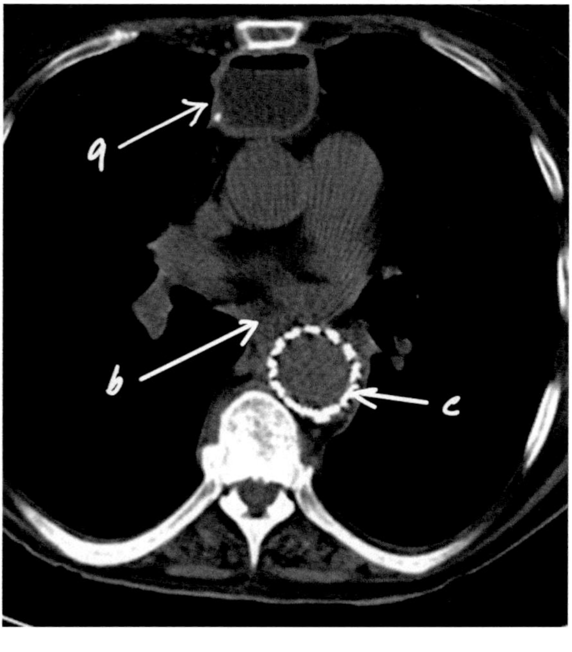

Fig. 12.28 CT scan two weeks after surgery showing the gastric conduit (a) lying centrally behind the sternum, a collapsed excluded oesophagus (b) and stent graft (c) without associated stranding

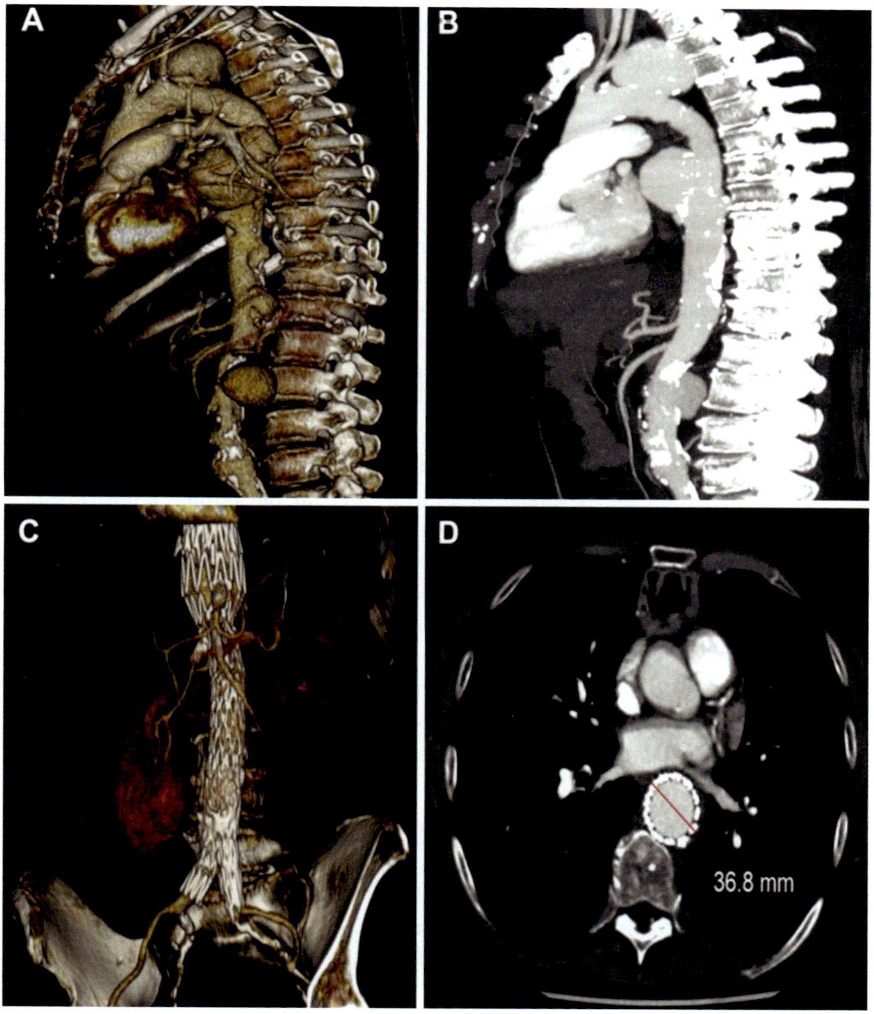

Fig. 12.29 CT angiograms before (A,B) and 30 months after stenting (C,D)

future access, if needed, to the oesophagus. The catheter provided egress for mucus and debris from the oesophagus and the output was monitored for any bleeding from the fistula. Against all expectations, the patient lived for four years.

12.10 Aorto-Oesophageal Fistula Following DXT and Oesophageal Stenting

12.10.1 Case Summary

A woman in her 60s presented with chest pain, systemic sepsis and haematemesis after failed attempts at removing a temporary oesophageal stent. She had undergone radical, definitive chemoradiotherapy for squamous cell carcinoma of the mid oesophagus 18 months previously and subsequent imaging had shown a complete metabolic response. She had a history of heavy alcohol intake. She developed a strictureat the site of the original oesophageal tumour and radiotherapy which required frequent dilatation. Because of recurrent stricturing, the decision had been taken to place a temporary oesophageal stent.

A CT scan showed the oesophageal stent with surrounding soft tissue thickening and a fistula between the oesophagus and the arch of the aorta 17 mm distal to the origin of the left subclavian artery and a further fistula at the midpoint of the oesophageal stent with active extravasation into the oesophagus (Fig. 12.30). The entire oesophagus was distended with blood clots. The stomach also contained large blood clots and the liver had an irregular contour with atrophy of the right lobe and oesophageal varices suggestive of cirrhosis and portal hypertension.

The thoracic aorta was stented to stop the bleeding (Fig. 12.31), and she was administered broad-spectrum antibiotics and antifungals. It was decided to perform an oesophageal bypass in view of the fistulation, to minimise stent infection.

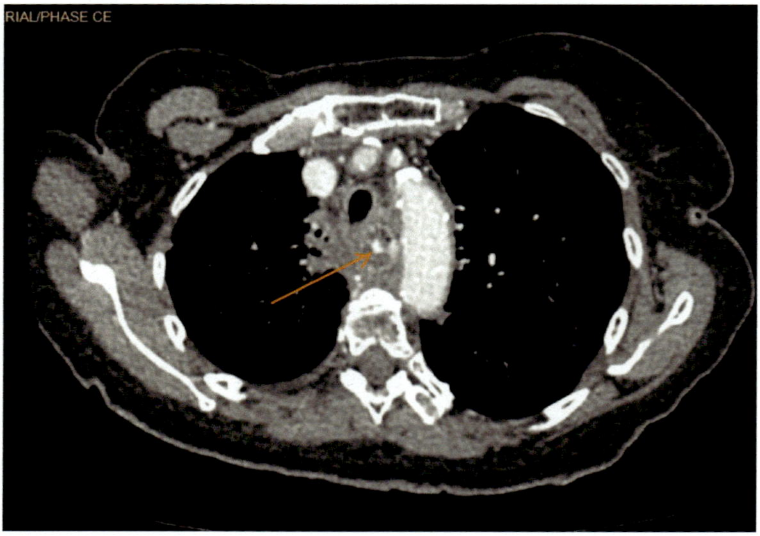

Fig. 12.30 CT angiogram showing a vascular blush into the oesophagus

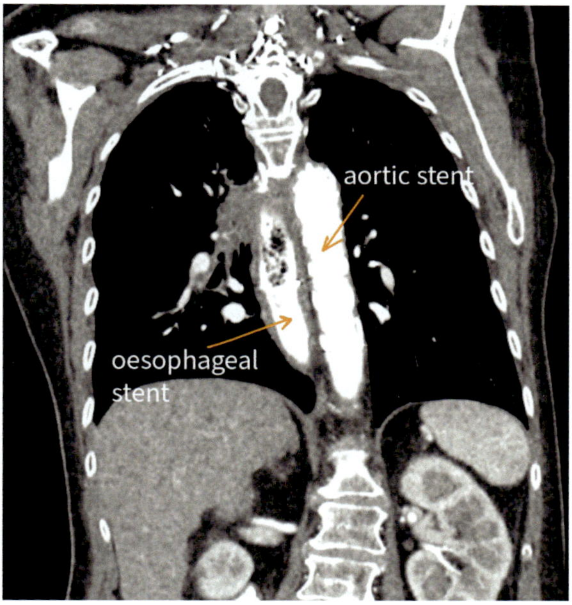

Fig. 12.31 CT scan with oral contrast after stenting of the aorta. The aortic stent is seen in position with contrast in the oesophageal stent

A lateral neck approach was used and the dissection was difficult due to intense fibrosis resulting in a blunting of the normal planes. It was necessary to perform a left thyroid lobectomy to gain sufficient access for dissection and mobilisation of the cervical oesophagus. The oesophagus was dissected into the mediastinum to the level of the top of the stent, where it was stapled off and the proximal end brought out for the cervical anastomosis. The stomach was mobilised, maintaining the gastroepiploeic arch and a conduit was created based on the greater curvature (Fig. 12.32). A Foley catheter was inserted to vent the lesser curvature of the stomach, which was retained to provide access to the oesophagus. A feeding jejunostomy was also placed. The gastric conduit was brought up to the neck through a retrosternal tunnel and anastomosed to the oesophageal stump (Fig. 12.33).

The patient made a slow but uncomplicated recovery (Figs. 12.34 and 12.35) and was discharged six weeks later with oral feeding and supplemental jejunostomy feeding, which was eventually removed. There was no further bleeding, as evidenced by the discharge from her venting gastrostomy tube. She succumbed to other conditions six months later.

12.10.2 Learning Points

Oesophageal stenting against a background of radiotherapy can give rise to fistulation into the aorta or the airways. In this case, the stent was meant to be temporary but had become embedded in the oesophagus because of the duration it had been left

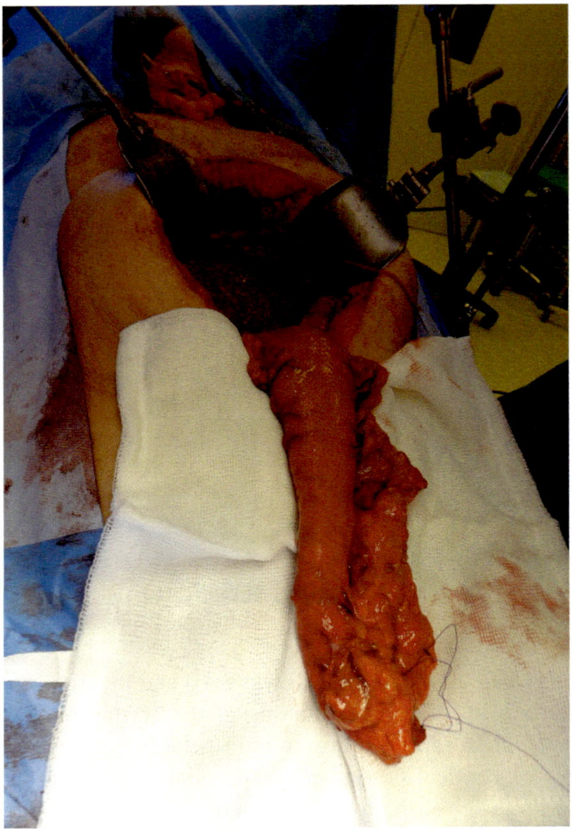

Fig. 12.32 Gastric conduit ready for transposition

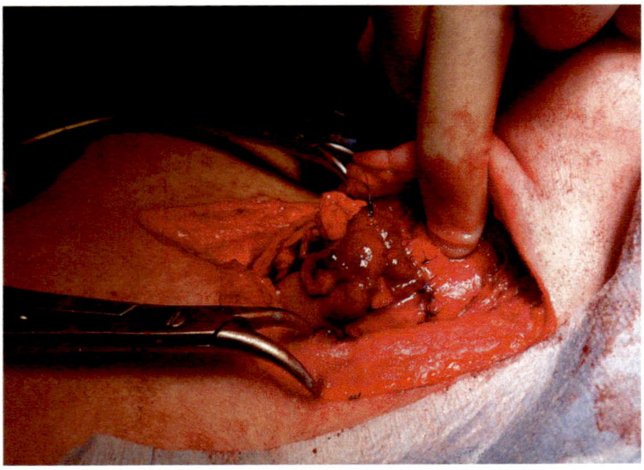

Fig. 12.33 Completed cervical anastomosis after left thyroid lobectomy

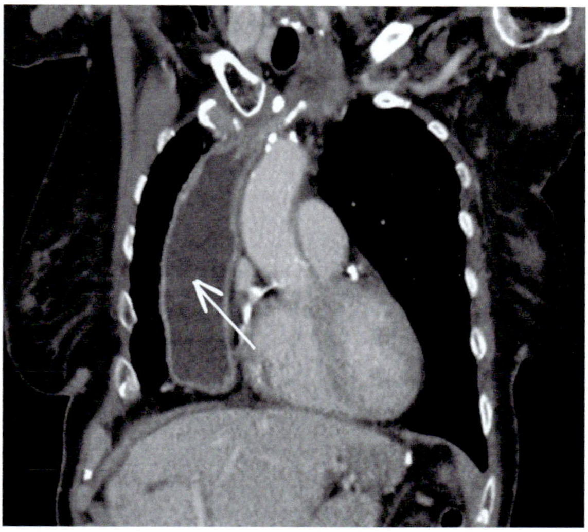

Fig. 12.34 CT scan one week later showing gastric conduit in place

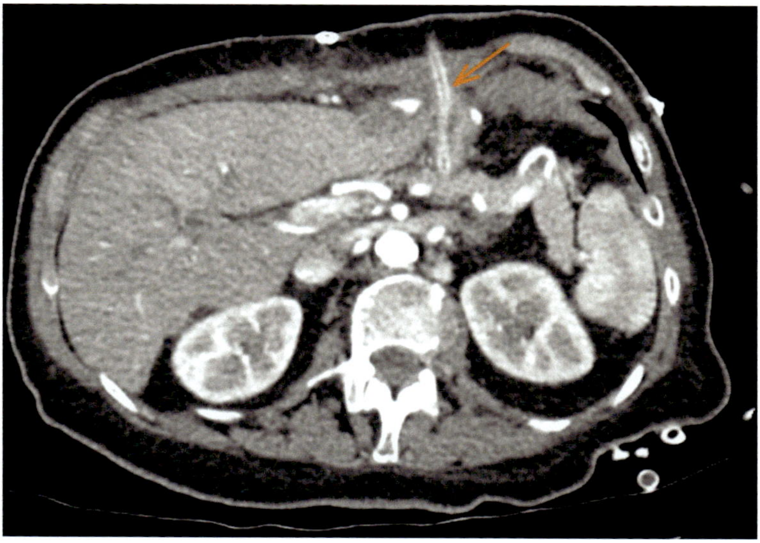

Fig. 12.35 CT showing Foley catheter draining the excluded oesophagus

in place. The stent could not be removed and attempts at dislodging it may have triggered bleeding from the aorta. This was managed with an aortic stent, but it was then necessary to exclude the oesophagus to minimise contamination of the aortic stent through the fistula to the oesophagus. A left thyroid lobectomy was performed to gain enough space to perform a cervical anastomosis, and this is a strategy that I have used on other occasions. It would have been too hazardous to try and remove the oesophageal stent or the oesophagus itself. Because the oesophagus was left in situ, the lesser curve of the stomach was retained after forming the gastric conduit and a Foley catheter was placed to drain the oesophagus and particularly to know if there was any further bleeding from the aorta into the oesophagus (see stomach portioning technique illustrated in Fig. 12.20).

12.11 Atrio-oesophageal Fistula

Atrio-oesophageal fistula (Fig. 12.36) is a serious complication of atrial ablation and carries a significant mortality. The incidence is underestimated because of misdiagnosis or underreporting but is likely to be between 0.03% and 0.08% [18]. Although it is rare, it is important to bear in mind because of the increasing application of ablation in the Western world with greater than 50,000 procedures performed annually in the USA. Fever, neurological, gastrointestinal and cardiac symptoms are the most common presentations. Symptoms present two to four weeks after the procedure but can occur up to eight weeks later.

Neurological symptoms (72%) include focal signs, seizure, confusion, loss of consciousness or non-specific features. The gastrointestinal manifestations (41%) include haematemesis, melaena, dysphagia or odynophagia, nausea and vomiting. Fever is one of the most common signs, being present in 73% of cases. Chest pain is also present in up to 30% of patients. CT of the chest is abnormal in 98% of cases, showing free air in the left atrium or pericardium. OGD can result in deterioration or death from air embolus and yet stenting has been used as the first line management of bleeding. It is recommended that if endoscopy is performed, minimal, if any, insufflation should be used.

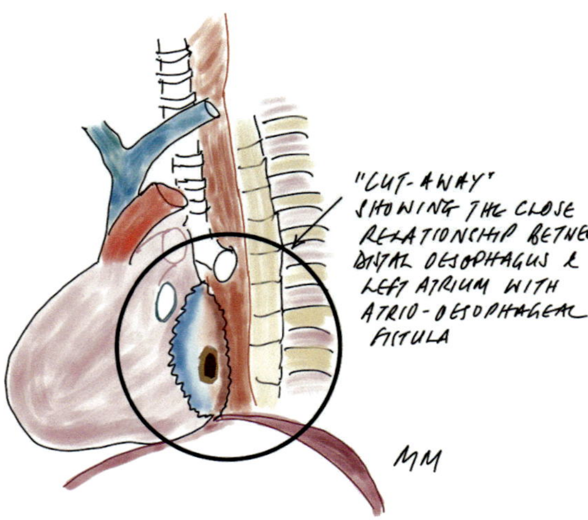

Fig. 12.36 Diagrammatic depiction of an atrio-oesophageal fistula

Neurological symptoms (OR 16) and gastrointestinal bleeding (OR 4.2) are strong predictors of mortality. Mortality without intervention is high, with an odds ratio of 24.9. In a review by Han 67% of the 70 patients who underwent surgery survived [19].

A systematic review of the surgical treatment of atrio-oesophageal fistula [20] has analysed the management of 219 patients. Overall survival was 47%. For those undergoing surgery, survival was 71.9%. Typically, a right thoracotomy was performed with a patch repair of the left atrium and primary repair of the oesophagus on cardiopulmonary bypass with an interposition flap between the two organs. The authors of this paper used a combination of sternotomy for the atrial repair and a right thoracotomy for the oesophageal repair.

Others have described a staged approach, starting with oesophageal stenting. The atrial defect was closed after resecting the fistula and the oesophagus was resected with the contained stent. Oesophageal reconstruction was performed at a second stage with a gastric pull-up through the right chest [21].

It is important that patients are managed jointly by cardiothoracic and Upper GI teams. The risk of atrio-oesophageal fistula may be reduced in the future by advances in ablation technology, including different ways of delivering RF energy and better localisation by using magnetic navigation. Other strategies include oesophageal temperature monitoring, cooling and posterior displacement of the oesophagus.

References

1. Pickering O, Pucher PH, De'Ath H, Abuawwad M, Kelly J, Underwood TJ, Noble F, Byrne JP. Minimally invasive approach in Boerhaave's syndrome: case series and systematic review. J Laparoendosc Adv Surg Tech. 2021;31(11):1254–61. https://doi.org/10.1089/lap.2020.0751.
2. Anundsen TK, Dag TF, Hans-Olaf J, Egil J. Outcome after stent and endoscopic vacuum therapy-based treatment for postemetic esophageal rupture. Scand J Gastroenterol 2023;1–6. https://doi.org/10.1080/00365521.2023.2248537.
3. Pattynama L, Wietse JE, Mattheus CBW, Roos EP. Successful endoscopic management of a large esophageal defect due to boerhaave syndrome with endoscopic vacuum therapy using vacuum sponge and vacuum stent. VideoGIE 2023;8(4):144–47. https://doi.org/10.1016/j.vgie.2022.12.001.
4. Ryom P, Jesper BR, Luit P, Susanne S, Maria GI, Peter S, Henrik K. Aetiology, treatment and mortality after oesophageal perforation in Denmark. n.d.
5. Markar SR, Hugh M, Tom W, Alan A, Omar F, Giovanni Z, George BH. Management and outcomes of esophageal perforation: a national study of 2,564 patients in England. Offic J Am Coll Gastroenterol ACG. 2015;110(11):1559. https://doi.org/10.1038/ajg.2015.304.
6. Ben-David K, Kevin B, Steven H, Georgios R, Angel C, Cristina C, Thomas C et al. Esophageal perforation management using a multidisciplinary minimally invasive treatment algorithm. J Am Coll Surg. 2014;218(4):768–74. https://doi.org/10.1016/j.jamcollsurg.2013.12.033.
7. Heiss MM, Clemens S, Christian AG. Editorial: endoscopic vacuum therapy (EVT) in the gastrointestinal tract—a paradigm shift in the surgical treatment and prevention of anastomotic insufficiencies and perforations. Front Surg. 2023;10. https://doi.org/10.3389/fsurg.2023.1222993.
8. Lange J, Kähler G, Bernhardt J, Knievel J, Dormann A, Hügle U, Eisenberger CF, Heiss MM. The VACStent trial: combined treatment of esophageal leaks by covered stent and endoscopic

vacuum therapy. Surg Endosc. 2023;37(5):3657–68. https://doi.org/10.1007/s00464-023-09861-7.
9. Sancheti MS, Fernandez FG. Surgical management of esophageal perforation. Oper Tech Thorac Cardiovasc Surg. 2015;20(3):234–50. https://doi.org/10.1053/j.optechstcvs.2016.02.002.
10. Shivanand G, Seemar S, Srivastava DN, Pande GK, Sahni P, Prasad R, Ramachandra N. Gastric volvulus: acute and chronic presentation. Clinic Imag. 2003;27(4):265–68. https://doi.org/10.1016/S0899-7071(02)00549-1.
11. Borchardt M. Zur Pathologie und Therapie des Magen Volvulus. Arch Klin Chir. 1904;74:243–60.
12. Lee RY, Leayn F, Nikhil IK, Kazunori K, Chukwumere N, Saikrishna Y, Hector RN, Gary YY. Aorto-esophageal fistula: a rare fatal case caused by Esophageal malignancy. J Gastrointestin Oncol. 2010;1(1):64–65. https://doi.org/10.3978/j.issn.2078-6891.2010.006.
13. Czerny M, Eggebrecht H, Sodeck G, Weigang E, Livi U, Verzini F, Schmidli J, et al. New insights regarding the incidence, presentation and treatment options of aorto-oesophageal fistulation after thoracic endovascular aortic repair: the European registry of endovascular aortic repair complications. Eur J Cardiothorac Surg. 2014;45(3):452–7. https://doi.org/10.1093/ejcts/ezt393.
14. Takeno S, Ishii H, Nanashima A, Nakamura K. Aortoesophageal fistula: review of trends in the last decade. Surg Tod. 2020;50(12):1551–9. https://doi.org/10.1007/s00595-019-01937-z.
15. Zhan Y, Zhaojun X. Massive hemorrhage from an aortoesophageal fistula caused by Esophageal stent implantation: a case report and literature review. Medicine. 2019;98(51):e18303. https://doi.org/10.1097/MD.0000000000018303.
16. Dorigo W, Pulli R, Azas L, Pratesi G, Alessi Innocenti A, Pratesi C. Early and long-term results of conventional surgical treatment of secondary aorto-enteric fistula. Euro J Vascul Endovascul Surg. 2003;26(5):512–18. https://doi.org/10.1016/S1078-5884(03)00379-4.
17. Chong D, Debra ST, Hamish H, Jason C, Meryl D, Muntzer M, Krasnodar I. Successful stent graft repair of multiple thoracoabdominal mycotic aortic aneurysms in the presence of kommerell diverticulum and complicated by aortoesophageal fistula. J Vascul Surg Cases 2015;1(3):197–200. https://doi.org/10.1016/j.jvsc.2015.05.003.
18. Han H, Francis JH, Prashanthan S, Ryan S, Andrew WT, David O, Omar F, Han SL. Atrioesophageal fistula: clinical presentation, procedural characteristics, diagnostic investigations, and treatment outcomes. Circul Arrhythmia Electrophysiol. 2017;10(11):e005579. https://doi.org/10.1161/CIRCEP.117.005579.a.
19. Han H, Francis JH, Prashanthan S, Ryan S, Andrew WT, David O, Omar F, Han SL. Atrioesophageal fistula: clinical presentation, procedural characteristics, diagnostic investigations, and treatment outcomes. Circul Arrhythm Electrophysiol 2017;10(11):e005579. https://doi.org/10.1161/CIRCEP.117.005579.
20. Amirkhosravi F, Azimuddin A, Nguyen DT, Chihara R, Chan EY, Graviss EA, Reul RM, Kim MP. Surgical treatment of atrioesophageal fistula: a systematic review. Ann Thorac Surg. 2023;116(2):421–8. https://doi.org/10.1016/j.athoracsur.2023.04.016.
21. Kamla C, Belyaev S, Hagl C, Angele M, Dashkevich A. Interdisciplinary management of the emergency treatment in an atrioesophageal fistula. Ann Thorac Surg. 2022;114(2):e149–51. https://doi.org/10.1016/j.athoracsur.2021.10.050.
22. Heits N, Stapel L, Reichert B, Schafmayer C, Schniewind B, Becker T, Hampe J, Egberts J-H. Endoscopic endoluminal vacuum therapy in esophageal perforation. Ann Thorac Surg. 2014;97(3):1029–35. https://doi.org/10.1016/j.athoracsur.2013.11.014.

Chapter 13
Corrosive Injuries of the Oesophagus and Stomach

Abstract Corrosive injuries to the oesophagus and stomach represent a significant medical challenge, with higher incidence rates in developing countries compared to Western nations. Alkaline substances, such as sodium hydroxide, are the primary causative agents in Western countries, leading to liquefactive necrosis and oesophageal injury, while acid injuries typically affect the stomach due to rapid transit. Initial management focuses on preventing life-threatening complications, with endoscopy playing a crucial role in grading injuries and guiding treatment. Long-term complications, including strictures and perforation, necessitate ongoing monitoring and intervention. Surgical options, including resection and reconstruction, may be required in severe cases, with careful consideration of individual patient factors and multidisciplinary collaboration essential for optimal outcomes. This chapter underscores the importance of prompt assessment, tailored management strategies, and ongoing support for patients with corrosive injuries to the upper gastrointestinal tract.

Keywords Corrosive injuries · Oesophagus · Stomach · Alkaline substances · Acid injuries · Endoscopy · Surgical complications · Perforation · Surgical options · Timing—CT · Timing—endoscopy · Timing of interventions · Multidisciplinary collaboration

Corrosive injuries to the oesophagus and stomach are uncommon but have a high morbidity and mortality. There is a higher incidence in developing countries where corrosive substances are more readily accessible, whereas in Western countries, with the incidence is estimated to be 5–15 cases per 100,000, per year [1].

Corrosive injuries are mainly caused by caustic substances, ingested accidentally or intentionally, with the most common agents being sodium hydroxide and hydrochloric acid. It is important to understand the difference between alkaline (caustic) and acid injuries. Alkaline agents cause liquefactive necrosis, with deeper penetration into tissues, whereas acidic injuries cause coagulative necrosis, with a limited depth of injury [2]. Muslim and colleagues have published an excellent expert review of corrosive injuries in adults [3].

M. Mughal, *Reconstructive Surgery of the Oesophagus and Stomach*,
https://doi.org/10.1007/978-3-031-66846-3_13

Alkaline materials account for most injuries in Western countries. Alkaline materials have a higher viscosity, resulting in prolonged contact with and injury to the oesophagus. Acid indigestion is less frequent and causes more damage to the stomach than the oesophagus because of rapid transit. Acids cause pyloric spasm resulting in accumulation in the stomach.

Common presentations include pain, drooling, and dysphagia. Oral burns and odynophagia are common, and some patients present with respiratory distress due to aspiration and injury to the airways. Late complications include strictures, perforation, and an increased risk of oesophageal carcinoma [4].

Initial management of corrosive injury is focused on managing life-threatening consequences, controlling damage, preventing an exacerbation of the injury and managing the systemic complications. Oesophageal strictures are a common complication in those who survive. A large study of 295 patients with aerodigestive tract corrosive injuries [5] showed that 55% had an oesophageal injury, 25% had an oesophagogastric injury, 19% had a gastric injury, and three patients had a pharyngeal injury. Thirteen patients with diffuse oesophageal injury underwent surgery, whereas most of the others were treated by dilatation, often self-dilatation. Dilatation was commenced by the third week provided inflammation had settled. If successful, patients were taught to self-dilate.

It is recommended that endoscopy should be performed as early as possible and ideally within 12 hours. It is important, however, that this is planned in conjunction with ENT surgeons. An ENT assessment of the mouth and pharynx is vital to plan management and endoscopy is contraindicated in third degree burns of the hypopharynx. Endoscopy is best avoided from the fifth to the fifteenth days after ingestion because the softening of the tissues during this time increases the risk of perforation.

Endoscopic grading of oesophageal injury is helpful in planning treatment and prognosis. The following system is widely used:

Grade 0: normal endoscopy
Grade 1: oedema, hyperaemia of the mucosa.
Grade 2a: friability, blisters, haemorrhages, erosions, exudate, and superficial ulceration
Grade 2b: grade 2a+ plus deep discrete or circumferential alterations
Grade 3a: small, scattered areas of multiple observations and areas of necrosis (brown black or grey discolouration)
Grade 3b: extensive necrosis
Grade 3c: perforation

Patients with an injury grade up to 3a can usually be managed without surgery in the acute phase, reserving it for refractory strictures.

Some studies have shown an increased risk of perforation with the use of steroids and no benefit with regard to stricture formation [6]. However, intra-lesional injection of corticosteroids can be effective in reducing the number of dilatations for refractory strictures [7].

Ananthakrishnan and colleagues reported on their experience of treating corrosive gastric injuries [8] in 109 patients. They classified corrosive injuries into five types, as follows:

Type I: short ring stricture of the stomach within one or two centimeters of the pylorus;
Type II: stricture extending proximally up to the antrum;
Type III: mid-gastric stricture involving the body of the stomach and sparing the proximal and distal parts of the stomach;
Type IV: diffuse gastric involvement producing a linitis plastica like appearance; and
Type V: gastric stricture associated with a stricture of the first part of the duodenum.

Over 80% of patients had an injury resulting in a pre-pyloric stricture, with only 3% of strictures affecting the pyloro-duodenal area. It was notable that 18% of patients also had an oesophageal injury causing a stricture that was severe enough to require an oesophageal bypass. For most gastric injuries, a limited resection or a gastroenterostomy was sufficient.

13.1 Acid Ingestion

13.1.1 Case Summary

A woman in her 30s was brought to the Accident and Emergency Department by her family, who had found her in severe abdominal pain. She had a history of depression and told them she had tried to end her life by drinking a litre of acid. It was unclear how long before the family found her that she had swallowed the acid. On examination, she had burns affecting her mouth, but her airway was clear, and she had unobstructed breathing. She was pyrexial with a temperature of 38.9, her blood pressure was 100/60, and her pulse was 110. The initial treatment was with intravenous fluids, oxygen and intravenous antibiotics. An urgent CT scan showed the oesophagus to be oedematous and non-enhancing (Fig. 13.1). There was a large left pleural effusion, free fluid in the abdomen, a non-enhancing oedematous stomach(Fig. 13.2), and enhancement of only a small part of the spleen (Fig. 13.3).

She was taken to theatre and underwent a gastroscopy, which showed oedematous oesophageal mucosa with several linear ulcers distributed above the GOJ, with pale mucosa in between. The gastro-oesophageal junction appeared necrotic, as was the stomach. A laparotomy was performed, which confirmed the stomach to be necrotic with a large perforation along the greater curvature (Fig. 13.4). The spleen was also necrotic and carbonised. The transverse mesocolon had an acid burn in its middle with thrombosis of the middle colic vessels (Fig. 13.5), but the transverse colon appeared well vascularised with adequate collateral circulation. The first part of the

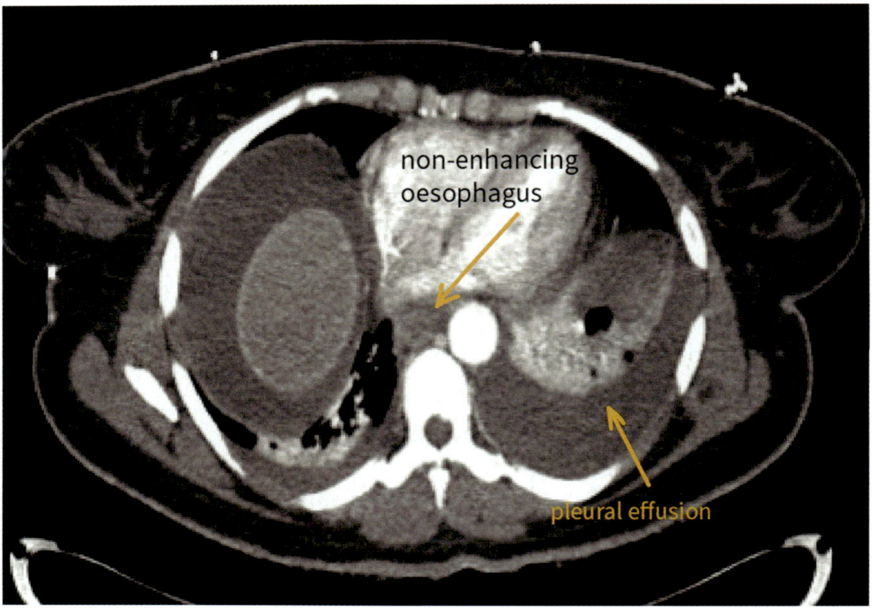

Fig. 13.1 CT showing bilateral pleural effusions and a non-enhancing distal oesophagus

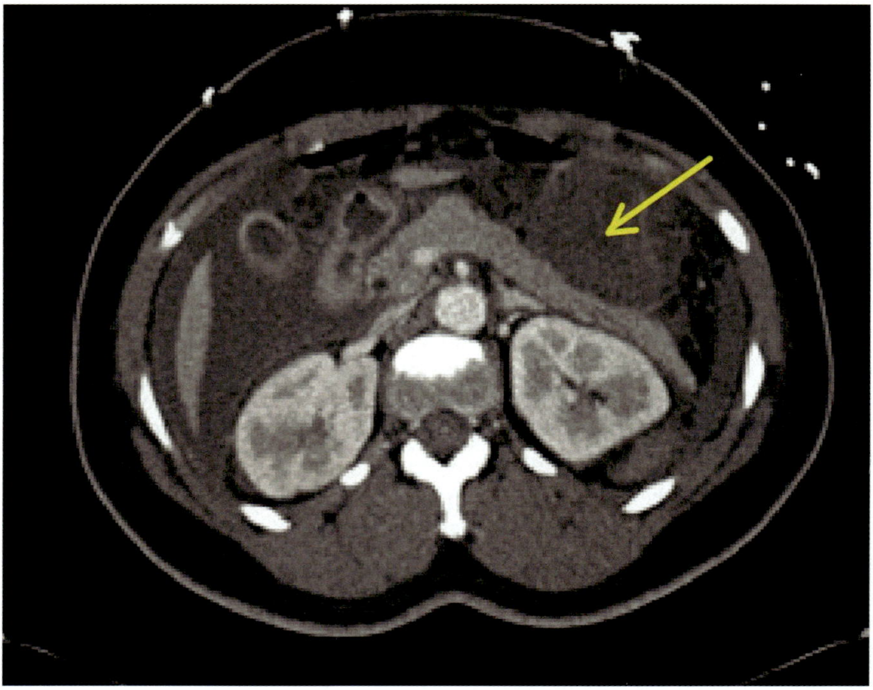

Fig. 13.2 CT showing a non-enhancing stomach

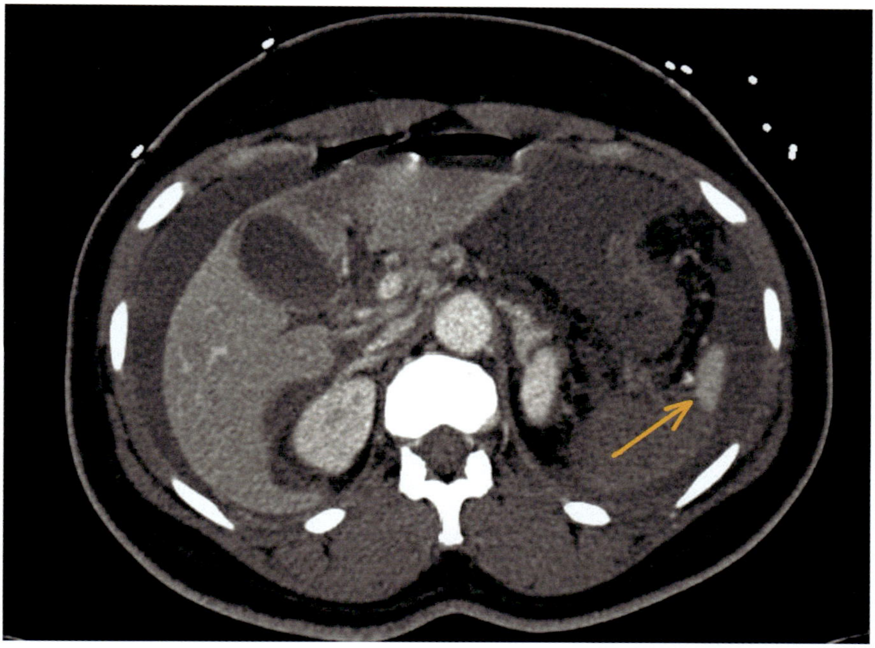

Fig. 13.3 CT showing only a small area of splenic enhancement

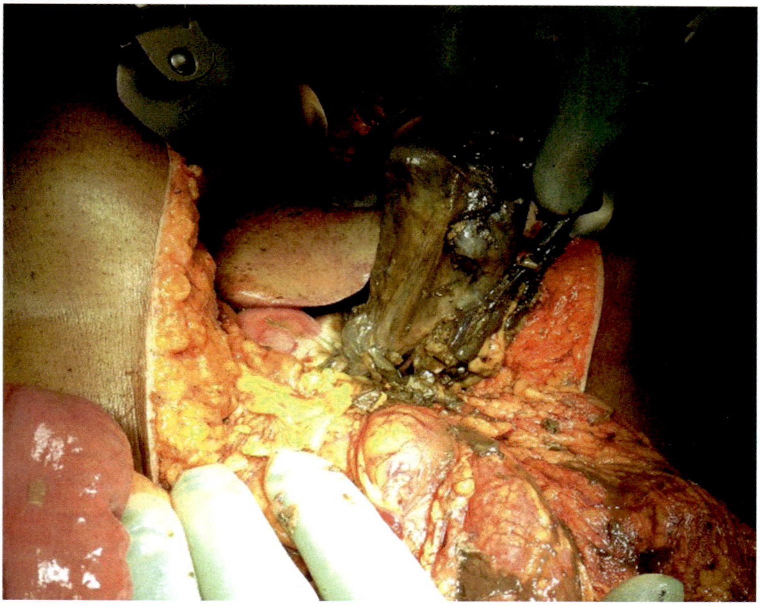

Fig. 13.4 Necrotic stomach

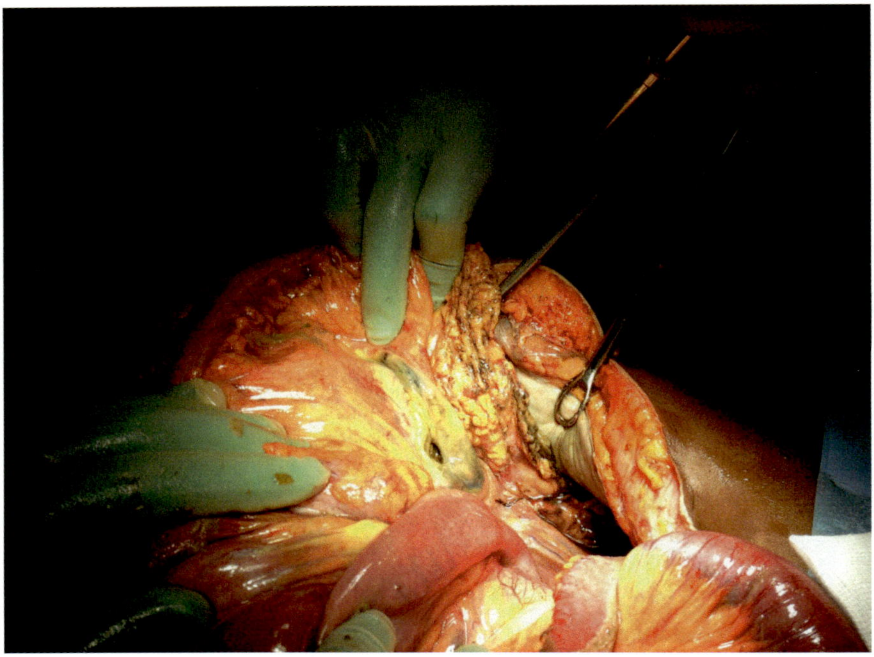

Fig. 13.5 Acid damage to the central part of the mesocolon

duodenum appeared undamaged. A total gastrectomy was performed by stapling the first part of the duodenum (Fig. 13.6) and transecting the oesophagus 3 cm above the necrotic GOJ. The spleen, which had been reduced to a black necrotic structure, was also excised (Fig. 13.7). A 28 Fr Robinson drain was placed into the oesophagus, which was closed with a No. 1 Vicryl purse string around it (Fig. 13.8). A feeding jejunostomy was also placed.

The patient made a slow but uncomplicated recovery, and the burns in the oropharynx were managed by the head and neck team and required staged reconstructions to restore her swallowing and voice. The oesophagus survived without permanent stricturing, and reconstruction was carried out with a Roux-en-Y oesophagojejunostomy four months later.

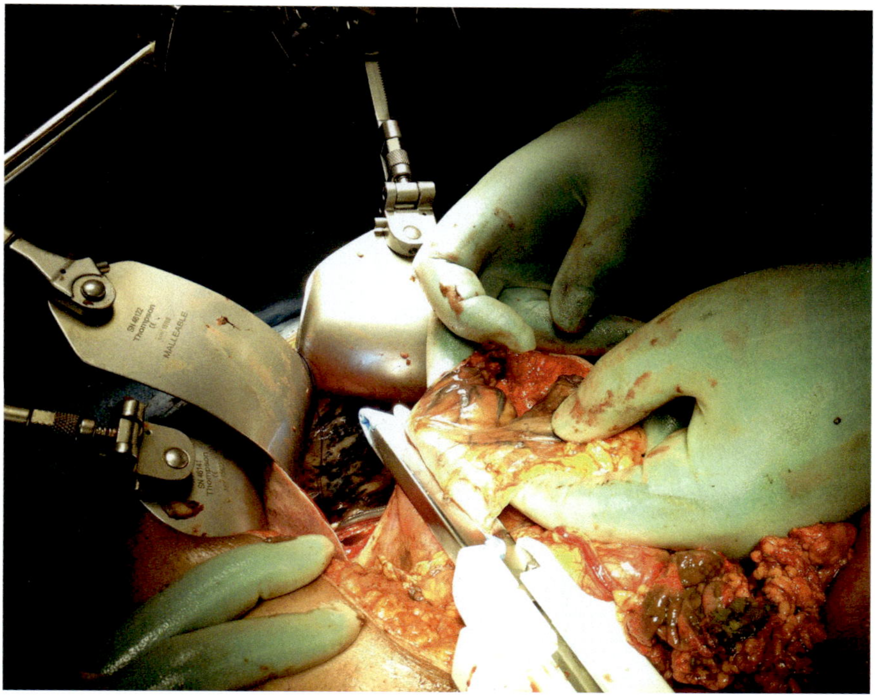

Fig. 13.6 Undamaged first part of the duodenum stapled-off

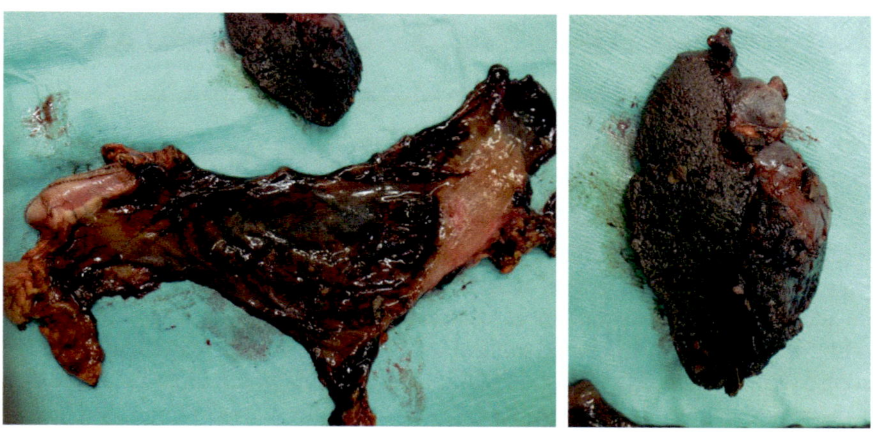

Fig. 13.7 Total gastrectomy and splenectomy specimens showing extent of damage

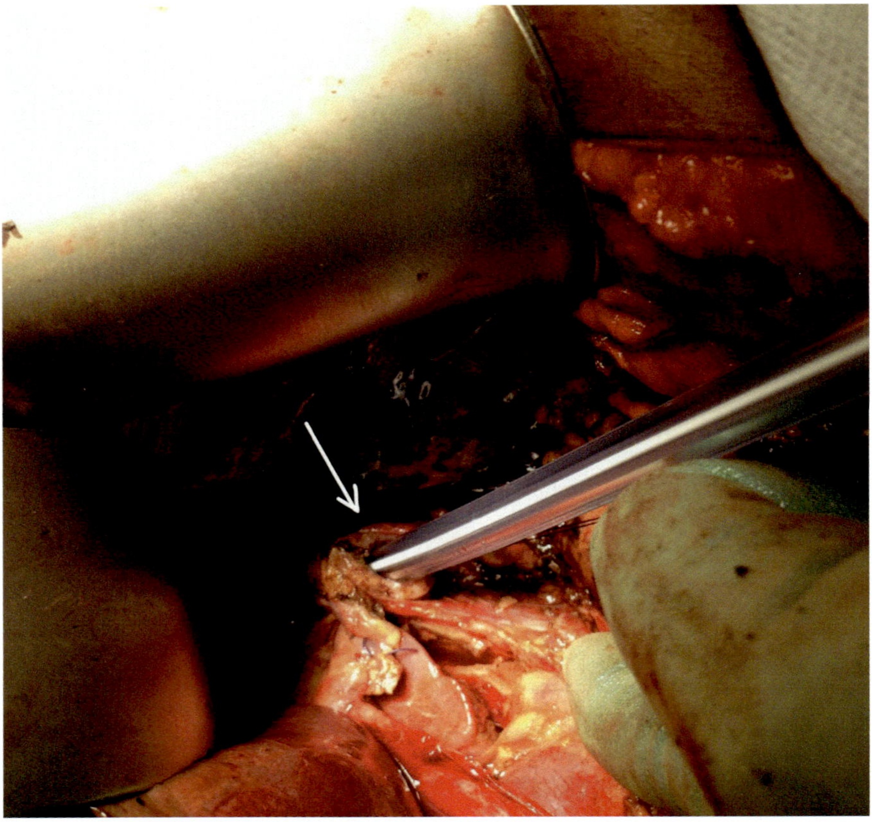

Fig. 13.8 28 Fr tube drain secured in the transected oesophagus with a purse-string suture

13.1.2 Learning Points

Resuscitation, including a detailed examination of the mouth, is very important in cases such as this. This patient was accompanied by a relative who was able to provide valuable information about what the patient is likely to have ingested and approximately when. A detailed clinical assessment, including examination of the oropharynx was carried out, followed by resuscitation, which included correction of metabolic acidosis. Although the stomach and spleen were almost completely destroyed by acid, the first part of the duodenum was spared, presumably due to pyloric spasm. The principles of damage-control surgery were followed in resecting the stomach and the spleen without a reconstruction. Reconstruction was carried out when the patient's condition had improved sufficiently. The delay also resulted in a better demarcation of the oesophageal damage, the extent of which was difficult to assess initially.

13.2 Caustic Injury to the Oesophagus

13.2.1 Case Summary

A woman in her 20s with a long psychiatric history, including schizophrenia, was admitted after ingesting caustic soda. She was brought to the hospital by an acquaintance. She had difficulty breathing and was drooling. She was administered PPIs, dexamethasone and broad-spectrum antibiotics and underwent endotracheal intubation and ventilation. An urgent CT scan showed a grossly oedematous oesophagusand stomach (Figs. 13.9 and 13.10).

An OGD was performed 48 h later, which showed mildly erythematous mucosa of the pharynx and proximal oesophagus but sloughing and widespread erythema of the distal two-thirds of the oesophagus. The stomach was erythematous with features of coagulative necrosis (black streaks). The first two parts of the duodenum were normal. A midline laparotomy was performed, which revealed serous fluid in the peritoneal cavity and an oedematous but viable stomach. A feeding jejunostomy was placed, and the patient was extubated 24 hours later. After she had recovered from surgery, she required a two-week stay under the psychiatrists to stabilise her mental condition and was then discharged with a feeding jejunostomy and liquid diet. She developed a long oesophageal stricture from 24 to 33 cm (Fig. 13.11).

It was serially dilated and managed with biodegradable stents (Fig. 13.12). However, the stricture recurred repeatedly and at best the patient was only able to swallow saliva and thin fluids. Eventually, it was decided to offer her a reconstruction three years later, after conservative measures to restore her swallowing had failed, and her mental condition was sufficiently stable for her to be counselled about the proposed surgery. A CT scan before surgery showed distal oesophageal stricturing with surrounding oesophageal/perioesophageal soft tissue thickening in contact with the carina, main bronchus, the ascending aorta, the azygous vein the posterior wall of the atrium and the inferior pulmonary vein. The stomach appeared to be normal (Figs. 13.13, 13.14 and 13.15).

She was counselled and consented for an oesophageal bypass in case it proved hazardous to resect her oesophagus because of the surrounding inflammation. At laparotomy, the stomach and its vasculature appeared normal, with no evidence of significant abnormality from the caustic injury. It was mobilised in the usual manner, maintaining the gastroepiploeic arch. At thoracotomy, dense perioesophageal inflammation was encountered as expected, particularly around the level of the azygous arch and the carina. Dissection was therefore kept to the perioesophageal plane to avoid damage to the surrounding structures. The oesophagus was resected, and a gastric conduit anastomosed to the upper oesophagus.

The patient made an uneventful post-operative recovery.

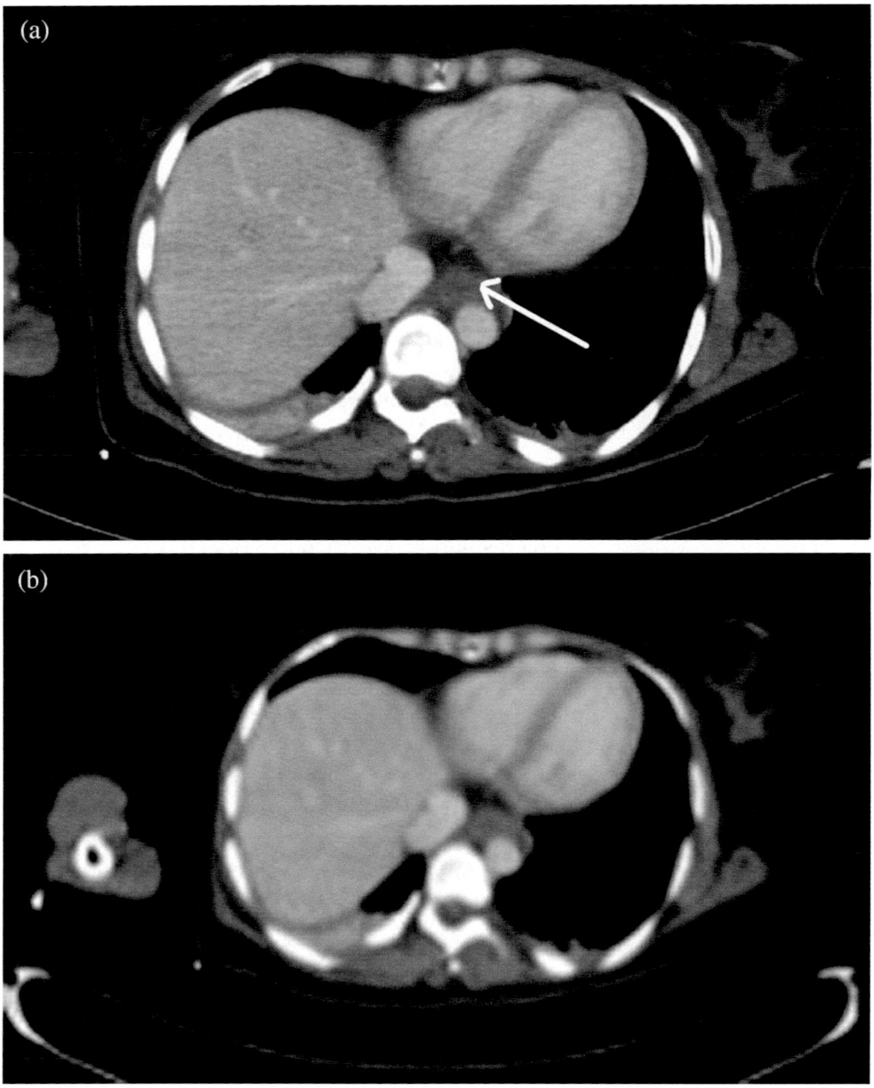

Fig. 13.9 CT sections showing non-enhancing distal oesophagus

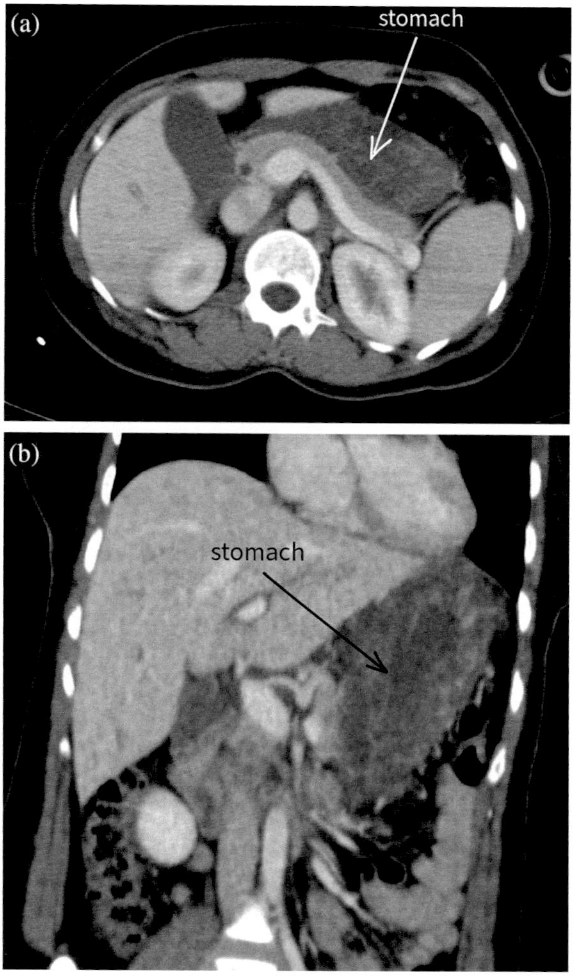

Fig. 13.10 Axial (a) and coronal (b) CT sections showing oedematous, poorly-enhancing stomach

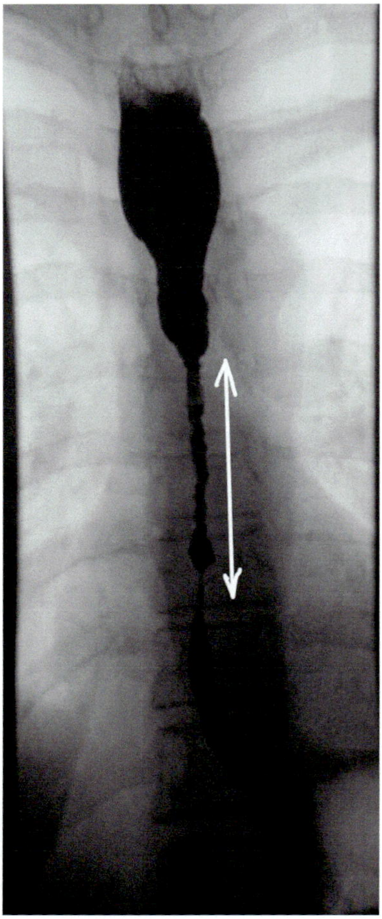

Fig. 13.11 Contrast swallow showing a long oesophageal stricture

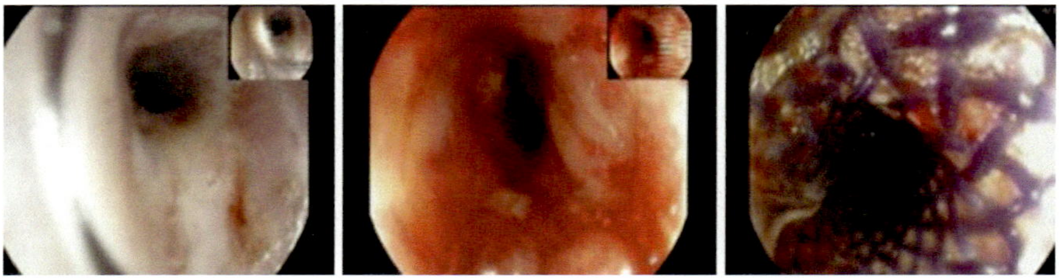

Fig. 13.12 OGD pictures showing a tight long stricture and deployment of a biodegradable stent

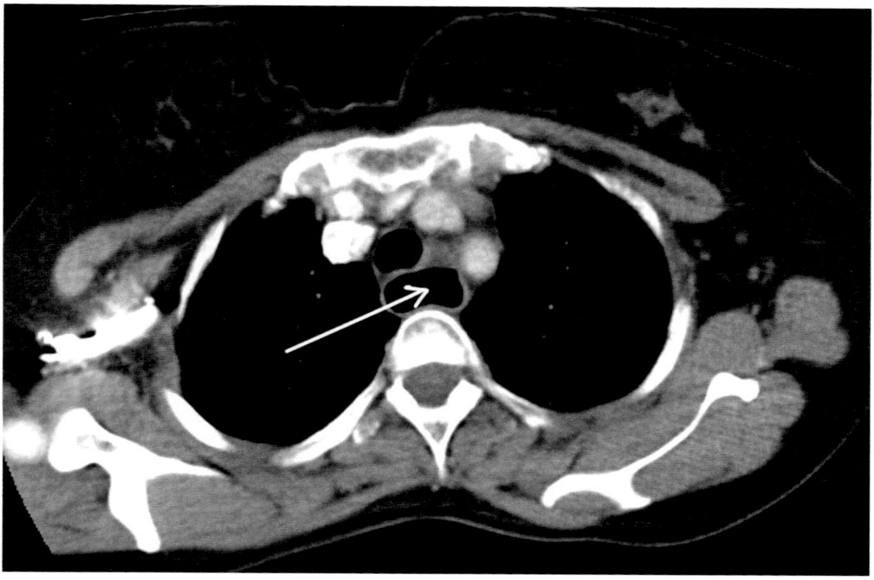

Fig. 13.13 CT showing a dilated proximal oesophagus with normal fat planes

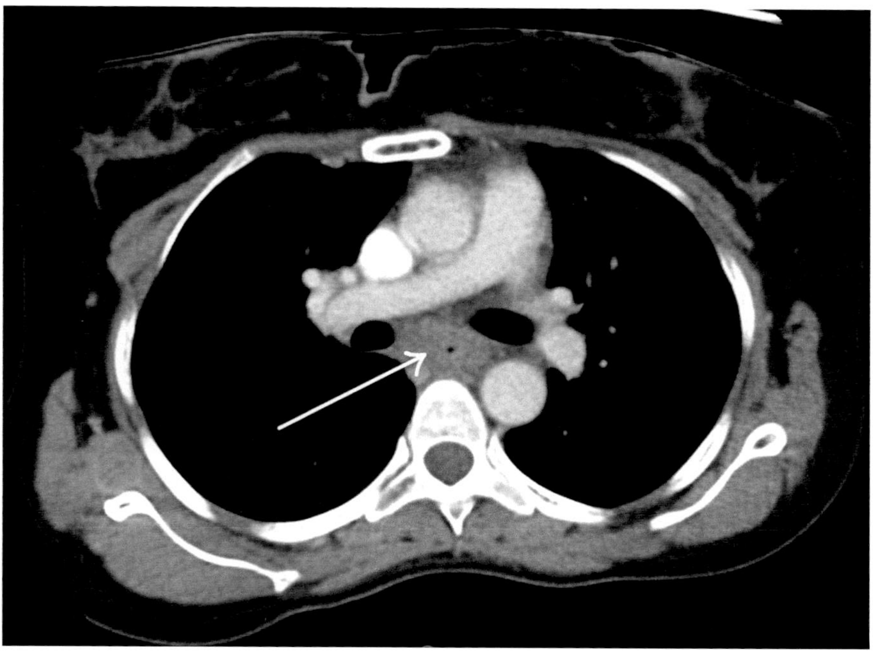

Fig. 13.14 CT section just below the carina showing thick-walled oesophagus with a tiny lumen surrounding and fibrosis

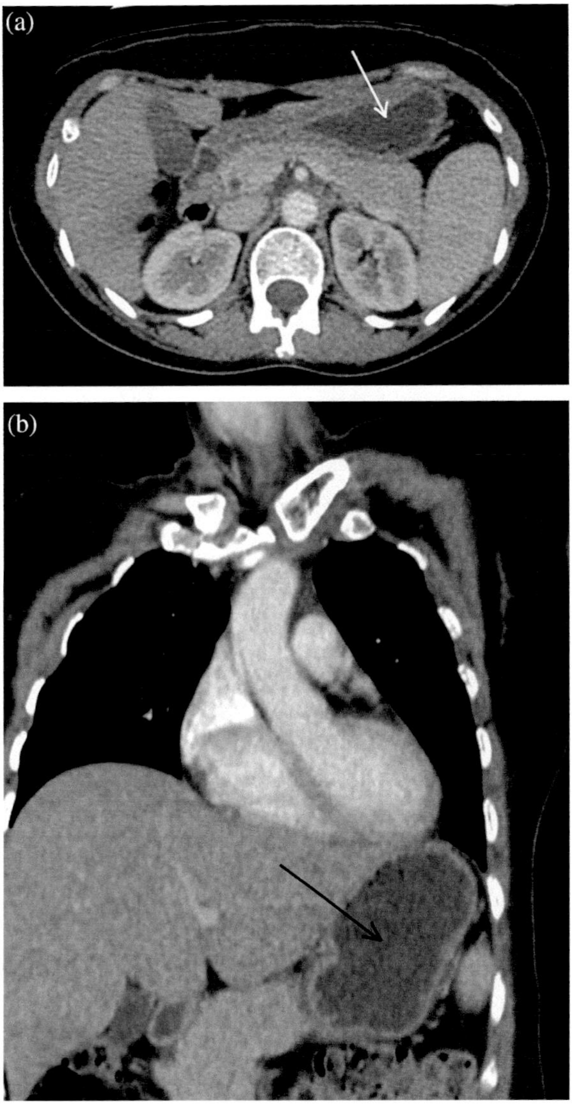

Fig. 13.15 Axial (a) and coronal (b) CT sections showing a normal stomach

13.2.2 Learning Points

Initial treatment with a caustic injury entailed securing the airway before the swelling worsened to a degree requiring a tracheostomy. Early treatment with steroids was directed towards minimising oedema of the airways. CT showed oedema of the oesophagus and stomach but no suggestion of perforation. An OGD was carried out 48 hours later to determine the extent of the mucosal injury, and a feeding jejunostomy was placed at the same time. Conservative methods of dealing with the long oesophageal stricture failed, and therefore an oesophagectomy and reconstruction were offered. A careful assessment was carried out, including a CT to determine the degree and extent of perioesophageal fibrosis and the state of the stomach to plan surgery. The patient was counselled for an oesophageal bypass in case an oesophagectomy proved hazardous to perform. However, oesophagectomy was safely performed by keeping the dissection very close to the wall of the oesophagus, considering that the resection was being performed for benign disease rather than cancer. The input of the psychiatric team in helping to improve the patient's mental condition was crucial so that she could be adequately counselled. It was important that she understood the risks and benefits of the proposed surgery and the expected quality of life.

References

1. Kochhar R, et al. Comparative evaluation of nasoenteral feeding and jejunostomy feeding in acute corrosive injury: a retrospective analysis. Gastrointest Endosc. 2009;70(5):874–80. https://doi.org/10.1016/j.gie.2009.03.009.
2. Showkat AZ et al. The role of fiberoptic endoscopy in the management of corrosive ingestion and modified endoscopic classification of burns. Gastrointestin Endoscop. 1991;37(2):165–69. https://doi.org/10.1016/S0016-5107(91)70678-0
3. Muslim A, et al. Corrosive injury to the gi tract in adults: a practical approach. Exp Rev Gastroenterol Hepatol. 2009;3(6):701–9. https://doi.org/10.1586/egh.09.56.
4. Mircea C, et al. Caustic ingestion. The Lancet. 2017;389(10083):2041–52. https://doi.org/10.1016/S0140-6736(16)30313-0.
5. Ravi SB, Dipankar R. Outcomes of the management of corrosive injuries of the upper digestive tract in a tertiary care center. Dis Esophagus. 2022;35(3):doab096. https://doi.org/10.1093/dote/doab096
6. Karnak et al. Combined use of steroid, antibiotics and early bougienage against stricture formation following caustic esophageal burns. J Cardiovascul Surg. 1999;40(2):307–10.
7. Rakesh K, Kuchhangi SP. Intralesional steroid injection therapy in the management of resistant gastrointestinal strictures. World J Gastrointestin Endoscop. 2010;2(2):61–8. https://doi.org/10.4253/wjge.v2.i2.61.
8. Ananthakrishnan N, Parthasarathy G, Vikram K. Chronic corrosive injuries of the stomach—a single unit experience of 109 patients over thirty years. World J Surg 2010;34(4):758–64. https://doi.org/10.1007/s00268-010-0393-8.

Chapter 14
Late Presentations of Catastrophic Conduit Complications

Abstract This chapter highlights the rare but potentially fatal consequences of oesophageal reconstruction with conduits, which can manifest many months or years after surgery. While literature reports on such occurrences are rare, the author describes a case of, acute dilatation and perforation of a colonic conduit resulting in cardiorespiratory collapse. It underscores the urgency of recognising and addressing these complications. In this instance, a 42-year-old man experienced severe chest pain and cardiorespiratory collapse due to a grossly distended and perforated colonic conduit, necessitating urgent thoracotomy and conduit resection. Despite aggressive treatment, the patient's condition rapidly deteriorated, resulting in death. The narrative emphasises the need for vigilance in monitoring conduit function post-surgery and underscores the potential gravity of late conduit-related complications, which demand prompt diagnosis and intervention to mitigate fatal outcomes.

Keywords Catastrophic conduit complications · Late presentations · Oesophageal reconstruction · Conduit surgery · Cardiorespiratory collapse · Colonic conduit · Perforation · Thoracotomy · Mediastinal sepsis · Conduit resection

Most serious complications of oesophageal reconstruction with conduits occur early, but catastrophic complications can occur many months or years later. There are very few reports in the literature [1], but I have encountered several cases, including acute dilatation causing cardiorespiratory collapse.

Although these complications are rare, it is important to be aware that deterioration can be rapid, and they can be fatal if not diagnosed and treated urgently.

M. Mughal, *Reconstructive Surgery of the Oesophagus and Stomach*,
https://doi.org/10.1007/978-3-031-66846-3_14

14.1 Late Perforation of a Colonic Conduit

14.1.1 Case Summary

A man in his 40s was admitted to his local hospital with severe chest pain and cardiorespiratory collapse. Only a limited history was available from an acquaintance who accompanied him. His general health was described as good, and there was a history of surgery that had been carried out in childhood. A CT scan of the chest and abdomen showed what appeared to be a grossly distended and perforated colonic conduit (Fig. 14.1).

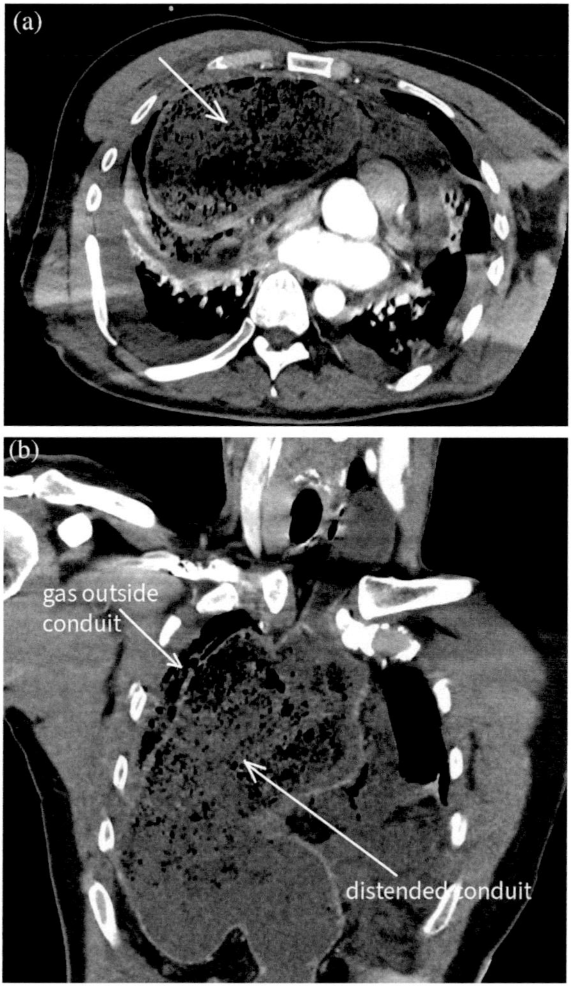

Fig. 14.1 Axial (a) and coronal (b) CT sections showing a massively dilated colonic conduit full of food with perforation and compression of the heart

He was transferred to our centre, by which time he was in extremis and on a high dose of inotropes. He underwent an urgent right thoracotomy, which revealed a grossly distended colonic conduit, that appeared to have been placed in the retrosternal plane. It was full of food and had perforated, causing widespread contamination of the right chest and mediastinum. The conduit was resected, and the chest closed after thorough debridement and drainage. A cervical oesophagostomy and feeding jejunostomy were performed, but the patient continued to deteriorate and died several hours later.

14.1.2 Learning Points

Colonic conduits have a propensity to become distended and sigmoid over time. Usually, this results in difficulty with the transit of food to the stomach and aspiration. This develops slowly and is usually managed by dietary manipulations, although surgery may be required to correct the redundancy [2]. However, acute on chronic dilatation can happen, resulting in sudden cardiorespiratory collapse either from distension preventing venous return or, as in this case, perforation with mediastinal and pleural sepsis. Unfortunately, this patient was in extremis before he was transferred to our unit for definitive treatment and died despite excision of the conduit and mediastinal debridement.

References

1. Jinsoo M, Young-Jae C. Non-surgical management of critically compromised airway due to dilatation of interposed colon. Tuberculosis Respirat Dis. 2016;79(2):98–100. https://doi.org/10.4046/trd.2016.79.2.98.
2. Strauss DC, Forshaw MJ, Tandon RC, Mason RC. Surgical management of colonic redundancy following esophageal replacement. Dis Esophag. 21(3):E1–5. https://doi.org/10.1111/j.1442-2050.2007.00708.x.

Chapter 15
Catastrophic Complications of Anti-reflux Surgery and Hiatal Hernia Repair

Abstract This chapter discusses the rarity of catastrophic complications following antireflux and hiatal hernia surgeries, citing an analysis of 5502 cases showing a low overall prevalence of life-threatening events. However, it emphasises the potential underreporting of such complications. A case study highlights a post-Nissen herniation leading to a perforated stomach, requiring emergency laparotomy and subsequent reconstruction. The case underscores the importance of prompt diagnosis through CT imaging in suspected complications, advocating for early surgical intervention to prevent necrosis and perforation. It also stresses careful chest drain placement to avoid gastric injury and the challenges of reduction of the distended stomach. This comprehensive overview provides vital insights into managing rare yet critical complications of antireflux surgeries, emphasising timely intervention to avoid the development of gastric ischaemia necessitating resection.

Keywords Antireflux surgery · Hiatal hernia repair · Catastrophic complications · Post-Nissen herniation · Perforated stomach · Emergency laparotomy · Reconstruction · Surgical intervention · Damage control surgery · Staged reconstruction

Catastrophic, life-threatening complications are uncommon after antireflux and hiatal hernia surgery. A paper by Rantanen et al. has reported on fatal and life-threatening complications of antireflux surgery in Finland, based on an analysis of 5502 antireflux operations performed from1987 to 1996 [1]. This included mainly open fundoplications (72.6%) compared with 21.1% laparoscopic fundoplications. They found that life-threatening complications had an overall prevalence of 0.8%. It was 0.6% in the open group, compared with 1.3% in patients who had a laparoscopic fundoplication. Complications included oesophageal perforation, gastric perforation, and haemorrhage and were ascribed to the learning curve of laparoscopic surgery.

The true incidence of catastrophic, life-threatening complications of antireflux surgery is unknown, as it is likely to be underreported. In my clinical and medicolegal practice, I have dealt with or given advice and/or an opinion in 15 cases over the last 12 months.

M. Mughal, *Reconstructive Surgery of the Oesophagus and Stomach*,
https://doi.org/10.1007/978-3-031-66846-3_15

15.1 Post-Nissen Herniation and Perforation

15.1.1 Case Summary

A woman in her 60s was admitted to the general surgical ward with chest pain five days after a laparoscopic Nissen fundoplication. She was short of breath on exertion, but her oxygen saturation was satisfactory on air. Her blood pressure and pulse were within normal limits, and an ECG was normal. Examination of the chest revealed decreased air entry at the left base and abdominal examination was unremarkable, with healing port sites. Her haemoglobin and white cell count were normal, but the CRP was moderately raised at 45. Her chest x-ray was reported as showing a raised left hemidiaphragm (Fig. 15.1).

She was initially treated with analgesia and physiotherapy. She became acutely unwell with tachypnoea, tachycardia, and hypotension 24 hours later, and a repeat chest x-ray showed deviation of the trachea to the right with an air-fluid level in the left lower chest and likely pneumothorax on that side (Fig. 15.2). A CT scan confirmed this, along with a large right hydropneumothorax (Fig. 15.3). A chest drain was inserted on the left side, which yielded a large amount of air and bile-stained fluid containing food matter with an improvement in her general condition.

A diagnosis of a hiatus hernia with a perforated stomach was made, and she underwent an emergency laparotomy. This revealed that one of the hiatal repair sutures had cut out, and the stomach had herniated into the chest with disruption of the wrap, necrosis of the body of the stomach with the perforation in it. The stomach was reduced into the abdomen, a distal gastrectomy was performed, and a venting Foley catheter was placed in the remnant (Fig. 15.4). It was decided not to carry out

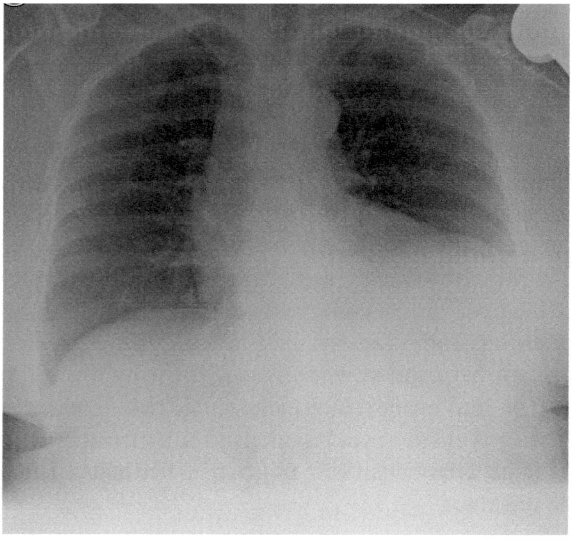

Fig. 15.1 CXR on admission showing raised left hemidiaphragm

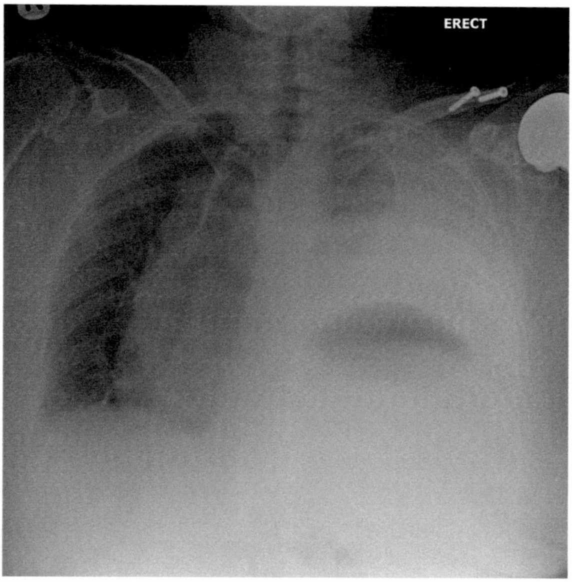

Fig. 15.2 CXR showing left hydropneumothorax with deviation of the trachea to the right

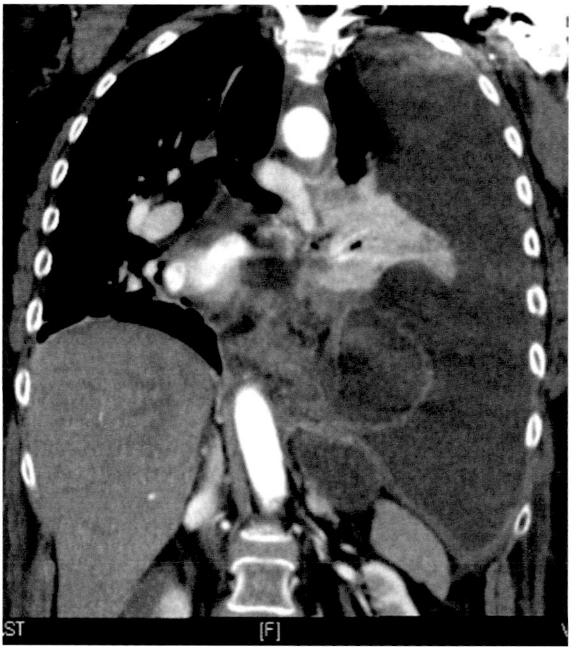

Fig. 15.3 CT section showing a large left hydropneumothorax with herniated stomach

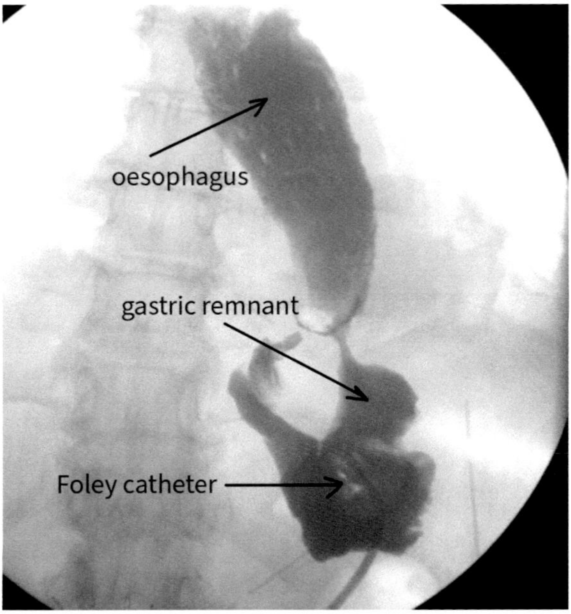

Fig. 15.4 Contrast swallow 10 days after surgery showing small stomach remnant drained by a Foley catheter

a reconstruction because of the adverse circumstances. A feeding jejunostomy was also performed.

The patient made a slow but uncomplicated post-operative recovery. She was discharged with a plan was to carry out an elective reconstruction after three months, but she presented 10 weeks later with vomiting after the venting Foley catheter had fallen out. This precipitated the reconstruction, which was carried out urgently, as the catheter could not have been replaced without a surgical approach, and the alternative would have been a nasogastric tube for a few more weeks until the date for the scheduled surgery.

A straightforward Roux-en-Y reconstruction was carried out, and she made an uneventful post-operative recovery.

15.1.2 Learning Points

Herniation of the stomach and fundoplication in the early postoperative period is a rare but well-known complication of antireflux surgery. A patient presenting with chest pain or respiratory symptoms soon after a fundoplication should be urgently investigated for this complication. A chest x-ray is often insufficient and, in my opinion, a CT scan of the chest and abdomen is essential. In this case, it is likely that herniation occurred very soon after the fundoplication but got worse over the subsequent days and eventually presented acutely.

A CT scan was only performed after the patient had deteriorated 24 hours after admission and provided the diagnosis. The initial chest Xray had not raised any concerns. Increasing pain and respiratory symptoms after fundoplication should be regarded as suspicious of herniation and merit an urgent CT scan. If herniation is diagnosed, a reoperation should be carried out urgently to prevent the chance of necrosis of the stomach or wrap, which can be trapped above a tight hiatal closure and result in a perforation. Furthermore, the sooner a reoperation is carried out after the original operation, the easier it is before worsening adhesions make dissection difficult and hazardous. Before surgery, it is important to place a chest drain to deal with any associated complications, such as a hydrothorax or pneumothorax. However, the drain should be placed with particular care to avoid damaging the stomach, which may be massively distended and occupying most of the chest cavity. I am aware of cases where a chest drain has been inserted into a distended, air-filled stomach which has been mistaken for a pneumothorax.

At operation, it proved difficult to reduce the stomach into the abdomen because it was firmly jammed at the hiatus and distended. Because any attempts at manual reduction of the migrated stomach carried a risk of tearing it, and it had been impossible to advance a nasogastric tube into the stomach, a small gastrotomy was made in the antrum, and the stomach decompressed through this. It was then possible to reduce the stomach without causing further damage. As the patient was very septic and on inotropes, once the stomach had been reduced then and the necrotic portion excised, it was decided not to reconstruct. Reconstruction was planned three months later but was precipitated by the venting gastrostomy falling out. It was coming up to the time for the planned reconstruction and we did not want to place a nasogastric tube or re-explore the abdomen simply for the purpose of replacing the venting gastrostomy.

Reference

1. Rantanen TK, Salo JA, Sipponen JT. Fatal and life-threatening complications in antireflux surgery: analysis of 5502 operations. BJS. 1999;86(12):1573–7. https://doi.org/10.1046/j.1365-2168.1999.01297.x.

Chapter 16
Late Complications of Mesh Repair of Hiatus Hernia

Abstract This chapter discusses the complications of meshes for repairing large hiatal defects when suture repair is inadequate. While many studies report the benefits of mesh repair in reducing the recurrence of hiatus hernia with a low complication rate, some complications can be catastrophic. Complications such as intraluminal mesh erosion can be difficult to manage and may require oesophageal resection. The chapter presents two cases illustrating these complications: one involving mesh causing pseudoachalasia, and another of mesh erosion into the oesophagus. These cases underscore the complexity of managing mesh-related issues, often requiring extensive surgical intervention to address symptoms and prevent further complications. Key learning points emphasize the importance of careful evaluation and surgical planning in such cases to mitigate risks and optimize patient outcomes.

Keywords Hiatus hernia · Mesh repair · Complications · Dysphagia · Intraluminal mesh erosion · Oesophagectomy · Pseudoachalasia · Mesh erosion · Surgical intervention · Patient outcomes

Meshes are commonly used for repairing large hiatal defects when suture repair is either impossible or unlikely to achieve a good long-term outcome. Many studies have shown the benefit of mesh repair over suture repair in treating hiatus hernia, and some guidelines have recommended the use of mesh [1]. Several long-term studies have shown low rates of hiatus hernia recurrence and good patient satisfaction up to 9 years after surgery [2]. Others have reported high long-term complication rates [3].

One study has shown that complications of mesh repair are more common than generally reported [4]. Through contacting other experienced oesophageal surgeons, the authors were able to find 26 patients with mesh -related complications in addition to their own two cases. Dysphagia was the main symptom in 22 of 26 patients, and the main re-operative finding was intraluminal mesh erosion in 17, oesophageal stenosis in six and dense fibrosis in five. Six patients required oesophagectomy. They did not find any relationship between the type and configuration of the mesh and the complications.

M. Mughal, *Reconstructive Surgery of the Oesophagus and Stomach*,
https://doi.org/10.1007/978-3-031-66846-3_16

I have dealt with several cases of mesh erosion into the oesophagus as well as stenosis presenting with features of achalasia.

16.1 Hiatal Mesh Causing Pseudoachalasia

16.1.1 Case Summary

A woman in her 50s who had no gastrointestinal symptoms underwent surgery for a pelvic fracture and subsequently developed symptoms of gastro-esophageal reflux, which were initially managed with PPIs. Her symptoms worsened despite treatment, and investigations showed a 4 cm hiatus hernia on endoscopy and pathological gastro-oesophageal reflux on 24-hour pH monitoring, she underwent a laparoscopic Nissen fundoplication and repair of hiatus hernia. Four years later, she had a mesh repair for a recurrent hiatus hernia. Her symptoms did not improve, and she was diagnosed with delayed gastric emptying. Prokinetics were ineffective, and she underwent a subtotal gastrectomy with a Roux-en-Y reconstruction. She also underwent a redo of the jejunojejunal anastomosis for reasons that are not clear. Her reflux symptoms improved, but she started to experience dysphagia. OGD did not reveal a mechanical cause, but manometry suggested outflow obstruction. She had several balloon dilatations of the GOJ without any benefit. A CT scan with intravenous and oral contrast showed a dilated distal oesophagus and radiopaque mesh encircling the GOJ for about 280° (Fig. 16.1). Gastrografin progressed normally into the stomach remnant, but the remnant emptied slowly.

Her case was discussed at the benign complex upper GI MDT meeting, and it was decided to offer her a laparotomy to determine if the mesh was implicated in the dysphagia and to remove it if that was the case.

At laparotomy, there were extensive adhesions in the upper abdomen, as expected. There was a small gastric remnant with an adequate gastrojejunal anastomosis. The jejunojejunostomy anastomosis had an excessively long ‘candy cane’ measuring almost 10 cm (Fig. 16.2), which was trimmed. The oesophageal hiatus was carefully dissected out, and a semi-circular piece of mesh was found with an intense fibrotic reaction around the oesophagus. A plane was carefully developed between the mesh and the oesophagus, and the mesh was removed (Figs. 16.3, 16.4 and 16.5). During this, no vagal trunks were found on careful inspection around the hiatus.

After removal of the mesh and mobilisation of the oesophagus, it was decided to perform a completion gastrectomy excising the small stomach remnant as well as the oesophagus with the fibrotic ring around it. The mesh was removed with care to preserve as much of the crura as possible. No attempt was made to repair the resultant hiatal defect. A hand-sewn oesophagojejunal anastomosis was carried out with interrupted 3/0 PDS (Fig. 16.6).

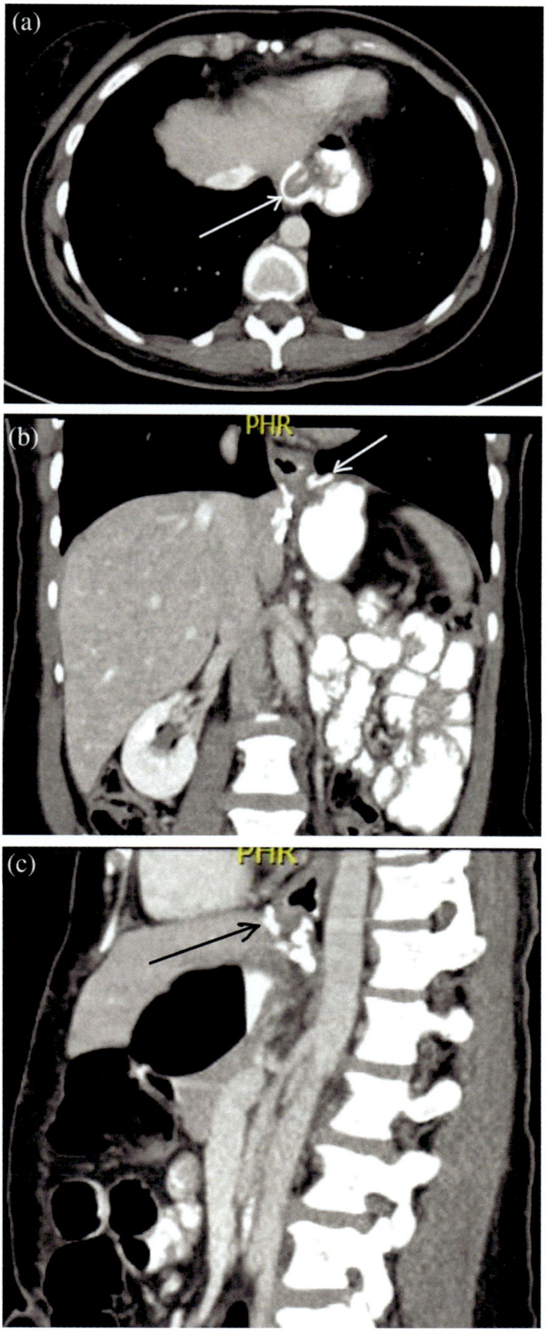

Fig. 16.1 CT sections showing mesh encircling the GOJ at the hiatus

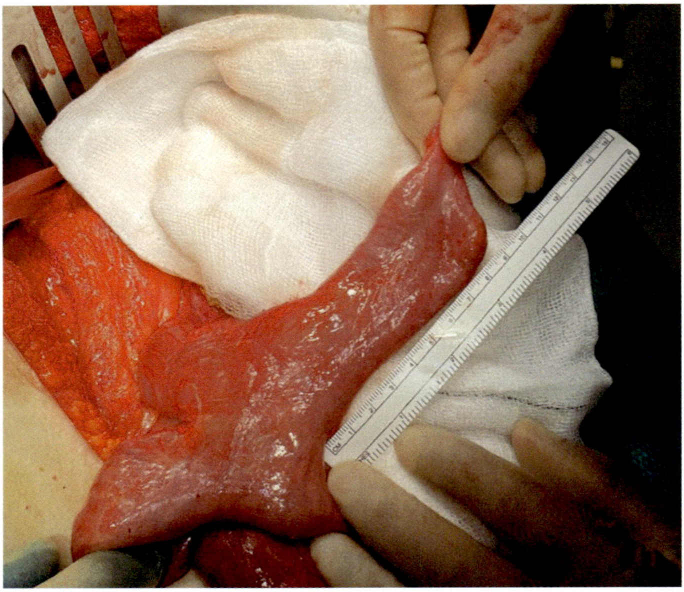

Fig. 16.2 Excessively long 'candy cane' at the jejunojejunostomy

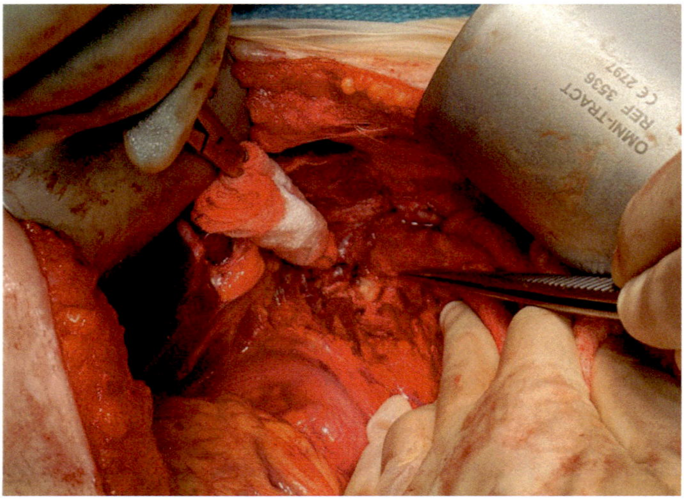

Fig. 16.3 Mesh at the hiatus pointed out with the forceps

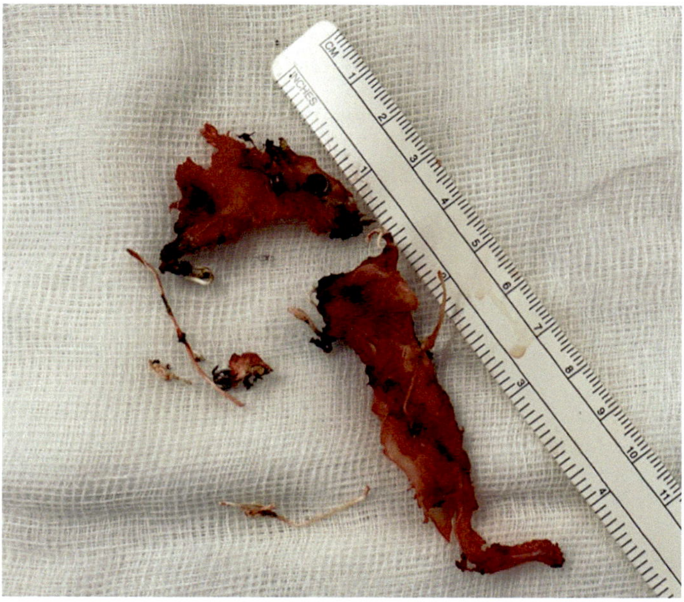

Fig. 16.4 Mesh and tackers removed from the oesophageal hiatus

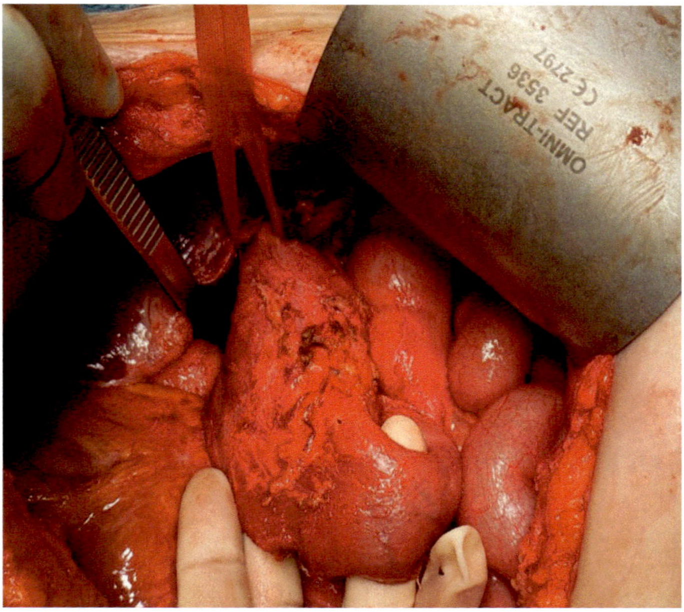

Fig. 16.5 Small stomach remnant shown with the nylon tape around the GOJ

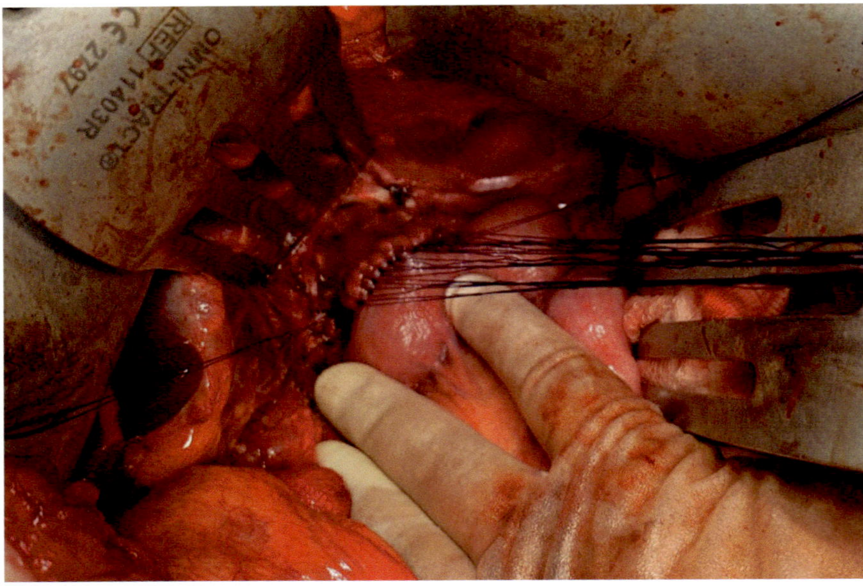

Fig. 16.6 Oesophago jejunostomy showing the anterior layer of sutures completed and ready to be cut

16.1.2 Learning Points

This patient had all her operations in another country, and no records were available to determine the rationale for the interventions. However, her symptoms at referral were dysphagia and regurgitation, which had not responded to balloon dilatation of the GOJ. She also complained of bloating and upper abdominal pain. The primary objective of the operation was to relieve her of the dysphagia, which was suggestive of pseudoachalasia on manometric criteria. Because there was also evidence of poor emptying of the small stomach remnant, it was decided to remove the mesh as well as carry out a completion gastrectomy.

16.2 Mesh Erosion into the Oesophagus

16.2.1 Case Summary

A man in his 50s who had undergone surgery abroad to repair a large diaphragmatic hernia was referred with mesh eroding into the oesophagus. The details were of previous operations were unclear, but the first repair was through a left thoracotomy when the hernia was reduced, and the defect was repaired with mesh. Within two months, there was a recurrence, and he underwent a right thoracotomy, and a further repair was performed. A few days after the second repair, there was a discharge of bile-stained fluid from the chest drain, and a CT scan with oral contrast showed a leak from the oesophagus. A gastroscopy showed erosion of the mesh into the oesophagus with a complex cavity leading into the right chest. This was managed with bilateral chest drains, venting gastrostomy and feeding jejunostomy. An oesophageal stent was also placed across the GOJ (Fig. 16.7). The patient was transferred to our unit for further management.

OGD showed a fluid-filled oesophagus and a free-floating stent across the GOJ. The stent was removed and revealed mesh eroding through the GOJ (Fig. 16.8). There was a large complex defect in the right wall of the oesophagus above the GOJ, with mesh sutured to the oesophagus and extending into the chest cavity. The proximal stomach was oedematous and fluid filled. A CT with oral and intravenous contrast showed a recurrent hiatus hernia with a grossly oedematous migrated stomach and extravasation of contrast into the left chest (Fig. 16.9).

A laparotomy was carried out after further drainage of loculated chest collections, treatment with antibiotics, and improvement of nutritional state. Dissection of the oesophageal hiatus was extremely difficult because of previous surgery and sepsis. Still, as much of the mesh as possible was excised, and the migrated stomach was removed by transhiatal dissection. The cervical oesophagus was dissected out through a neck incision, and as much as possible of the intrathoracic oesophagus was removed, leaving a small stump for the reconstruction. The right colon was chosen as a conduit,

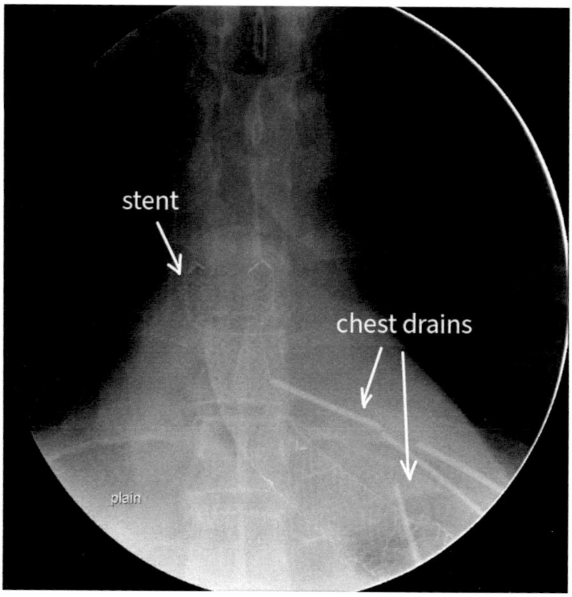

Fig. 16.7 Chest Xray showing stent and chest drains in place

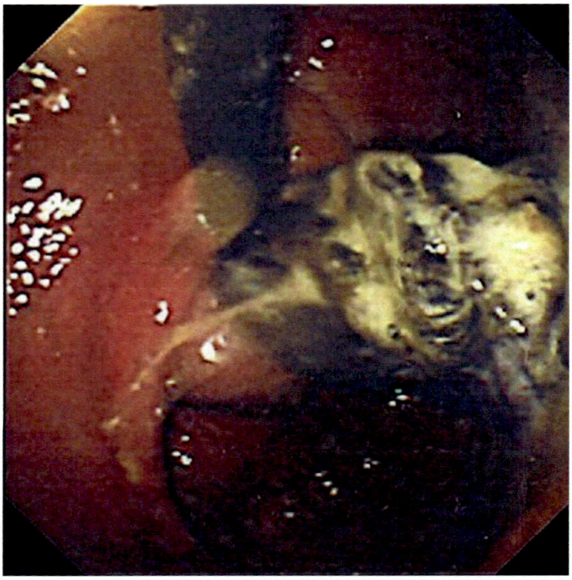

Fig. 16.8 Mesh seen on J-manoeuvre at OGD

and after preparation with its vascular pedicle, a retrosternal tunnel was created, and the conduit was brought up through it into the neck. The oesophageal remnant was anastomosed to the ileum, and the distal end of the colonic conduit was anastomosed to the jejunum 25 cm distal to the DJ flexure. A contrast study one week later showed no leaks (Fig. 16.10).

The patient was discharged after two weeks but was readmitted six weeks later with chest pain and pyrexia. A CT scan showed a collection in a small remnant of the oesophagus in the mediastinum. This was drained under radiological guidance. The pigtail stent was kept in place for two months and eventually removed after a tubogram had shown that the remnant had reduced considerably in size and the output was minimal.

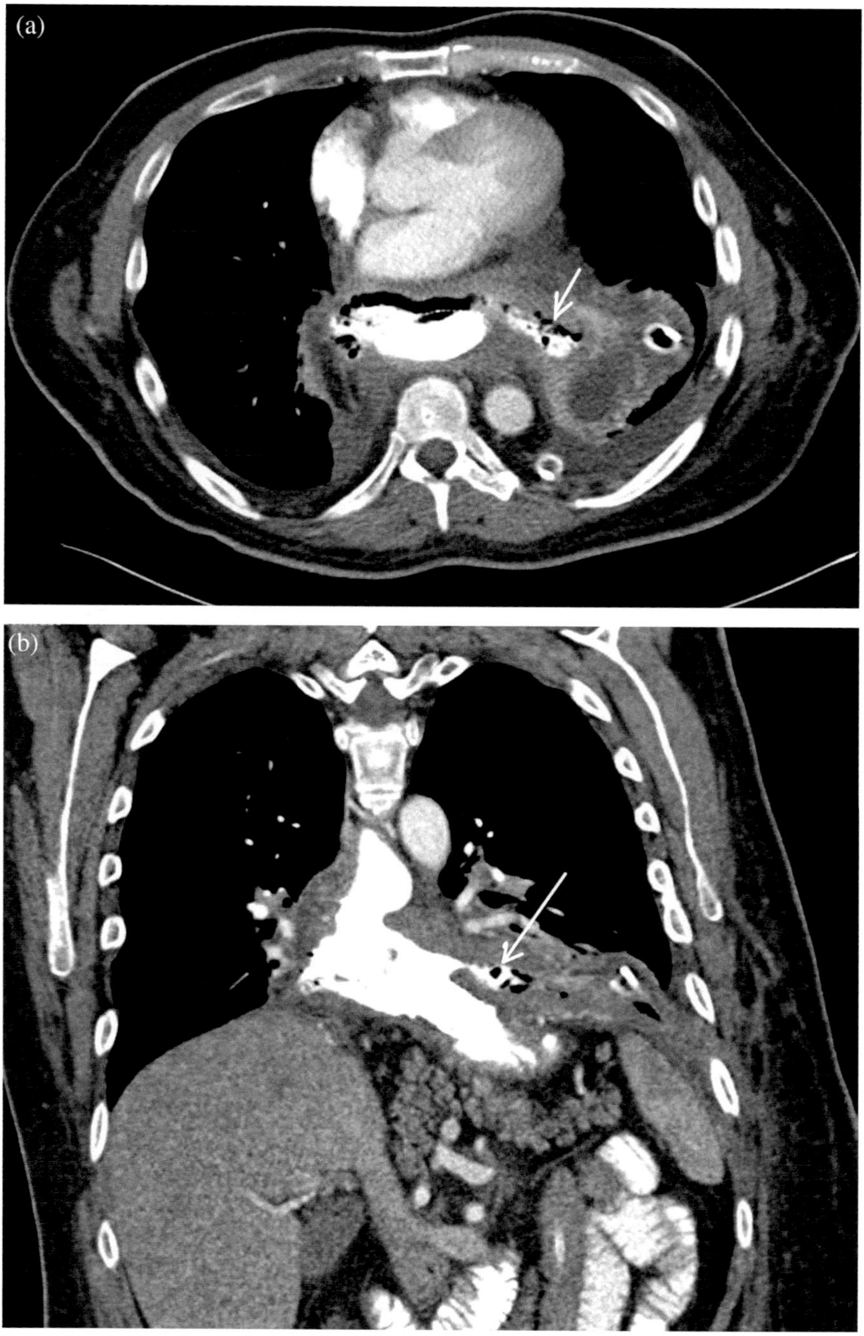

Fig. 16.9 Axial (a) and coronal (b) CT sections showing a recurrent hiatus hernia with contrast leaking from it into the left chest

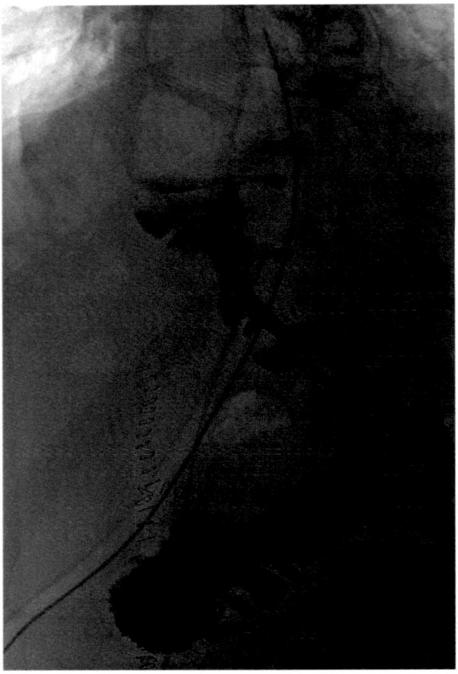

Fig. 16.10 Contrast swallow 7 days after surgery showing transit through the colonic conduit with no leaks

16.2.2 Learning Points

This was a particularly complex situation because the bilateral thoracotomies with subsequent chronic mediastinal sepsis meant that a further thoracotomy would have been extremely difficult and potentially hazardous. It was, therefore, decided to carry out as much of the excision of the mesh, the involved stomach and the oesophagus through the hiatus and from the neck. Under normal circumstances, dissecting the oesophagus for at least 10 to 15 cm into the mediastinum through a neck approach is possible. This was achieved in this case, but a small length of oesophagus in the mid chest could not be safely removed from the neck or the abdomen as it was intimately adherent to the surrounding structures. This resulted in a small remnant, possibly with a small portion of the mesh attached being retained in the chest, causing post-operative sepsis. The 'collection' which was drained was actually in the lumen of the remnant and necessitated the pigtail drain to stay in place for a long time with periodic control studies which showed a gradual decrease in its volume. The lumen eventually became obliterated, and no further intervention was required once the final drain was removed three months later. Because almost the entire stomach had to be removed, reconstruction was carried out with the colon routed through the retrosternal space, which was straightforward.

References

1. For the SAGES Guidelines Committee, Geoffrey PK, Raymond RP, Steven RM, Jörg Z, Oliver JM, Ziad A et al. Guidelines for the management of hiatal hernia. Surgic Endoscop. 2013; 27(12):4409–28. https://doi.org/10.1007/s00464-013-3173-3.
2. Gordon AC, Gillespie C, Son J, Polhill T, Leibman S, Smith GS. Long-term outcomes of laparoscopic large hiatus hernia repair with nonabsorbable mesh. Dis Esophagus. 2018;31(5):dox156. https://doi.org/10.1093/dote/dox156.
3. Priego P, Perez De Oteyza J, Galindo J, Carda P, García-moreno F, Rodríguez Velasco G, Lobo E. Long-term results and complications related to crurasoft^sup ^ mesh repair for paraesophageal hiatal hernias. Hernia. 2017;21(2):291–98. https://doi.org/10.1007/s10029-016-1486-6.
4. Stadlhuber RJ, Amr El S, Sumeet KM, Robert JF, Michael Brunt L, John GH, Tom RD, Lee LS, Daniel Smith C, Charles JF. Mesh complications after prosthetic reinforcement of hiatal closure: a 28-case series. Surgic Endoscop. 2009;23(6):1219–26. https://doi.org/10.1007/s00464-008-0205-5.

Chapter 17
The 'Short' Oesophagus

Abstract The "short" oesophagus presents a significant challenge in the surgical management of large hiatus hernias, as the gastro-oesophageal junction (GOJ) cannot be brought below the diaphragm after mobilisation. Whether congenital or acquired due to chronic gastro-oesophageal reflux disease, the diagnosis of true oesophageal length can only be established at operation. Thorough dissection and mobilisation of both the oesophagus and the GOJ are essential for accurate diagnosis and effective treatment. Although techniques such as Collis gastroplasty have been described for lengthening the oesophagus and restoring the GOJ below the diaphragm, the procedure is difficult with variable outcomes and postoperative complications. This underscores the need for careful patient counselling and planning including thorough mobilisation of the oesophagus before considering a gastroplasty. While postoperative dysphagia and reflux remain concerns, meticulous surgical approaches offer the best chance for successful management of the short oesophagus in large hiatus hernias.

Keywords Short oesophagus · Hiatus hernia · Surgical management · Gastro-oesophageal junction (GOJ) · Collis gastroplasty · Oesophageal mobilisation · Intraoperative assessment · Reflux disease · Dysphagia · Surgical complications · Patient counseling

The 'short' oesophagus is a term used to describe an oesophagus of reduced length such that the GOJ cannot be brought down below the diaphragm after mobilisation. It poses significant challenges in the surgical management of large hiatus hernias. Restoring the gastro-oesophageal junction below the diaphragm is crucial for effective treatment of hiatus hernia particularly if an antireflux procedure is also required.

A short oesophagus may be congenital or acquired because of chronic gastro-oesophageal reflux disease, leading to fibrosis and shortening. The only way to determine whether there is true shortening of the oesophagus is to fully mobilise the oesophagus. Although preoperative evaluation with endoscopy, barium swallow, and oesophageal manometry may indicate oesophageal shortening, whether the

M. Mughal, *Reconstructive Surgery of the Oesophagus and Stomach*,
https://doi.org/10.1007/978-3-031-66846-3_17

oesophagus is truly short can only be determined during surgery, and even then, the assessment is subjective [1].

It is essential that a thorough dissection and full mobilisation is carried out of not just the oesophagus but also of the GOJ. This requires a thorough dissection of the oesophagus in the mediastinum at least up to int inferior pulmonary vein. In addition to this, a full reduction of the hernia sac and division of the short gastric vessels gains extra length. In one study of 220 laparoscopic fundoplications, only 16% (4% of the study population) of those suspected preoperatively to have a short oesophagus turned out to have one after thorough dissection [2]. Bochkarev and colleagues have reported their experience of laparoscopic antireflux surgery in 106 patients with short oesophagus diagnosed on a barium swallow. With diligent mobilisation, up to 18 cm into the mediastinum, they were able to achieve a mean oesophageal elongation of 2.65 cm and restore the GOJ below the diaphragm in all cases without the need for a Collis gastroplasty [3]. Post-operative barium swallows showed no recurrence of hiatus hernia.

A variety of surgical techniques have been developed to address the short oesophagus, including the Collis gastroplasty, Hill gastropexy, Roux-en-Y oesophagojejunostomy, the Merendino procedure and intrathoracic fundoplication. Poor outcomes have been reported for the Merendino operation for failed antireflux surgery [4] and for intrathoracic fundoplication [5]. It is widely acknowledged that a Collis gastroplasty is the treatment of choice for the true short oesophagus, although variable outcomes have been reported [2, 6]. In one study, postoperative dysphagia was reported in 11–26% of cases, symptomatic reflux in 3–26% and objective evidence of pathological reflux in up to 50% [1]. Although a Collis gastroplasty with a fundoplication (Fig. 17.1) is currently the best strategy to deal with a short oesophagus, it is not a perfect operation, and patients should be carefully counselled regarding this.

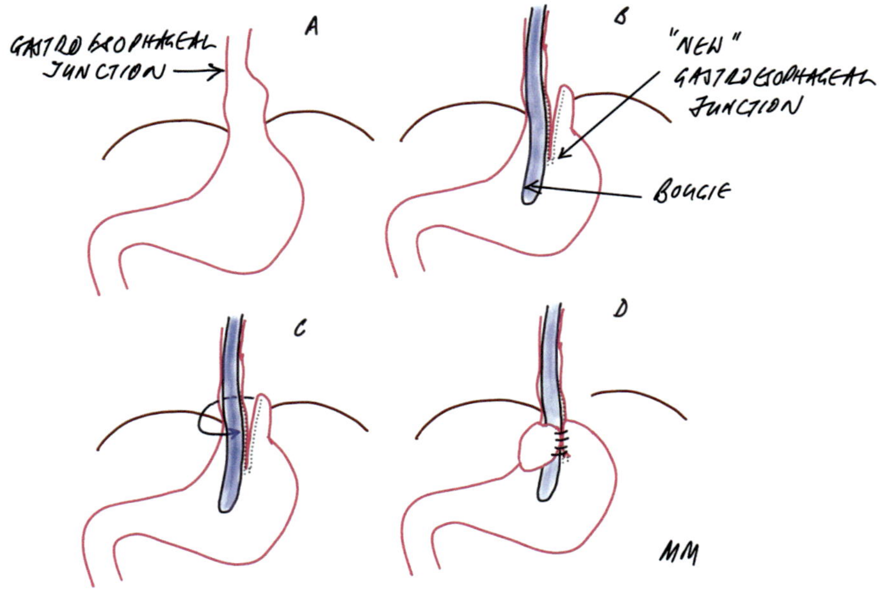

Fig. 17.1 Principle of Collis gastroplasty with a Nissen fundoplication. After mobilisation of the GOJ which cannot be brought down into the abdomen (A), a 54 Fr bougie is placed in the oesophagus and the stomach transected parallel to it with a stapler (B). The new GOJ is at the distal extent of the transection. The fundus is then brought round the oesophagus (C) and used to create a fundoplication (D)

References

1. Horvath KD, Swanstrom LL, Jobe BA. The short esophagus: pathophysiology, incidence, presentation, and treatment in the era of laparoscopic antireflux surgery. Ann Surg. 2000;232(5):630–40. https://doi.org/10.1097/00000658-200011000-00003.
2. Johnson A, et al. Laparoscopic collis gastroplasty and nissen fundoplication a new technique for the management of esophageal foreshortening; n.d.
3. Bochkarev V, Yong Kwon L, Michelle V, Dmitry O. Short esophagus: how much length can we get? Surgic Endoscop. 2018;22(10):2123–27. https://doi.org/10.1007/s00464-008-9999-4.
4. Analatos A, Mats L, Ioannis R, Peter E, Lars L, Magnus N, Andrianos T, Jon AT. Evaluation of resection of the gastroesophageal junction and jejunal interposition (Merendino Procedure) as a rescue procedure in patients with a failed redo antireflux procedure. a single-center experience. BMC Surg. 2018;18(1). https://doi.org/10.1186/s12893-018-0401-8.
5. Mansour KA, Burton HG, Miller JI, Hatcher CR. Complications of intrathoracic nissen fundoplication. Ann Thorac Surg. 1981;32(2):173–8. https://doi.org/10.1016/S0003-4975(10)61027-2.
6. Swanstrom LL, Daniel RM, Gil QG. Laparoscopic collis gastroplasty is the treatment of choice for the shortened esophagus. n.d.

Chapter 18
Recalcitrant Benign Oesophageal Strictures

Abstract This chapter discusses recalcitrant benign oesophageal strictures, commonly caused by gastro-oesophageal reflux disease or radical radiotherapy for squamous cell cancer of the oesophagus. While most strictures respond to acid suppression and dilatation, long strictures resistant to non-surgical measures may necessitate resection or reconstruction. The case presented involves a 52-year-old female with strictures from chemoradiotherapy, requiring frequent dilatations and experiencing complications like perforation. Due to fibrotic changes and previous interventions, oesophageal bypass was chosen over resection. Using a gastric conduit placed retrosternally, successful reconstruction was achieved, emphasising the importance of careful patient selection and surgical planning in managing such challenging cases.

Keywords Recalcitrant benign oesophageal strictures · Gastro-oesophageal reflux disease · Radiotherapy · Oesophageal reconstruction · Surgical management · Antireflux surgery · Chemoradiotherapy · Oesophagectomy · Gastric conduit · Retrosternal placement

Benign oesophageal strictures are most commonly caused by gastro-oesophageal reflux disease and most of these can be satisfactorily managed with a combination of acid suppression and dilatation. Some patients with severe reflux may also require antireflux surgery. It is rare, therefore, to have to resect such strictures. The strictures likely to require resection are those that are long and where non-surgical measures have failed. In my experience, these have been commonly due to corrosive injury [1] or the result of radical radiotherapy for squamous cell cancer of the oesophagus. Even with long strictures, combinations of conservative interventions can achieve a good symptomatic result. This includes serial dilatations with or without the injection of steroids, temporary stenting and educating the patient on self-dilatation [1]. When all these interventions have failed, oesophageal reconstruction may be the only option.

M. Mughal, *Reconstructive Surgery of the Oesophagus and Stomach*,
https://doi.org/10.1007/978-3-031-66846-3_18

18.1 DXT Related Recalcitrant Oesophageal Stricture

18.1.1 Case Summary

A woman in her 50s was referred with recalcitrant oesophageal strictures at 20 and 32 cm. These had resulted from definitive radical chemoradiotherapy for squamous cell carcinoma of the oesophagus three years previously. The strictures had been dilated and stented several times, and although she had been trained to self-dilate, this was abandoned because of bleeding. She had also developed a perforation at the site of the proximal stricture during a dilatation which was successfully treated with antibiotics and parenteral nutrition. At the time of referral, the patient was requiring dilatations every two weeks. CT scan showed no evidence of recurrent tumour or metastatic disease but considerable thickening and fibrosis of the oesophagus at the level of the carina and the GOJ (Figs. 18.1 and 18.2).

Given the fibrotic changes in the oesophagus, previous radiotherapy and oesophageal perforation, it was decided to bypass rather than attempt resection of the oesophagus, which may have been hazardous. A laparotomy was carried out, and the stomach was noted to be suitable for use as a conduit.

After mobilisation of the stomach a 4 cm wide conduit was created based on the greater curvature of the stomach taking care to preserve the gastroepiploic arch. The partitioned lesser curve of the stomach was left attached to the GOJ, and was retained. Its tip was hitched up to the abdominal wall and intubated with a Foley catheter to provide access to the excluded oesophagus and for drainage of mucus. The cervical

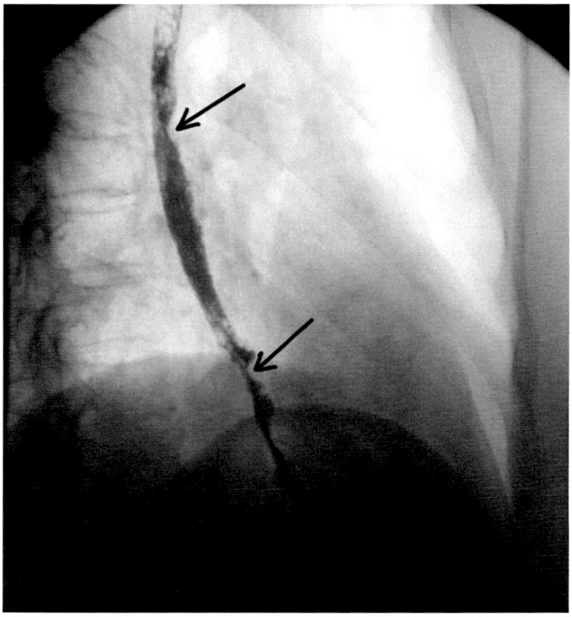

Fig. 18.1 Contrast swallow showing proximal and distal oesophageal strictures

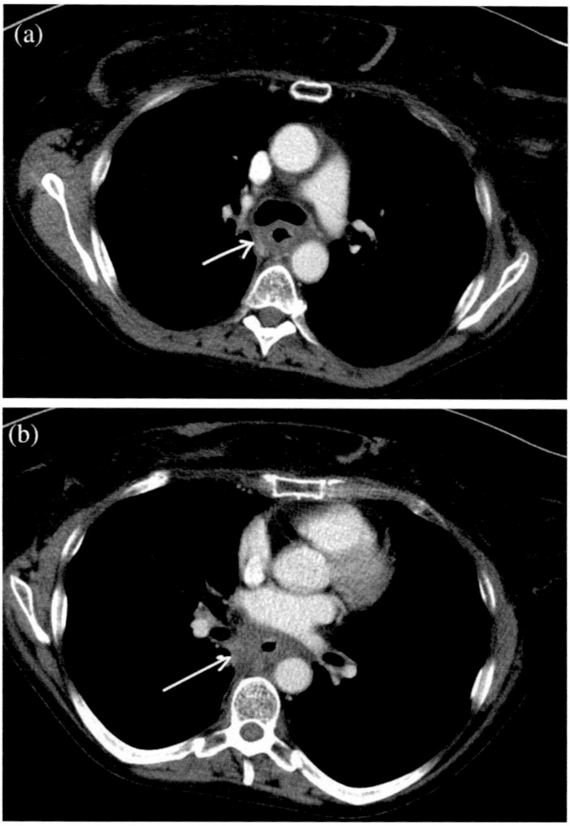

Fig. 18.2 CT sections at the level of the carina and pulmonary veins showing a thick-walled oesophagus with loss of fat planes

oesophagus was dissected out through an incision along the anterior border of the left sternomastoid muscle. Once encircled, the oesophagus was mobilised as far down into the superior mediastinum as possible and transected, and the distal end was ligated with PDS. A retrosternal tunnel was then made, and the stomach conduit was brought up through this and anastomosed to the oesophageal stump in the neck. Postoperative appearances are shown in Figs. 18.3, 18.4 and 18.5. The patient made an uneventful post-operative recovery and was eventually able to swallow normally. She was placed on long-term PPI. She reported discharge of between 200 and 300 mL of mucus daily from the Foley catheter.

The catheter had to be replaced several times because of blockage. She sometimes noticed coffee ground in the Foley catheter bag, indicating inflammation of the excluded oesophagus or the attached lesser curve of the stomach. This responded to a temporary increase in the dose of PPIs and insillation of sucralfate through the Foley catheter.

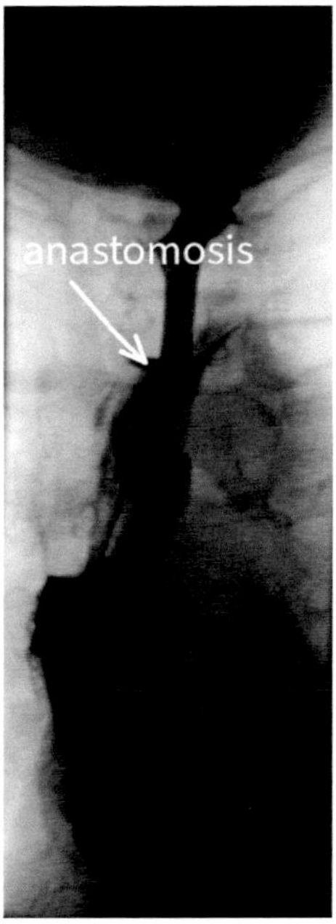

Fig. 18.3 Contrast swallow 7 days after reconstruction

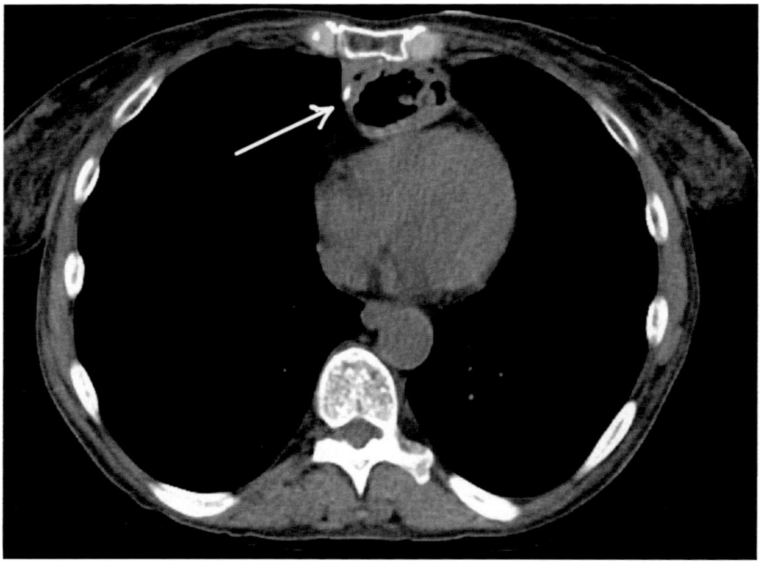

Fig. 18.4 Post-op CT scan showing retrosternal conduit

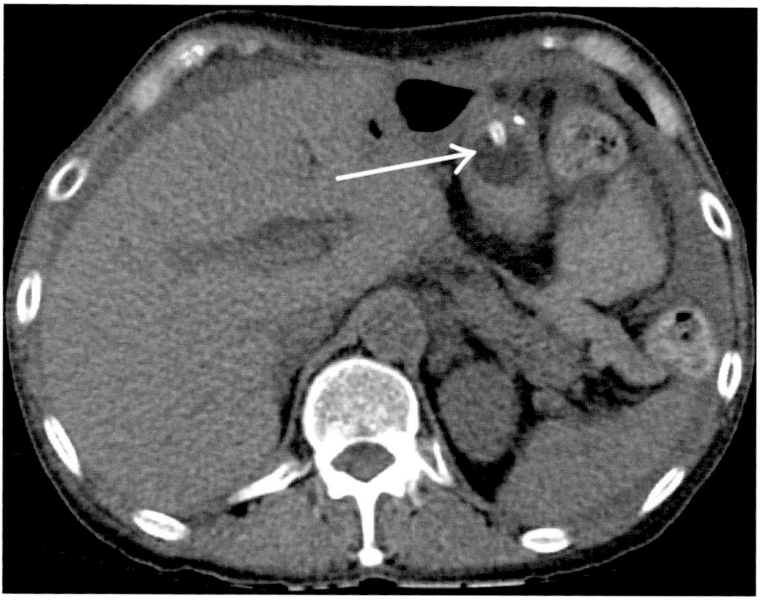

Fig. 18.5 CT scan showing Foley catheter in the partitioned lesser curve of stomach

18.1.2 Learning Points

It is not uncommon for definitive chemoradiotherapy for squamous cell cancer of the oesophagus to achieve a complete response, but also to cause strictures that are difficult to manage. In this patient, the strictures required repeated dilatations with increasing frequency, which raised the risk of complications. It was not surprising, therefore, that she suffered a perforation. Self-dilatation can be an effective strategy, but this had to be abandoned after an episode of bleeding. In considering surgery, it was essential to determine that she was clear of cancer. In this case, reconstruction was not considered until three years after her cancer treatment and then only after she had undergone a CT and PET scan to exclude a recurrence of metastatic disease. Having decided on reconstruction, it was then a question of whether the oesophagus should be resected or bypassed. Had investigations shown recurrent tumour, the correct decision would have been to carry out an oesophagectomy despite the risks associated with a salvage operation against a background of mediastinal radiotherapy and a history of oesophageal perforation. In my experience, the main risk of an oesophagectomy with previous radiotherapy is damage to the airways that can be rendered fragile, almost like tracheomalacia. However, in this case, as there was no suspicion of a recurrence, it was decided to bypass the oesophagus. It was decided to place the gastric conduit retrosternally since a thoracotomy was not required.

Because a substantial part of the oesophagus was left in situ, it was important to ensure that it was drained to allow the escape of mucus. We decided to do this by keeping the separated lesser curvature of the stomach attached to the oesophagus and drained with a Foley catheter. We have used this strategy successfully in several cases when bypassing the oesophagus.

Reference

1. Karnak I, Tanyel FC, Buyukpamukcu N, HiCsonmez A. Combined use of steroid, antibiotics and early bougienage against stricture formation following caustic esophageal burns. J Cardiovascul Surg. 1999;40(2):307–10.

Chapter 19
Leaks Following Bariatric Surgery

Abstract The chapter discusses leaks following bariatric surgery, particularly from gastric sleeves, which can have severe consequences compared to complications of gastric bypass. Management strategies depend on factors like leak size and timing of diagnosis, ranging from conservative measures with antibiotics to more invasive interventions like laparoscopy with washout and drainage, endoscopic suturing, stenting, and even innovative techniques such as septotomy. The presented cases highlight the challenges in managing a leak from a gastric sleeve in a morbidly obese patient, necessitating multiple surgical interventions including laparotomy, thoracotomy, and eventual completion gastrectomy with oesophagostomy. Complications like fistula formation and subsequent lung infection underscore the complexity of treating such leaks and the importance of a multidisciplinary approach. Learning points emphasise the need for timely intervention and consideration of alternative surgical techniques in challenging cases to achieve successful outcomes.

Keywords Bariatric surgery · Gastric sleeve · Leaks · Surgical complications · Surgical management · Laparoscopy · Endoscopic suturing · Stenting · Septotomy · Multidisciplinary approach

Bariatric surgery is now generally extremely safe and effective. Nevertheless, complications do occur even though they are rare [1]. Because bariatric operations are being performed in increasing numbers in the Western world, we are beginning to see patients with serious, often life-changing and sometimes life-threatening complications. The leak rate from gastric sleeves is between one and 3% and its consequences are worse than complications of gastric bypass [2].

Leaks most commonly develop at the top of the staple line just below the angle of His [3].

The management depends on the timing of the diagnosis, the size of the leak and the systemic manifestations. Small leaks can be managed conservatively with antibiotics and stopping oral intake. Larger leaks may also require a laparoscopy with washout and drainage and others can be effectively treated with a combination of endoscopic suturing and stents as well as EVT (Endoluminal Vacuum Therapy).

M. Mughal, *Reconstructive Surgery of the Oesophagus and Stomach*,
https://doi.org/10.1007/978-3-031-66846-3_19

Pigtail stents have been used for drainage of a para-gastric cavity back into the stomach, and internal drainage is also the rationale for the intriguing technique of septotomy.

As with many of the scenarios covered in this book, it is important to use a multidisciplinary approach to decide which of the many different interventions is most appropriate in a particular case.

In this book, I am only going to cover those complications that are relevant to oesophagogastric reconstruction. In my experience, this is usually due to serious complications from gastric sleeve leaks, when all other interventions have failed. These have been leaks that have been defined as "malignant" by some groups [4], i.e., those that could not be successfully treated by first-line endoscopic treatment and those complicated by either generalised peritonitis, anatomical abnormalities, gastric fistula or chronic leaks, which persisted for more than four weeks. Such leaks may require several different, and sometimes concurrent interventions, and, rarely, radical surgery.

There are some intriguing and innovative techniques, such as septotomy, which has been successful in difficult cases of persistent leaks after first-line treatment [5]. This entails the enlargement of the defect in the staple line by a combination of septotomy and dilatation, thereby allowing for internal drainage of the adjacent abscess cavity.

19.1 Gastric Sleeve Leak 1

19.1.1 Case Summary

A morbidly obese (BMI 55) woman in her 40s was readmitted with abdominal pain a week after a straightforward sleeve gastrectomy. A CT scan showed a leak from the staple line below the GOJ, and she underwent a laparoscopy with a washout and the placement of a drain. She was treated with antibiotics and nasojejunal feeding but was still leaking three weeks later. Endoscopy showed a 1 cm diameter perforation 2 cm below the GOJ, which was treated with a covered stent (Figs. 19.1, 19.2 and 19.3).

Gastrografin swallow a week later showed a leak, and oral feeding was commenced. She developed a fever and a left pleural effusion. A repeat contrast study showed a persistent leak. A laparotomy was performed with drainage of the collection in the left upper quadrant, stent removal, balloon dilatation of the pylorus and a feeding jejunostomy. Gastrografin swallow six days later showed an ongoing leak. She developed a recurrence of the left pleural effusion, which was drained and revealed bile. A further laparotomy was carried out, the left upper quadrant collection was drained, and the perforation in the upper part of the sleeve was intubated with a T-tube. A contrast study through the T-tube two weeks later showed no leak. The T-tube was clamped, oral nutrition was recommenced and she was discharged. She was readmitted with a fever and a cough after two weeks. Imaging revealed a

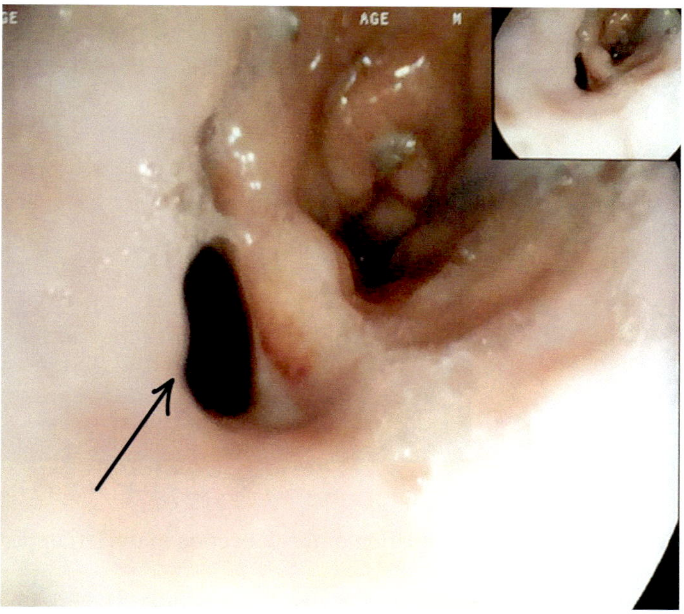

Fig. 19.1 OGD showing a leak at the GOJ

Fig. 19.2 Deployment of stent to cover the leak

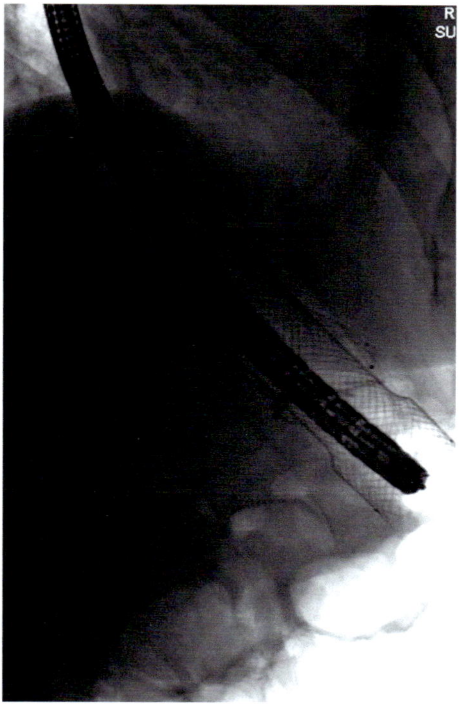

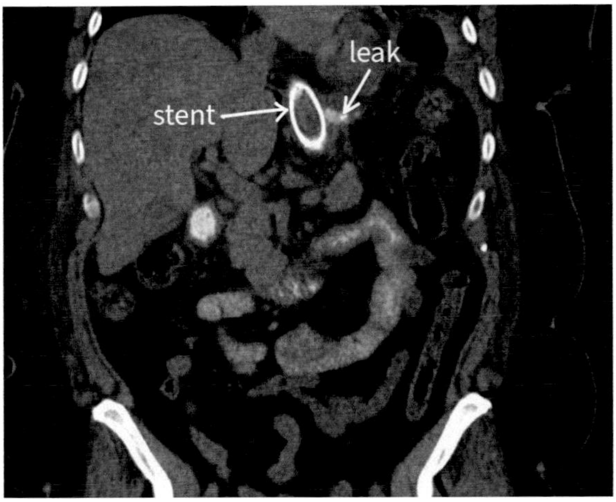

Fig. 19.3 CT section showing stent in position with ongoing extravasation of contrast

left pleural effusion and re-accumulation of the collection in the left upper quadrant (Fig. 19.4).

Another laparotomy was performed, the collections drained, and a completion gastrectomy was performed, stapling off the oesophagus above the GOJ with the placement of a T-tube through the oesophageal stump to provide drainage of saliva (Fig. 19.5). Two days later, she suffered a significant bleed through her abdominal drain. CT angiography showed the cause to be a pseudoaneurysm of the phrenic artery, which was successfully embolised (Fig. 19.6).

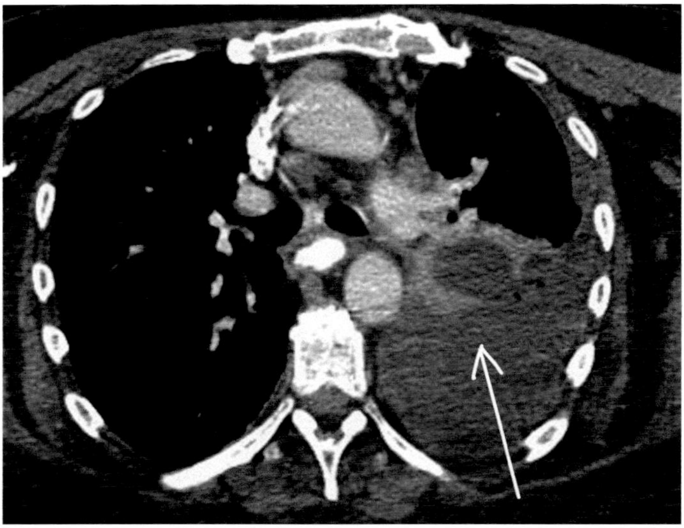

Fig. 19.4 CT showing complex chest collection from an ongoing leak

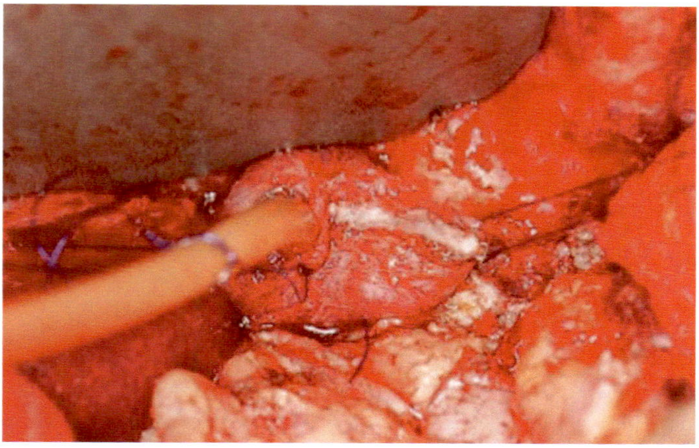

Fig. 19.5 T-tube placed in the transected oesophagus after a completion gastrectomy

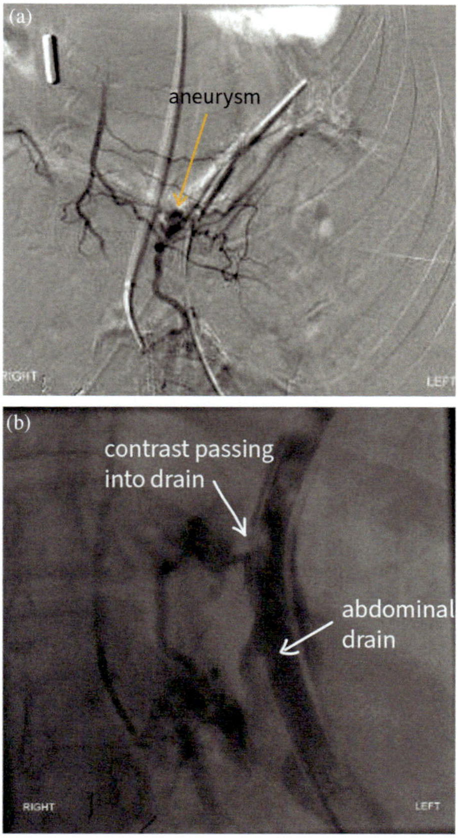

Fig. 19.6 Angiogram showing aneurysm of the phrenic artery (a) with extravasation of contrast through the drain (b)

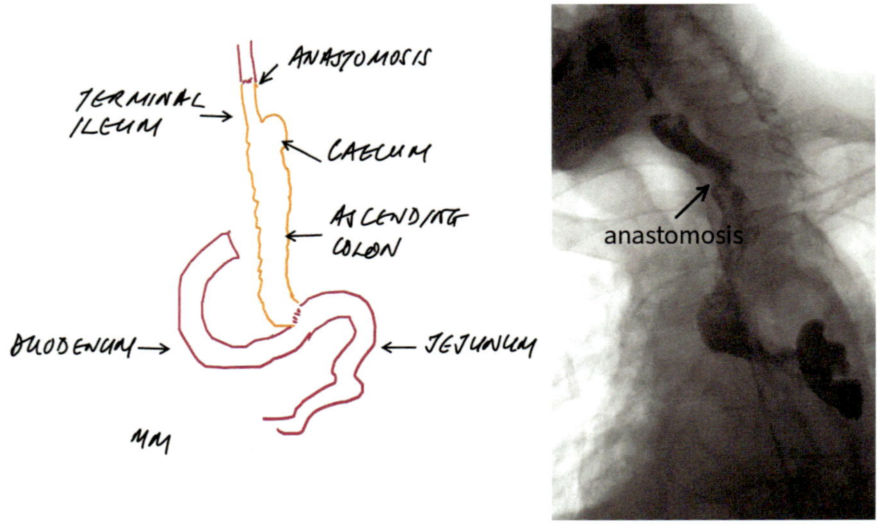

Fig. 19.7 Diagram showing reconstruction and contrast swallow 7 days post-operatively

She continued to have mediastinal sepsis with saliva draining through the T-tube as well as the paraoesophageal drain inserted through the hiatus. It was therefore decided to carry out a cervical oesophagostomy, transecting the cervical oesophagus with a stapler and bringing out the proximal end as a stoma in the neck. This finally resolved the sepsis.

Four months later, after the patient had recovered fully, a reconstruction was carried out using the right colon, which was brought up retrosternally to the neck, and the cervical oesophageal stump was anastomosed to the ileum. The distal end of the colonic conduit was anastomosed to the jejunum 25 cm distal to the DJ flexure (Fig. 19.7).

The patient developed a small but persistent leak at the cervical anastomosis, which was treated with endocopic application of a clip and Tisseel (a fibrin sealer) (Fig. 19.8). The leak healed but resulted in an anastomotic stricture, which responded to serial dilatation and she was eventually able to swallow normally. Endoscopic appearances of the anastomosis and colonic conduit are shown in Fig. 19.9.

She had a small, retained portion of the oesophagus in the chest, which was seen as a fluid-filled remnant on subsequent CTs. The remnant did not appear to change in size on serial scans over the subsequent three years. She did not describe any symptoms that could be ascribed to the remnant. She remained well, eating nearly normally until the last follow up four years after the reconstruction.

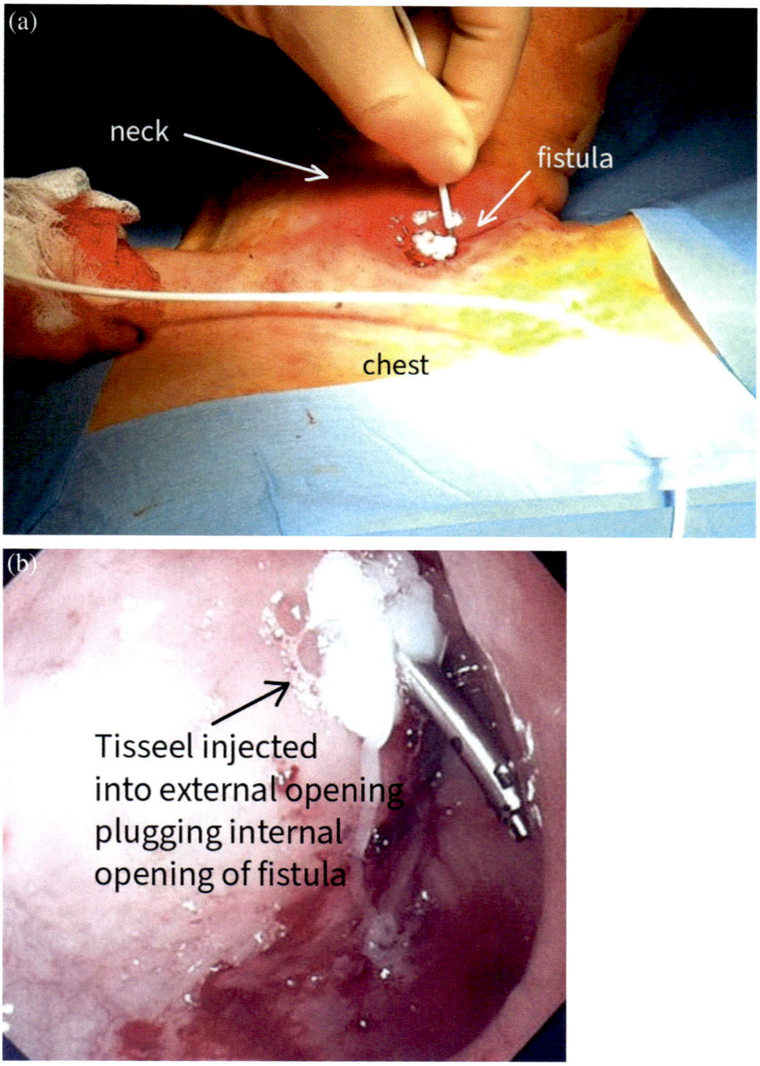

Fig. 19.8 Tisseel was applied to the cervical fistula (a), which was clipped endoscopically (b)

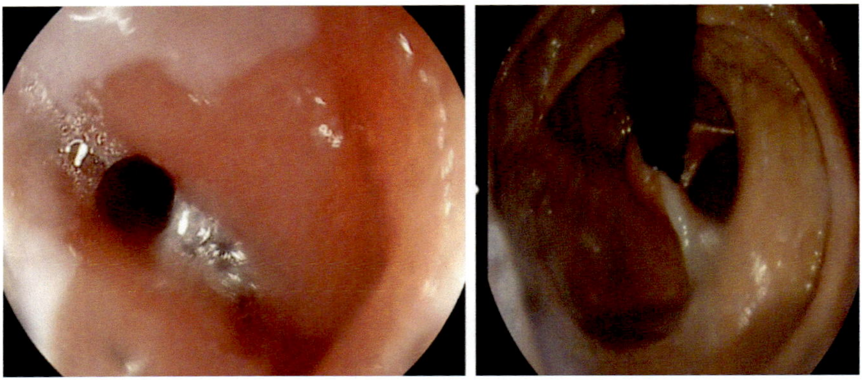

Fig. 19.9 Healed leak and patent anastomosis after several dilatations on the left. Retroflexion view showing the ileocaecal valve on the right

19.1.2 Learning Points

Leaks from gastric sleeves can be extremely troublesome and difficult to treat. In this case, all the usual approaches were tried in a timely and appropriate sequence. The chest component of the sepsis meant that when, finally, a completion gastrectomy was carried out, but the conditions were not suitable for reconstruction with a Roux-en-Y jejunal conduit. And because a diversion oesophagostomy proved essential to deal with ongoing sepsis, the only way of reconstruction was to use a colonic conduit. This was complicated by a small leak at the cervical anastomosis, which failed to settle with conservative treatment because of the development of a fistula through the cervical scar. Application of a clip and Tisseel was successful and the patient was kept nil by mouth and jejunostomy feeding was maintained until the leak had healed. As expected, a stricture developed at the cervical anastomosis, which responded to serial dilatation. Eventually, the patient was able to resume oral feeding. CT scans to monitor the mediastinal remnant of the oesophagus showed a fluid-filled structure that remain static. In some patients, the remnant can become chronically infected and require prolonged use of pigtail drains. However, the fibrosis resulting from chronic infection often results in the obliteration of the lumen, transforming the remnant into a small solid structure.

It is important to be aware of the possibility of false aneurysms complicating chronic sepsis, which can result in life-threatening bleeding, as in this case. Interventional radiology is critical in the diagnosis and treatment of such bleeds and highlights the benefits of treating such cases in centres that have not only the depth and range of expertise, but also the necessary infrastructure and ready access to appropriate equipment and operating theatres.

19.2 Gastric Sleeve Leak 2

19.2.1 Clinical Summary

A 24-year-old female underwent a sleeve gastrectomy which was revised for years later because of weight gain. This was complicated by a leak, which was initially treated with antibiotics and stenting. She remained unwell and developed a significant persistent cough. CT scan showed a chronic proximal gastric sleeve leak associated with a gastrobronchial fistula (Figs. 19.10 and 19.11).

Endoscopy confirmed a leak from the proximal end of the staple line 2 cm below the GOJ. There also appeared to be a twist within the sleeve.

She was transferred to my care three months after the diagnosis of the leak. Repeat imaging showed a significant leak from the gastric sleeve with an adjacent collection, which appeared to have penetrated the diaphragm, forming a supradiaphragmatic abscess and a fistula into the bronchial tree. Gastroscopy showed the fistula opening just above the GOJ and bronchoscopy showed inflammation in the second-level branches of the right main bronchus (Fig. 19.12).

Initially, attempts were made to treat the leak and fistula with the EsoSponge. As the gastric opening of the fistula was only 6 mm in diameter, it was difficult to cut the sponge to size and deploy it sufficiently deeply into the adjacent cavity. Therefore, a laparotomy was performed, and a chronic abscess cavity was entered in the left upper quadrant. As the cavity was debrided, a low-volume air leak became apparent through the left hemidiaphragm. A T-tube was placed in the defect in the sleeve, and omentum was used to packed round it to manage the air leak. After the operation, the patient did not tolerate extubation and returned to the intensive-care unit ventilated. The

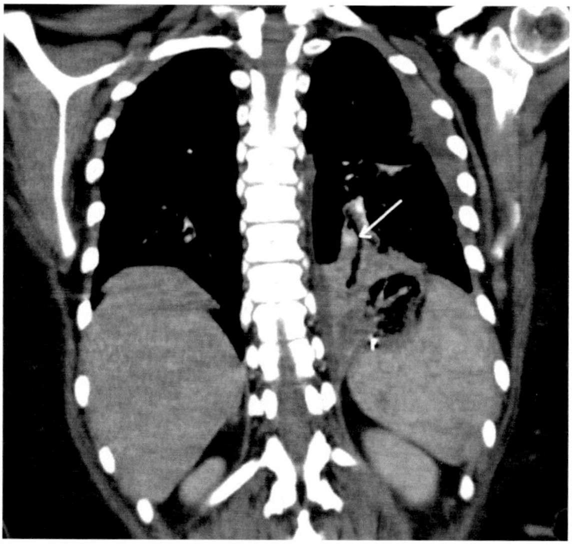

Fig. 19.10 CT section showing sleeve leak communicating with the peripheral airways

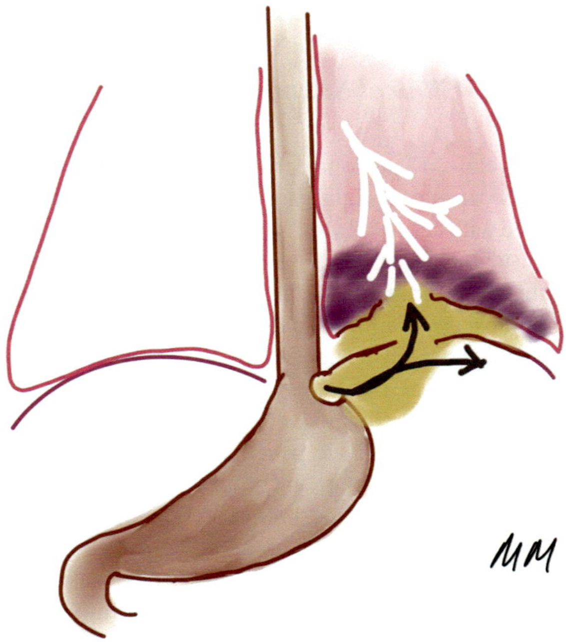

Fig. 19.11 Diagrammatic representation of the sleeve leak communicating through a sub-diaphragmatic collection with the peripheral airways

leak continued through the abdominal drain, which was connected to an underwater seal chest drain bottle. She remained septic and was treated with antibiotics and antifungal agents based on blood and drain cultures.

Further imaging showed persistent collapse/consolidation of the lower lobe of the left lung. After a period of stabilisation of her general condition, it was decided to reoperate as she had a continuing air leak from subdiaphragmatic drain. A left thoracotomy was performed and revealed a grossly infected, spongy lower lobe of the lung. As much as possible of the affected part of the lung was excised, leaving a small, basal portion that was densely adherent to the attached to the diaphragm (Fig. 19.13). This area was debrided, and the chest was closed with basal and apical drains. The patient was then turned to the supine position perform a laparotomy. The left upper quadrant abscess cavity was entered and debrided. The plan had been to perform a completion gastrectomy, but this was abandoned because of hostile conditions due to collections around the oesophageal hiatus and communicating with the chest. Instead, the gastric sleeve was dissected below the leak and stapled across its entire width with a non-cutting stapler, leaving the stomach in continuity but isolating the leak from the distal stomach. Through a collar incision, the cervical oesophagus was dissected out and tied off with a No 1 Vicryl suture as low as possible in the superior mediastinum. A Foley catheter was inserted into the through an oesophagotomy above the tie and secured with a purse-string suture (Figs. 19.14 and 19.15).

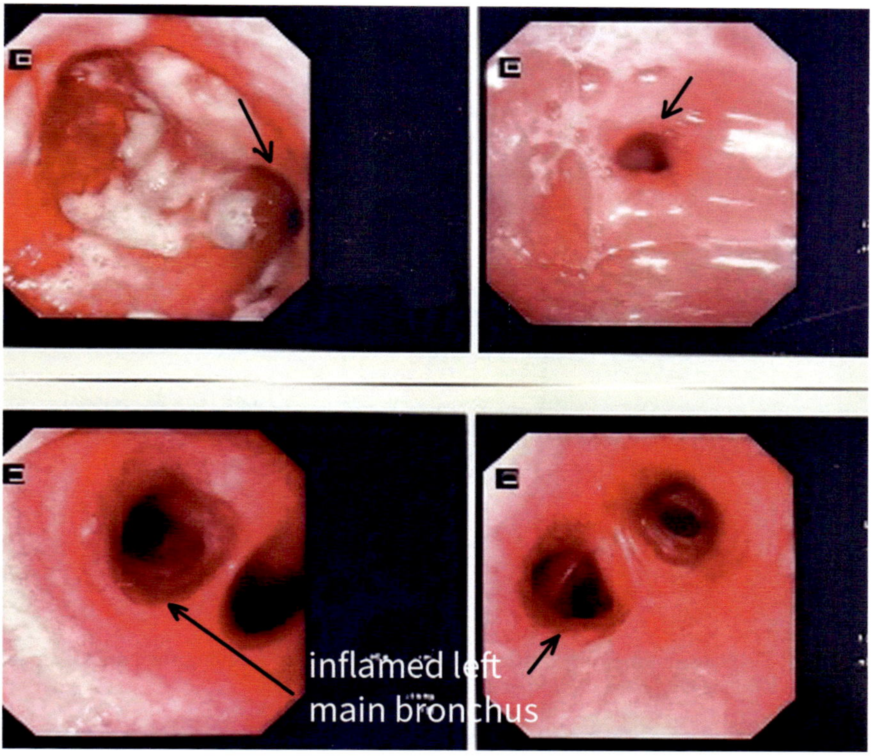

Fig. 19.12 OGD (upper two pictures) showing the opening of the fistula at the GOJ and bronchoscopy images (lower two pictures)

Fig. 19.13 CT scan showing staple line through the left lower lobe with a residual cavity below

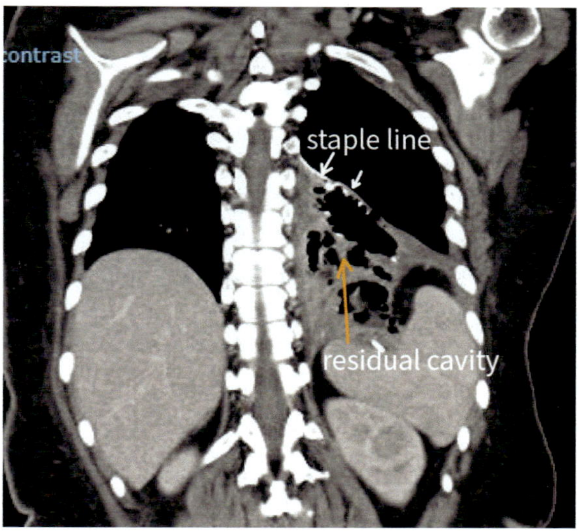

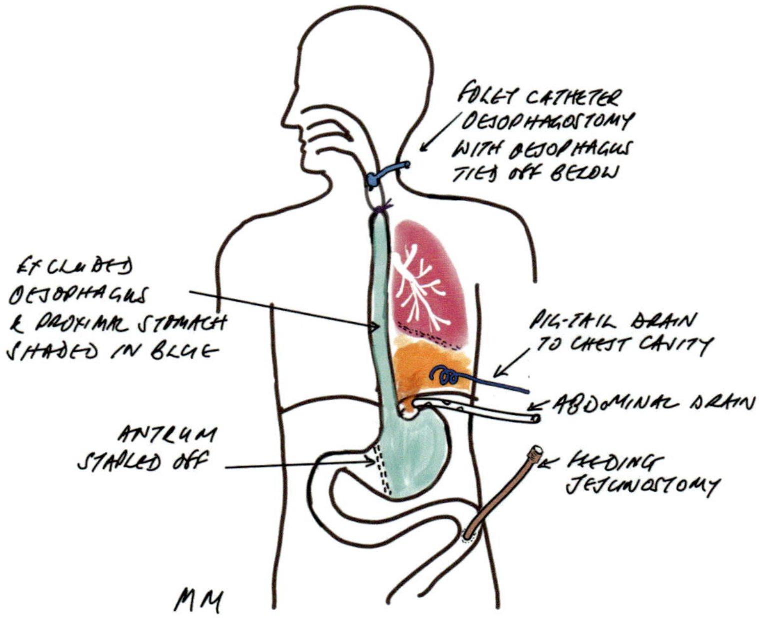

Fig. 19.14 Diagram showing Foley catheter oesophagostomy, gastric stapling, stapling of the lower lobe of the left lung disconnecting it from the necrotic basal segment

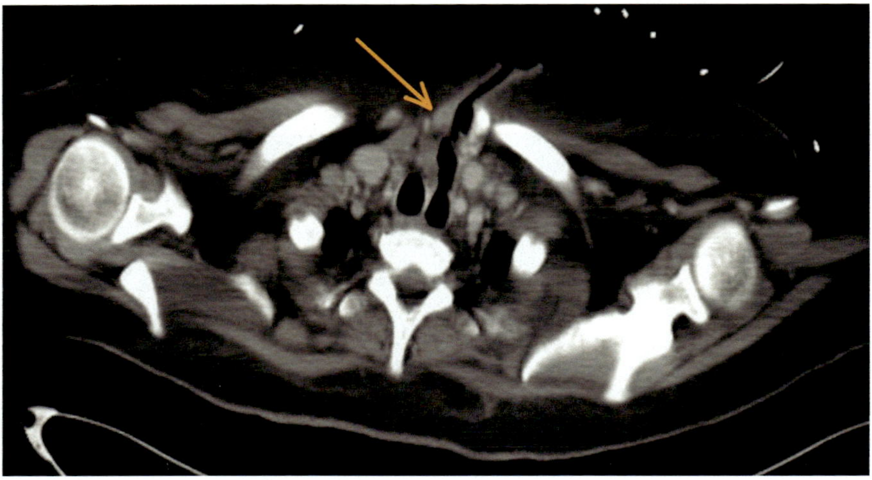

Fig. 19.15 CT section showing Foley catheter oesophagostomy

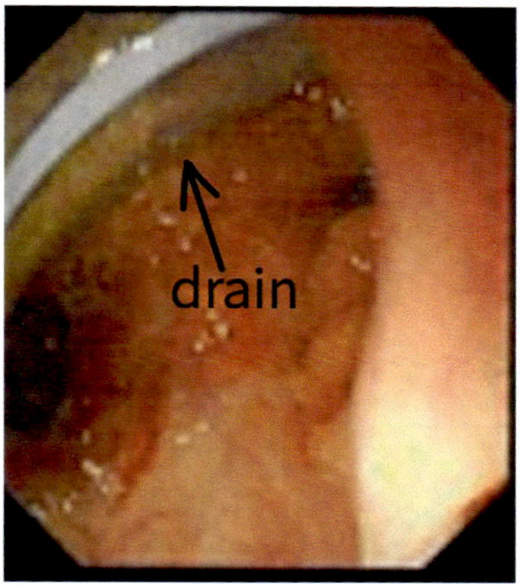

Fig. 19.16 Endoscopic view of abdominal drain with tip in the lumen of the GOJ

Following this, the patient started to improve, with near resolution of the sepsis in the left chest and abdomen. Six weeks later, a contrast swallow showed continuity of the oesophagus across the site of the Vicryl ligature, which had resorbed. This resulted in controlled, low-volume, salivary fistula through the abdominal drain which had been left adjacent to the hole in the sleeve, but had migrated into it (Fig. 19.16).

A laparotomy was performed, and, on this occasion, due to the resolution of the abdominal sepsis, it was possible to resect the sleeve and perform a Roux-en-Y oesophagojejunostomy. After a contrast swallow five days later, which showed a patent oesophagojejunal anastomosis without a leak, the Foley catheter was spigotted, the balloon partially deflated, and the patient was started on oral fluids. A week later, the Foley catheter was removed, and once the residual fistula had dried up five days later, she gradually progressed to a regular diet. She was discharged six weeks later and continued to make a good recovery as an outpatient. CT scan two months after discharge showed low-grade inflammatory changes in the left lower chest, but she was asymptomatic with normal inflammatory markers. The scan also showed a small diverticulum of the oesophagus in the neck at the site of the tube oesophagostomy (Fig. 19.17).

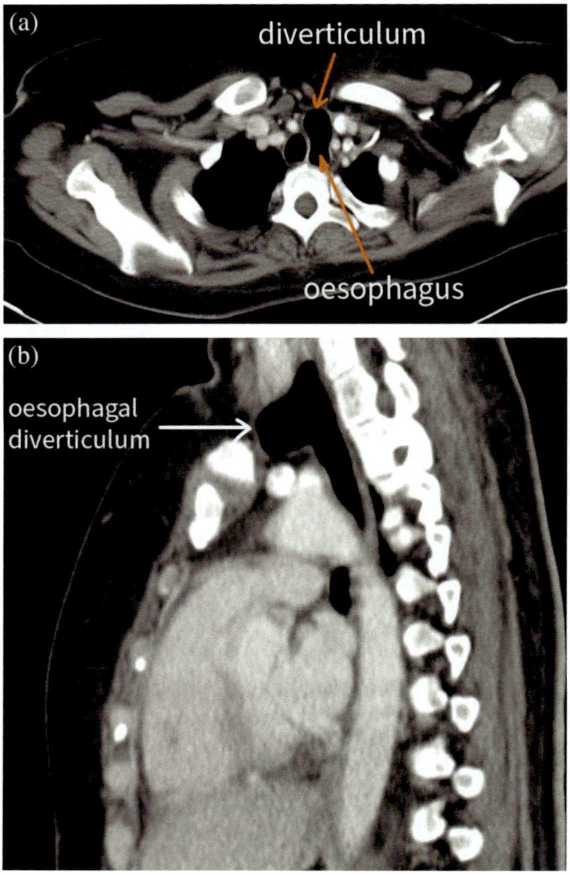

Fig. 19.17 Diverticulum at the site of the tube oesophagostomy shown in axial and sagittal CT sections

19.2.2 Learning Points

This patient was referred after several months of treatment with antibiotics and drainage for a chronic gastric sleeve leak. By the time she came under my care, she had a well-established gastro bronchial fistula with a chronically infected (bacterial and fungal infection) lower lobe of the left lung. It is likely that the fistula from the sleeve was to the peripheral airways as only a small track of oral contrast was seen on CT and bronchoscopy revealed inflammation but no bile in the distal bronchial tree. The initial operation was performed with the aim of disconnecting the fistula and placing a T-tube into the gastric defect. However, a moderate air leak started after disconnecting the fistula, as a result of positive pressure ventilation. Had it been possible to extubate the patient after the operation was completed, the air leak through the abdominal drain would have resolved. However, the continued need for ventilation and the resultant air leak necessitated a further operation within a short time. The plan had been to resect the lower lobe of the left lung and the sleeve, but neither was possible. The lower lobe was disconnected from the rest of the lung as usual by stapling across the fissure, but it proved impossible to resect the basal art of the lower lobe as it was densley adherent to the diaphragm. Attempts to excise it completely would have resulted in the loss of part of the diaphragm. The adherent portion was debrided by diathermy and curettage. Technically, the sleeve could have been excised but the collections in the surrounding abscess cavity. However, this would not have been conducive to a safe anastomosis. It was therefore decided to disconnect the distal part of the sleeve by stapling it below the leak. It was decided to carry out a temporary oesophagostomy to maintain oesophageal continuity. In this way, the sleeve leak was excluded from saliva and bile reflux. The temporary oesophageal exclusion provided a sufficient window of time to improve the condition of the patient and for the collections to resolve. It was then possible to carry out a completion gastrectomy without the need for reconstruction of the oesophagus that would have been necessary with a formal oesophagostomy.

References

1. Collazo-Clavell ML, Shah M. Common and rare complications of bariatric surgery. Endocrinol Metab Clin North Am. 2020;49(2):329–46. https://doi.org/10.1016/j.ecl.2020.02.003.
2. Antoine AR, Melkart B, Hicham EM. Gastric leaks post sleeve gastrectomy: review of its prevention and management. World J Gastroenterol: WJG. 2014;20(38):13904–10. https://doi.org/10.3748/wjg.v20.i38.13904.
3. Galloro G, Simona R, Teresa R, Donato AT, Mario M, Marco M, Raffaele M. Staple-line leak after sleve gastrectomy in obese patients: a hot topic in bariatric surgery. World J Gastrointestin Endoscop. 2015;7(9):843–46. https://doi.org/10.4253/wjge.v7.i9.843.
4. Caiazzo R, Marciniak C, Wallach N, Devienne M, Baud G, Cazauran J-B, Kipnis E, Branche J, Robert M, Pattou F. Malignant leakage after sleeve gastrectomy: endoscopic and surgical approach. Obes Surg. 2020;30(11):4459–66. https://doi.org/10.1007/s11695-020-04818-4.
5. Mahadev S, Vivek K, Josemberg C, Manoel GN, Mouen K, Yamile C, Marc B, Tamas G. Endoscopic septotomy: an effective approach for internal drainage of sleeve gastrectomy-associated collections. Endoscopy. 2017;49(05):504–8. https://doi.org/10.1055/s-0042-122012.

Chapter 20
Challenges of Primary and Secondary Reconstruction

Abstract This chapter explores the challenges and considerations in primary and secondary reconstruction, focusing on alternatives to the gastric pull-up conduit, such as colon and jejunal interposition. Colon interposition, while reliable, entails a higher morbidity compared to gastric pull-up, with reported leak and necrosis rates. Jejunal interposition poses challenges in obtaining a long, well-vascularized pedicled loop, although techniques like supercharging have shown promise.

Keywords Oesophagectomy · Reconstruction · Gastric pull-up · Colon interposition · Jejunal interposition · Case summaries · Patient selection

20.1 Choice of Conduit After Oesophageal Resection for Cancer: Alternatives to Gastric Pull-Up

Although early oesophageal cancer can be treated by endoscopic resection and invasive squamous cell cancer by chemoradiotherapy, resection and reconstruction are required in most cases. The gastric pull-up is the most common conduit choice; however, in cases where the stomach is unavailable due to previous surgery or resection, alternative conduits must be considered. This chapter discusses the pros and cons of various alternatives, namely the colon and jejunal interposition.

Colon interposition is a reliable method for oesophageal replacement. The choice of the right colon or left colon depends on the clinical situation and the individual patient. Although the surgical procedure is complex, DeMeester's group have reported that colon interposition can provide good functional results and quality of life [1]. In their report of 79 patients followed up for between 10 and 23 years, seven required reoperation for colonic redundancy. However, colonic conduits have a higher morbidity than gastric pull-ups and the authors of one study reported an anastomotic leak rate of 30% and conduit necrosis rate of 9% [2].

Jejunal interposition is another alternative to a gastric conduit. However, it is challenging to obtain a long, well-vascularised pedicled loop for a cervical anastomosis because of the need to preserve the second-order mesenteric arcades [3]. This

M. Mughal, *Reconstructive Surgery of the Oesophagus and Stomach*,
https://doi.org/10.1007/978-3-031-66846-3_20

can be overcome by supercharging a long loop by augmenting its blood supply by microvascular anastomosis between the vessels at the distal end of the loop and one of the neck vessels. Good functional results have been reported with this technique [4].

20.2 Completion Gastrectomy and Colonic Conduit for R1 Resection of the GOJ

20.2.1 Case Summary

A man in his 60s was diagnosed with a T3 N1 M0 adenocarcinoma of the gastro-oesophageal junction extending 2 cm into the stomach, as seen on retroflexion at OGD. PET scan showed activity in the distal oesophagus and no other suspicious uptake (Fig. 20.1).

After neoadjuvant chemotherapy, he underwent an Ivor-Lewis oesophagectomy and made an uneventful post-operative recovery. Resection histology showed extensive, poorly differentiated diffuse adenocarcinoma. It extensively involved the fundus and body of the resected stomach, involving the distal resection margin. There was

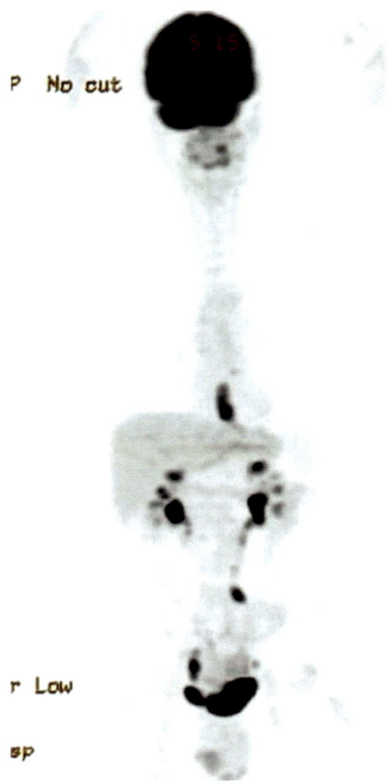

Fig. 20.1 PET scan image showing activity in the oesophagus

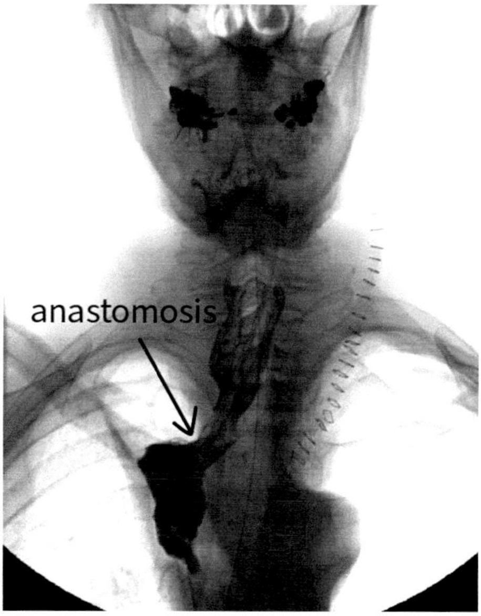

Fig. 20.2 Contrast swallow 7 days post showing free flow and no leak

no evidence of regression from the neoadjuvant chemotherapy. The pathological staging was ypT3 N1 (1/25) R1 (at the gastric resection margin). He made an uneventful post-operative recovery. His case was discussed in the oesophagogastric cancer MDT meeting following the resection. Several options were considered, including proceeding with the planned adjuvant chemotherapy followed by close surveillance. However, as it was clear from the resection histology that the neoadjuvant treatment had not had much benefit, this option was dismissed. Another option was to consider chemoradiotherapy, but the entire staple-line of the conduit would have to be irradiated with no guarantee that the tumour would be eradicated. It was therefore decided that the best option was to carry out a completion gastrectomy. The patient was counselled about the various options and chose the preferred option of the MDT.

Six weeks after his oesophagectomy, a right thoracotomy was performed, mobilising the conduit and remaining oesophagus from the apex of the chest to the diaphragm. The chest was closed with a drain, and the patient was repositioned supine. A laparotomy was performed, and a suitable loop of the right colon, based on the middle colic vessels, was isolated. Through a collar incision, the cervical oesophagus was mobilised and transected. The gastric conduit was pulled down into the abdomen with the attached oesophagus and resected, transecting the duodenum through its first part. The colonic loop was passed through the chest into the neck and anastomosed to the oesophageal stump. The distal end of the colon was anastomosed to the jejunum 25 cm distal to the DJ flexure, and a feeding jejunostomy was placed 20 cm distally.

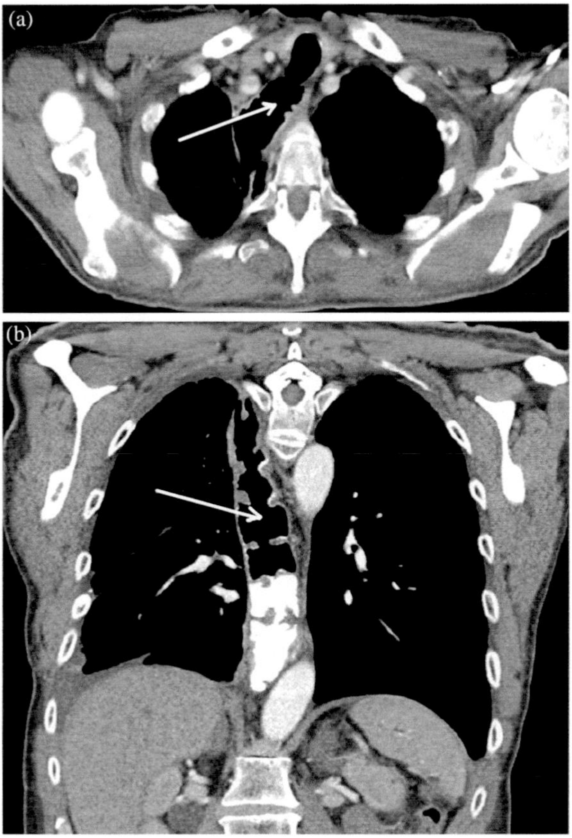

Fig. 20.3 Axial (a) and coronal (b) CT sections 6 months post-op showing colonic conduit

The patient developed a low-volume leak from the cervical anastomosis, which healed without intervention (Figs. 20.2 and 20.3). Resection histology showed residual, poorly differentiated diffuse adenocarcinoma around the anastomosis and extending into the gastric conduit along the lesser curvature.

20.2.2 Learning Points

Although the tumour involved the gastro-oesophageal junction, it was thought to be a Siewert Type II tumour, and a PET scan had shown no activity below the GOJ in the stomach. At operation, there was no macroscopic evidence of tumour in the part of the stomach chosen to create the conduit. Unfortunately, the distal resection margin turned out positive in this case. If it had been suspected on preoperative imaging that the distal margin was likely to be threatened, a frozen section would have been carried out, therefore avoiding an R1 resection. After an MDT discussion, the patient chose to have a completion gastrectomy. It was felt that the oesophageal stump was too high to consider a straightforward jejunal loop, and therefore, a colonic conduit was the only option. The operation was relatively straightforward, and the conduit was routed through the mediastinum to the neck.

20.3 Poor Gastric Emptying and Reflux Following Previous Gastric Surgery

20.3.1 Clinical Summary

A woman in her 60s with a complex history of several operations for a hiatus hernia was referred with severe gastroesophageal reflux and poor gastric emptying. She had undergone a laparoscopic repair of a hiatus hernia and a Watson operation for reflux 10 years previously. Her reflux symptoms returned a year later, and investigations showed a recurrence of the hiatus hernia and reflux. She was managed with a combination of lifestyle measures and PPIs but continued to have significant symptoms. She underwent a laparoscopy with the intention of repairing the hiatus hernia with a revision antireflux procedure. However, dense adhesions were found at the hiatus, partly related to the Watson operation, which entails suturing the lower oesophagus to the crura. After dividing the adhesions, the hiatus hernia was reduced, and a crural repair as well as a partial anterior fundoplication was performed.

She continued to experience reflux associated with bloating. OGD showed grade B oesophagitis above a small recurrent hiatus hernia and a large amount of food residue and bile in the stomach despite the usual fasting period before the procedure. Gastric emptying studies showed markedly delayed emptying, ascribed to damage to the vagus nerves from repeated surgery at the oesophageal hiatus. Her treating team decided to perform a duodenal switch without symptomatic benefit. A laparoscopic repair of the residual hiatus hernia was attempted in the hope that this would at least deal with the reflux. However, it proved impossible to safely dissect out the gastro-oesophageal junction due to dense adhesions and the procedure was abandoned.

She was referred to our unit and underwent a gastrografin contrast swallow and meal. This showed large volume gastro-oesophageal reflux and delayed emptying with no anastomotic or downstream stricture associated with the duodenal switch (Figs. 20.4 and 20.5).

It was decided that the best option was to perform a total gastrectomy. This was carried out as an open procedure, and, as expected, the hiatal dissection was difficult, but after careful division of adhesions, it was possible to mobilise the distal oesophagus. After disconnection of the alimentary limb from the stomach and transecting the oesophagus just above the GOJ, the alimentary limb was anastomosed to the oesophagus. The previous Roux-en-Y anastomosis was left undisturbed. The patient made an uneventful post-operative recovery and remains well and asymptomatic two years later.

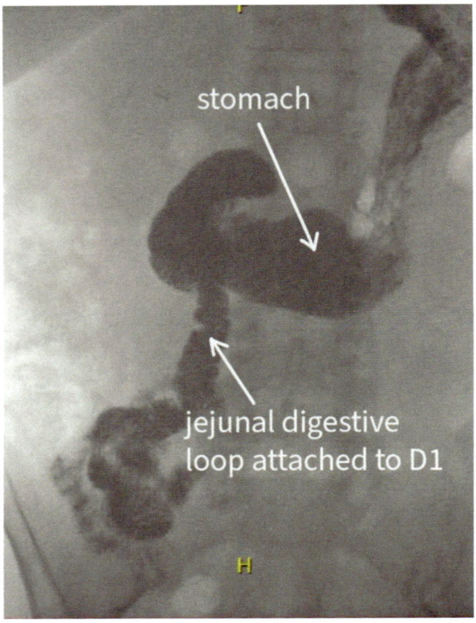

Fig. 20.4 Contrast swallow showing the anatomy of the duodenal switch

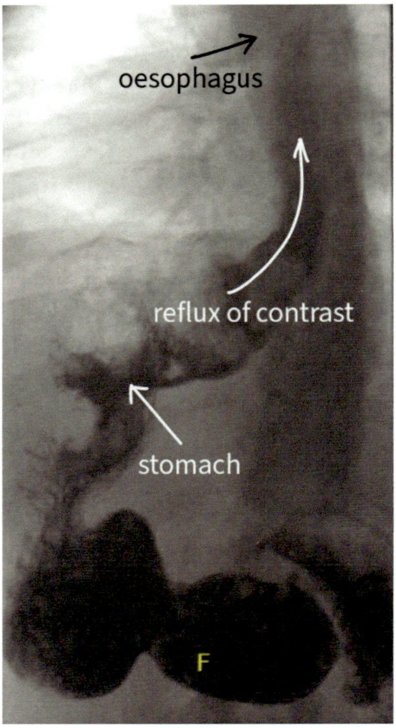

Fig. 20.5 Contrast swallow showing free gastroesophageal reflux

20.3.2 Learning Points

After the first two operations, this patient had been left with a recurrent hiatus hernia and gastroparesis due to likely vagal damage during repeated, difficult hiatal dissections. She had severe symptoms from delayed gastric emptying and gastro-oesophageal reflux. As it had not been possible to perform an effective antireflux procedure due to a hostile hiatus, the surgeon managing her care had decided to opt for the duodenal switch procedure to divert bile from the stomach. Unfortunately, this did not improve her symptoms as the underlying problem was poor gastric emptying, exacerbating the gastro-oesophageal reflux. This combination can be challenging to treat and responds poorly to medical treatment because of the lack of effective long-term drugs for poor gastric emptying. Total gastrectomy was difficult, but led to an excellent symptomatic outcome in this case.

References

1. Greene CL, DeMeester SR, Augustin F, Worrell SG, Oh DS, Hagen JA, DeMeester TR. Long-term quality of life and alimentary satisfaction after esophagectomy with colon interposition. Ann Thorac Surg. 2014;98(5):1713–20. https://doi.org/10.1016/j.athoracsur.2014.06.088.
2. Klink CD, Marcel B, Mark S, Kerstin O, Volker S, Mark J. Operative outcome of colon interposition in the treatment of esophageal cancer: a 20-year experience. Surgery. 2010;147(4):491–96. https://doi.org/10.1016/j.surg.2009.10.045
3. Cooper WA, Miller JI. Jejunal interposition for esophageal replacement. Oper Tech Thorac Cardiovasc Surg. 1999;4(3):239–51. https://doi.org/10.1016/S1522-2942(07)70120-4.
4. Baker CR, Matthew JF, James AG, Ng R, Mason RC. Long-term outcome and quality of life after supercharged jejunal interposition for oesophageal replacement. Surg. 2015;13(4):187–93. https://doi.org/10.1016/j.surge.2014.01.004

Chapter 21
Aerodigestive Fistulae (ADF)

Abstract This chapter explores the complexity and challenges associated with aerodigestive fistulae, highlighting their often unknown incidence and diverse aetiology. Some fistulae present with minimal symptoms, and some are diagnosed post-mortem. However they are generally associated with high mortality and morbidity. Fistulae can occur between the oesophagus and any part of the airways or the lung. Fistulae can also occur between the stomach and the lung as well as peripheral airways. Oesophageal and lung cancers, along with various medical procedures or inflammatory conditions, contribute to their development. The chapter presents a series of cases managed with stents or surgical repair, underscoring the importance of a comprehensive treatment algorithm considering fistula size, site, and etiology. Despite successful closure in some cases, challenges like post-operative strictures or persistent fistulae highlight the complexity of management, necessitating innovative surgical techniques and careful post-operative care.

Keyword Aerodigestive fistulae · Aetiology · Classification · Oesophagus · Stenting · Fistula closure · Surgical techniques · Case summaries · Surgical complications · Reconstruction · Post-operative complications

The incidence of aerodigestive fistulae is unknown. Some are only diagnosed post-mortem, in association with other diseases. Others may cause minimal symptoms. Most reports indicate that they are associated with high mortality and morbidity.

ADF fistulae most commonly occur between the oesophagus and the airways, typically involving the trachea or bronchi. However, they can also occur between the stomach, through the left hemidiaphragm to the lung itself or the peripheral airways. I have encountered several such cases, usually as a result of a chronic gastric sleeve leak with a 'collar-stud' abscess cavity on both sides of the left hemidiaphragm.

Oesophageal and lung cancers are the most common causes in adults. In these cases, the fistulae usually result from direct tumour invasion or as a complication of treatment, such as radiotherapy, chemotherapy, stenting and anastomotic leak after oesophagectomy [1].

M. Mughal, *Reconstructive Surgery of the Oesophagus and Stomach*,
https://doi.org/10.1007/978-3-031-66846-3_21

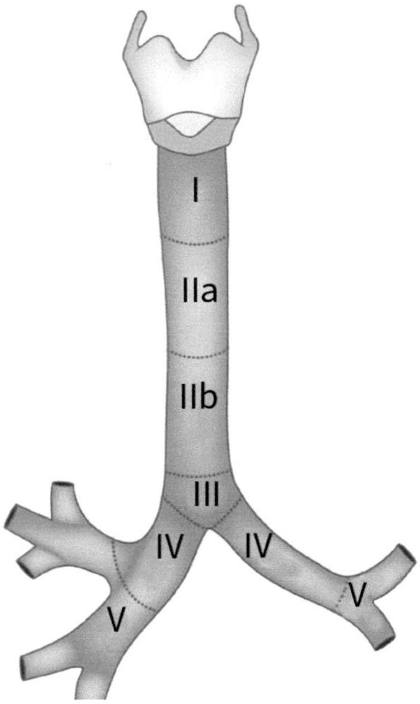

Fig. 21.1 Classification of ADFs according to Qureshi et al. [1]

Proximal tracheo-oesophageal fistulae (TOF) may occur as a complication of medical procedures, such as tracheostomy, oesophageal stenting, or prolonged mechanical ventilation. Inflammatory and infectious conditions, such as tuberculosis, histoplasmosis, or mediastinitis, can also lead to the development of TOFs.

We have found that most proximal fistulae have a benign aetiology, whereas the distal fistulae arise from malignant disease.

We have reported a series of 48 patients diagnosed with an ADF. The majority were managed with tracheal and/or oesophageal stents. We repaired eight ADFs, some of which had a benign aetiology and others where the malignancy had been treated, and restaging had indicated that they were tumour-free. The fistula was closed successfully in all cases, and seven patients were eating normally after a median follow-up of 32 months.

We have proposed a classification system based on the site and size of the fistula as well as the aetiology and have suggested a treatment algorithm taking these factors into account (Fig. 21.1). Survival was best for Type V fistula, followed by Types I, II, IV and III, in that order. ADFs over 20 mm in diameter were associated with poorer survival as was the previous use of radiotherapy.

21.1 TOF Following Chemoradiotherapy for B-Cell Lymphoma

21.1.1 Clinical Summary

A woman in her 40s with CREST syndrome presented dysphagia and was found to have a large, deep ulcer in the mid-oesophagus, a biopsy from which showed a large B-cell lymphoma. CT showed bulky disease in the posterior mediastinum with a fistulous tract from the oesophagus to the left main bronchus. She was given R-CHOP chemotherapy with a good response while fed through a nasojejunal tube. On completion of treatment, she was followed up with serial CT scans and bronchoscopy. These showed some reduction in the size of the fistula over the next six months. However, ten months after treatment, there was still a 5 mm diameter fistula in the proximal left main bronchus adjacent to the carina (Fig. 21.2). There was no evidence of recurrent disease on CT and biopsies from the fistula. Her general condition and nutritional status had improved sufficiently for surgery to be considered to close the fistula.

The operation commenced with a right thoracotomy and division of adhesions to free up the lung. The azygous arch was ligated and divided, and the oesophagus was mobilised above and below the level of the fistula. It was then transected just above and below the fistula, leaving a small rim attached to the left main bronchus. The bronchial defect was closed with interrupted 4/0 PDS sutures placed through the fibrous oesophageal tissue left around the rim of the bronchial opening. An intercostal flap was then mobilised and placed over the repair. After closing the chest, the patient was repositioned for a laparotomy. The distal oesophagus, which had been mobilised during the thoracotomy, was pulled down into the abdomen and removed. A gastric conduit was formed by stapling from the fundus to the incisura, keeping 4 cm parallel to the greater curvature. A feeding jejunostomy was placed. The cervical oesophagus

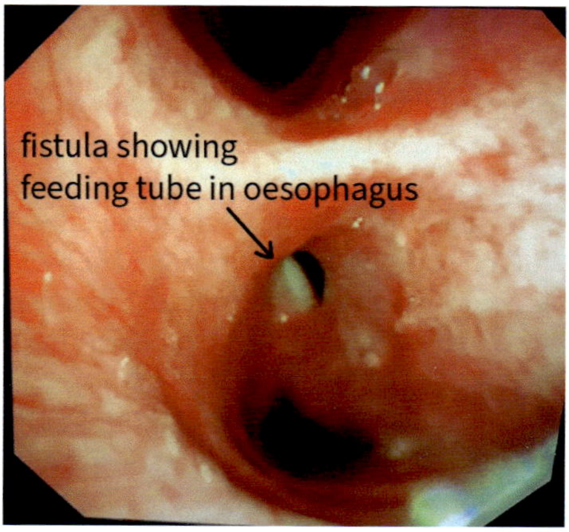

Fig. 21.2 Fistula seen at bronchoscopy

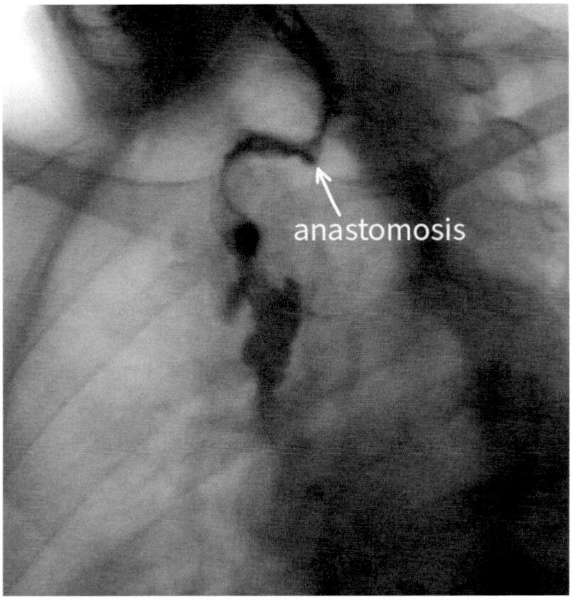

Fig. 21.3 Contrast swallow 10 days after surgery post-op showing good flow through the anastomosis and no leak

was mobilised through a collar incision after identifying and safeguarding the left current laryngeal nerve. The proximal, transected oesophagus was pulled up into the neck. A retrosternal tunnel was created, and the gastric conduit was pulled up through this and anastomosed to the cervical oesophagus (Fig. 21.3).

The patient made an uneventful post-operative recovery but developed a tight stricture at the anastomosis that could not be negotiated with a guidewire at endoscopy with image intensification. A contrast swallow showed a complete block at the anastomosis (Fig. 21.4).

It was decided to re-operate and perform a hybrid procedure jointly with our gastroenterology colleagues. The anastomosis was exposed by careful dissection through the previous neck incision, and the gastric conduit was exposed through a limited laparotomy. A paediatric gastroscope was introduced through a gastrotomy, just above the pylorus in the conduit and passed up to the anastomosis. The anastomosis was carefully separated from the trachea to avoid injury during the dilatation and in case a stricturoplasty was required. Another endoscope was passed through the mouth to the anastomosis and a guide wire was passed through it after a cut-down with a dual knife from above guided by the light from the gastric endoscope. The anastomosis was then dilated to 7 mm using Savary dilators passed over the guide wire and a 10 Fr nasogastric tube was finally placed across the anastomosis and the wounds closed (Fig. 21.5).

The patient was well two years after follow-up but was still requiring oesophageal self-dilatation two or three times a week.

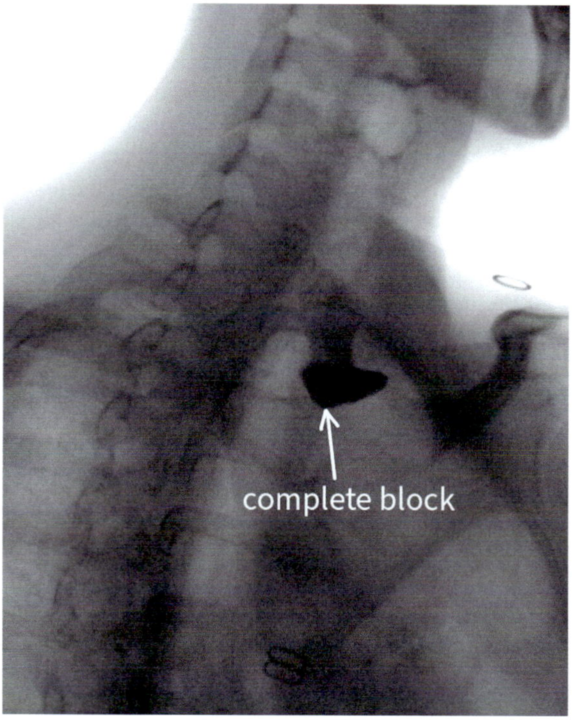

Fig. 21.4 Contrast swallow showing complete block at the cervical anastomosis

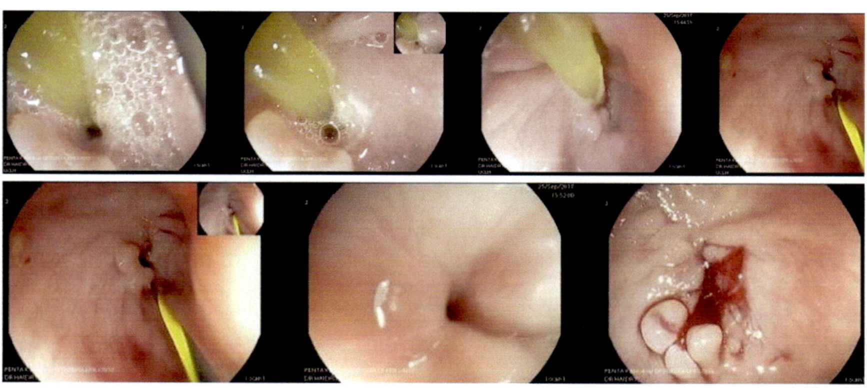

Fig. 21.5 Endoscopic views from the oesophageal side showing the tight anastomosis and placement of guide wire (first image, lower row) followed by nasogastric tube (first three images upper row)

21.1.2 Learning Points

This patient was found to have a tiny fistula between the oesophagus and the left main bronchus at the initial staging scan for her B-cell lymphoma. There was no other option at this stage but to proceed with the necessary treatment after the placement of a nasojejunal tube and stopping oral intake. As expected, the fistula became larger as her disease responded to treatment. It was important to wait six months after treatment completion to determine whether she was clear of disease and to see if the fistula would close spontaneously. As the fistula did not close and she remained disease-free, surgery was undertaken. Leaving part of the oesophagus attached to either the bronchus or trachea in dealing with a fistula allows stitches to be placed through this tissue, which is more robust than the airway. It is, of course, important that this is only done when no malignant disease exists in the attached oesophagus. In this case, the gastric conduit was brought up retrosternally and not through the right chest, which would have been a more direct and more straightforward route. It has been my preference to either close the fistula and perform a reconstruction later or if it is feasible to reconstruct simultaneously, to keep the conduit out of the chest. I have adopted this policy to ensure that if there are complications such as a persistent air leak or chest sepsis from the airway closure, the conduit is not compromised either as a direct result or from any thoracic interventions that may be required, such as drainage or VATS procedures.

The patient developed an impassable structure, even though the anastomosis had not leaked. Although strictures are not uncommon at the cervical anastomosis, in my experience, it is unusual to develop such a tight structure, as in this case, without a significant leak. Furthermore, it proved impossible to safely traverse the stricture with an antegrade deployment of the guide wire. It was, therefore, necessary to re-operate to facilitate a rendezvous procedure to approach the anastomosis from both sides. By doing so and first dissecting out the anastomosis from the trachea, it was possible to avoid tracheal injury and assist in the passage of the guide wire visually and by palpation. I have only rarely needed to use this approach. It is not without risks, particularly in the neck, including damage to the recurrent laryngeal nerves.

21.2 DXT Related TOF

21.2.1 Case Summary

A woman in her 50s was referred with a proximal tracheo-oesophageal fistula as a complication of treatment for a T3 N1 M0 squamous cell carcinoma from 22 to 29 cm in the oesophagus. This was treated with radical chemoradiotherapy and she developed a tight stricture at the site of the original disease. Several endoscopies confirmed the absence of recurrence on biopsy of the tumour site. The stricture was treated by a succession of temporary stents following which she developed a 2 mm diameter tracheo-oesophageal fistula at 20 cm. Bronchoscopy showed the fistula with an oesophageal stent eroding through it and causing a 50% tracheal obstruction. After an MDT discussion and detailed counselling, she was offered surgery.

This commenced with a laparotomy and the GOJ and proximal stomach were mobilised taking care not to damage the gastroepiploeic vessels. A venting gastrostomy was formed high on the lesser curve of the stomach using a 20 Fr Foley catheter which was then used to hitch the stomach onto the abdominal wall. A feeding jejunostomy was placed and the abdomen closed. Through a collar incision, the right strap muscles were mobilised and detached from the hyoid bone to be used as a pedicled flap. The oesophagus was transected just above the fistula, and the stent was removed. The oesophagus below the fistula was transected, leaving in situ the isolated portion of the oesophagus which was fistulating into the trachea. A T-tube was placed in the proximal oesophageal stump to drain it (Figs. 21.6, 21.7 and 21.8).

The patient made an uneventful post-operative recovery and underwent a reconstruction nine months later. The neck was re-explored, and the T-tube was removed from the oesophageal remnant. However, the remnant had fibrosed to the degree that it was no longer suitable for an anastomosis. Through a laparotomy, the previously mobilised stomach was dissected free, safeguarding its blood supply. A 4 cm wide gastric conduit was fashioned by stapling parallel to the greater curvature and resecting the lesser curve including the venting gastrostomy. The conduit was pulled up into the neck through a retrosternal tunnel. A longitudinal incision was made at the junction from the cricopharyngeus into the middle constrictor and used to anastomose the gastric conduit (Figs. 21.9, 21.10 and 21.11).

Post-operative imaging revealed healing of the anastomosis but showed a leak, probably from the site of the previous T-tube oesophagostomy communicating with

Fig. 21.6 Diagram showing relationship of the TOF and to the oesophageal stent

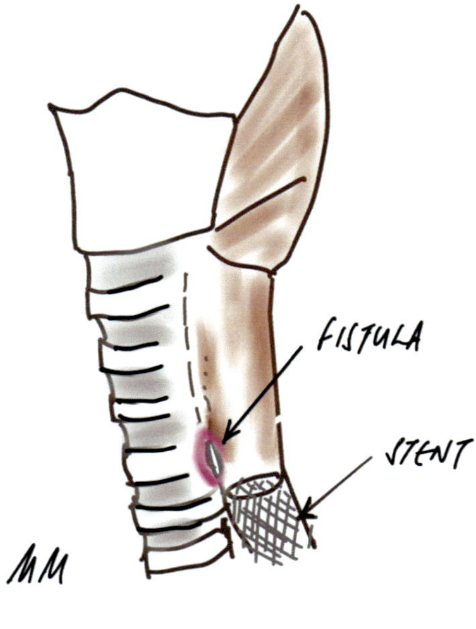

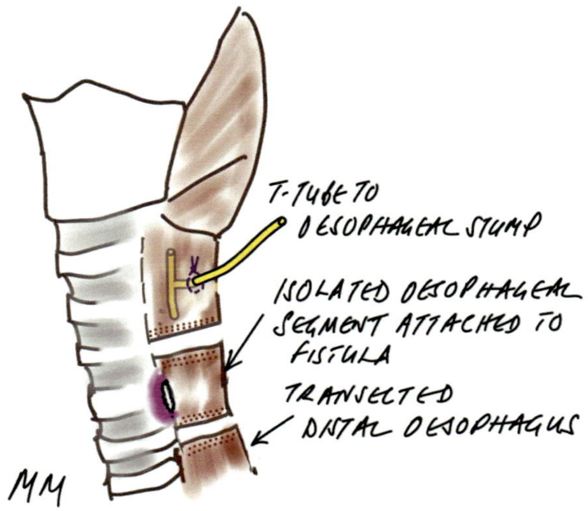

Fig. 21.7 Diagram showing isolation of fistula and T-tube to drain the short oesophageal stump

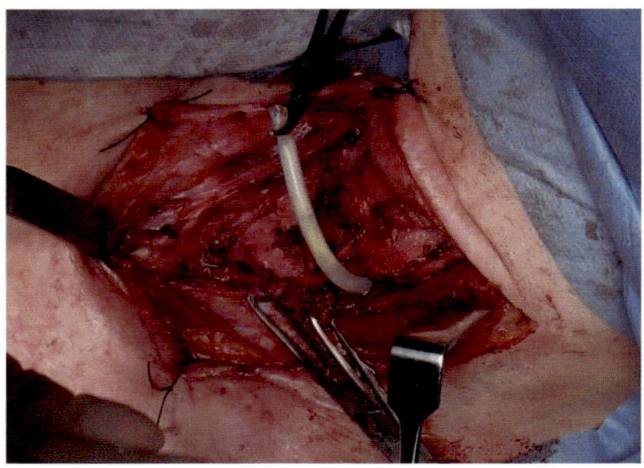

Fig. 21.8 Neck dissection showing T-tube in oesophageal stump

the trachea at the level of the clavicles. Oral intake was withheld and feeding continued via the jejunostomy. Combined gastroscopy and bronchoscopy six months later showed a persistent fistula from the oesophageal stump just above the anastomosis to the gastric conduit to the trachea 4 cm distal to the original proximal fistula (Fig. 21.12). A contrast study suggested that the isolated segment of the oesophagus left in situ at the site of the fistula had spontaneously re-anstomosed to the proximal oesophagus (Fig. 21.13). This probably resulted from the development of an abscess breaking through between the adjacent transected ends (Fig. 21.14).

Attempts at closing the fistula from the oesophageal side with tissue glue and clipping failed. The patient succumbed to respiratory complications 18 months after the reconstruction.

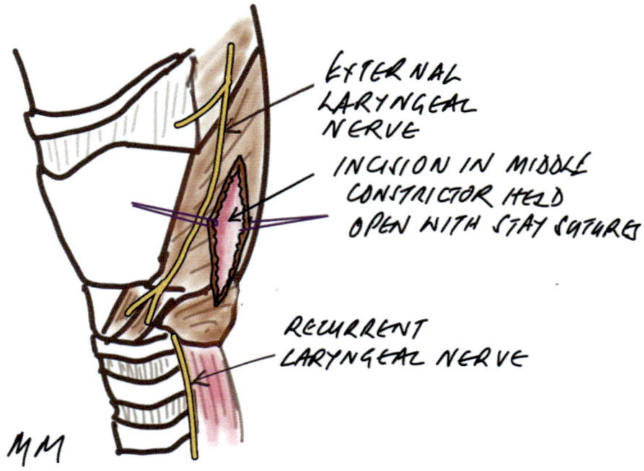

Fig. 21.9 Diagram showing the incision through the middle constrictor for the anastomosis

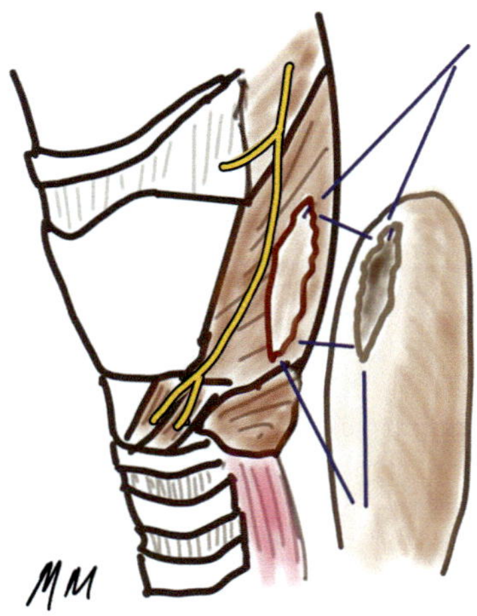

Fig. 21.10 Diagram showing anastomosis to the pharynx

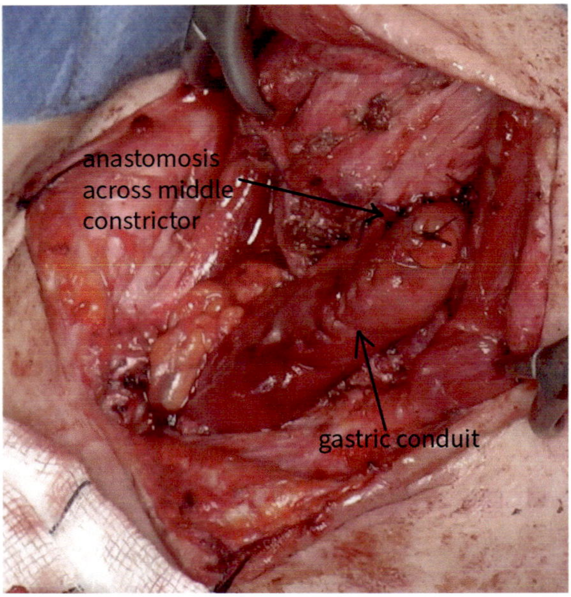

Fig. 21.11 Completed anastomosis of the gastric conduit to the pharynx

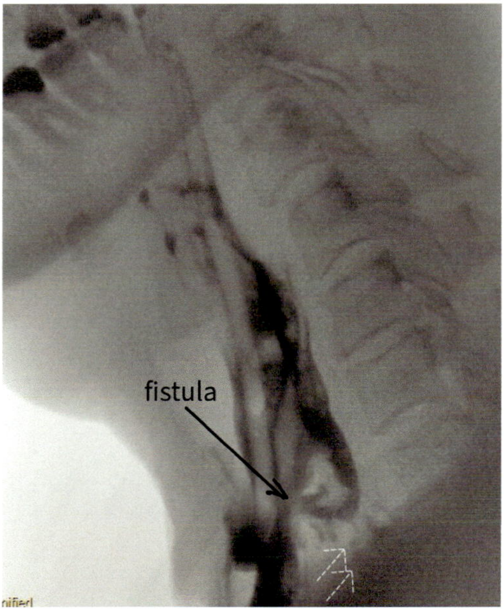

Fig. 21.12 Contrast swallow showing re-establishment of the fistula

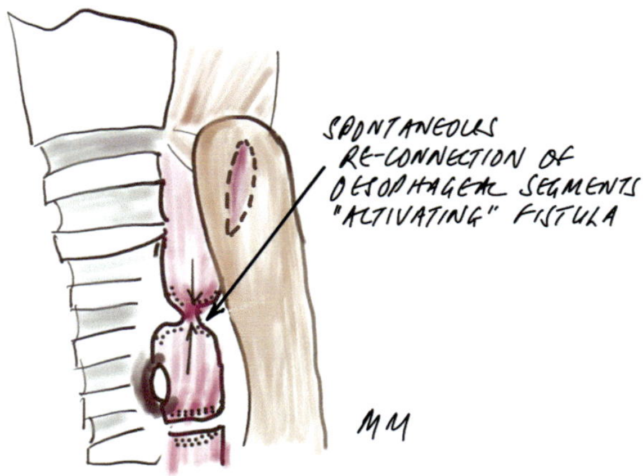

Fig. 21.13 Diagram showing the presumed mechanism for the re-establishment of the TOF

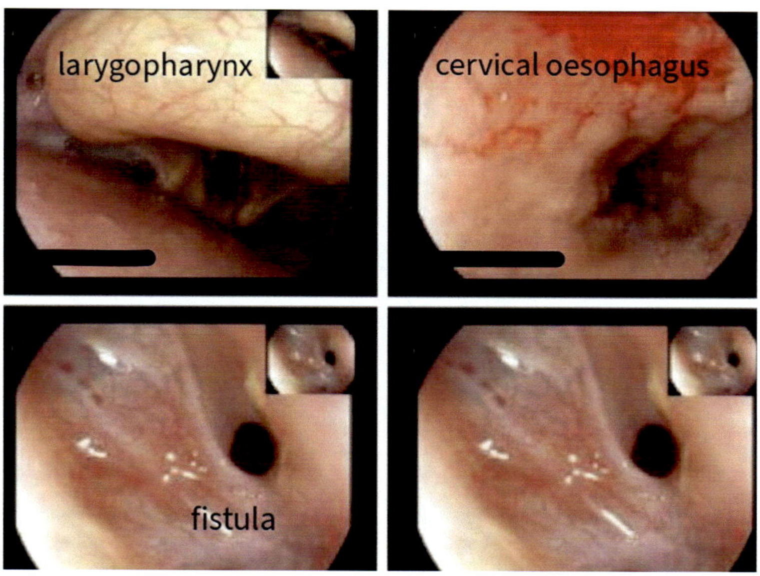

Fig. 21.14 OGD showing the opening in the oesophageal stump

21.2.2 Learning Points

This was a particularly difficult case. At the initial operation, there was a considerable amount of fibrosis around the site of the proximal tracheo-oesophageal fistula. As the initial bronchoscopy to, and beyond the carina, had only shown one proximal fistula, it was decided not to explore the trachea distal to this at the initial operation because of the risk of damaging the irradiated trachea. It is likely that the staple line of the proximal oesophageal stump had leaked and 'reconnected' with the isolated segment attached to the tracheal opening. Although the oesophageal end of the fistula was small, it proved impossible to close it endoscopically. A clip could not be deployed because of its position, and tissue glue was unsuccessful.

Reference

1. Qureshi YA, Muntzer Mughal M, Fragkos KC, Lawrence D, George J, Mohammadi B, Dawas K, Booth H (2018) Acquired adult aerodigestive fistula: classification and management. J Gastrointest Surg. 2018;22(10):1785–94. https://doi.org/10.1007/s11605-018-3811-0.

Chapter 22
Oesophago-Airways Fistula Complicating Oesophageal Stenting

Abstract This chapter discusses oesophago-airway fistula (OAF) complicating oesophageal stenting. This is a rare but serious complication of oesophageal stenting, with rates reported around 15% after stenting for oesophageal cancer. Factors contributing to OAF include stent-related pressure on the airway, migration, ischaemic injury, and malignancy progression. Management involves multidisciplinary team (MDT) discussion, considering factors like fistula aetiology, airway/ lung status, and patient condition. Ill-advised interventions can exacerbate the fistula. Two case summaries illustrate surgical approaches: one involving staged repair of a tracheo-oesophageal fistula (TOF) followed by reconstruction, and another detailing a combination of oesophagostomy and constructing an access loop for the use of EsoSponge deployment to manage persistent leakage and aspiration. Learning points emphasise careful stent use, staged repair strategies, and comprehensive MDT decision-making.

Keywords Oesophago-airway fistula · Oesophageal stenting · Multidisciplinary team · Tracheo-oesophageal fistula · Surgical repair · Non-surgical strategies · Stent-related pressure · Ischaemic injury

Oesophageal stenting is a commonly used intervention for the management of oesophageal strictures, malignancy-related obstruction, perforations and leaks. However, oesophago-airway fistula (OAF) can occur as a rare but serious complication of oesophageal stenting.

The true incidence of this complication is unknown, with rates reported to be around 15% after stenting for oesophageal cancer [1]. OAFs can cause significant morbidity and mortality, emphasising the importance of early diagnosis and intervention. Aetiological factors include pressure exerted by the stent on the airway wall, stent migration, ischaemic injury to the tissue due to impaired blood supply. Progression of the underlying malignancy is another factor. I share the experience of others [2], that stenting of an oesophageal stricture resulting from radical radiotherapy of oesophageal cancer is not an uncommon cause of a fistula. In many cases, there has been a complete oncological response to the tumour, leaving the patient with a difficult complication to manage.

M. Mughal, *Reconstructive Surgery of the Oesophagus and Stomach*,
https://doi.org/10.1007/978-3-031-66846-3_22

The management of such fistulae should be through MDT discussion. Factors such as the aetiology of the fistula, the state of the airways and the lungs and the patient's general condition must be considered in planning management. Ill-advised attempts at managing the fistula by placing more stents can both exacerbate the fistula and complicate surgical repair. Non-surgical options, in poor-risk patients and those with active malignancy, may include stenting of the airways and injection of tissue sealants, amongst others.

22.1 TOF Complicating Stenting for Boerhaave's Syndrome

22.1.1 Case Summary

A man in his 30s underwent a right thoracotomy and repair of spontaneous perforation of the oesophagus. He developed a recurrent leak and underwent a laparotomy and a fundoplication to cover the defect, as well as a feeding jejunostomy. This was complicated by a stricture at the site of the repair, for which he had three covered oesophageal stents a year later (Figs. 22.1 and 22.2). Following this, he developed

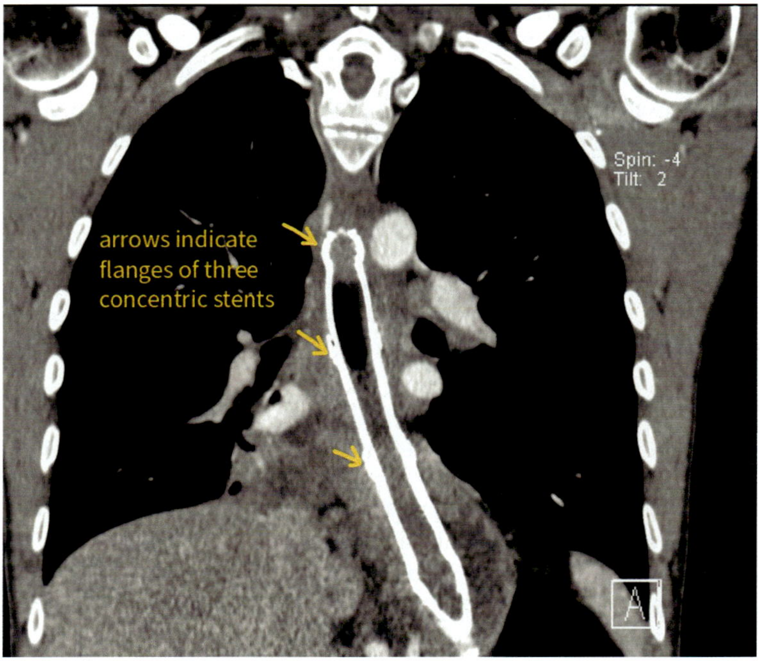

Fig. 22.1 Coronal CT image showing oesophageal stents in place

a tracheo-oesophageal fistula, for which he underwent a venting gastrostomy and feeding jejunostomy.

On referral to our unit, he underwent a general fitness assessment and a bronchoscopy which showed a 2.5 cm defect in the trachea just above the carina which was covered by the oesophageal stent (Fig. 22.3).

Surgery was performed with the assistance of thoracic surgical colleagues. A right thoracotomy through the sixth intercostal space revealed the lung to be extensively adherent to the chest wall. It was separated from the chest wall, and the azygous arch,

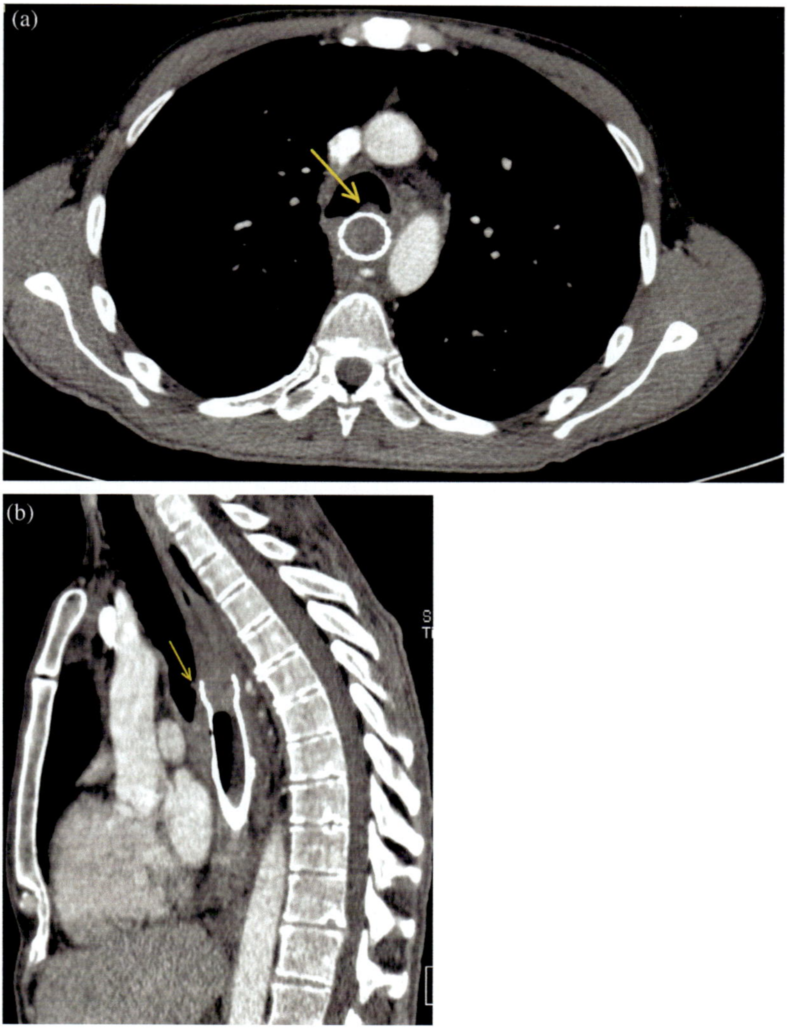

Fig. 22.2 Axial (a) and sagittal (b) CT sections showing the oesophageal stents with a small bulge into the trachea at the level of the top flange, marking the site of the fistula

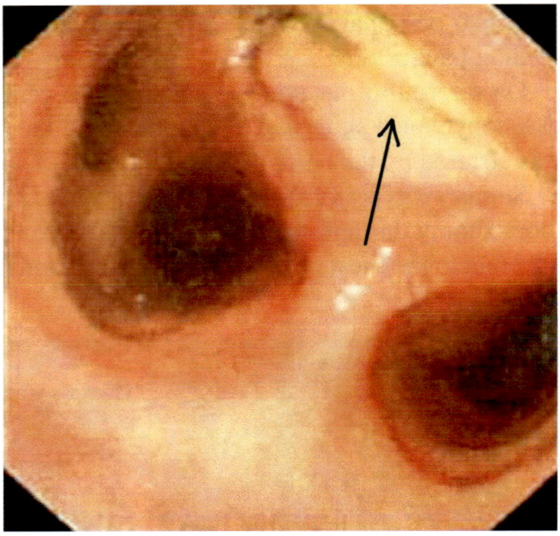

Fig. 22.3 Bronchoscopy showing the tracheal defect just above the carina, covered by the stent

which was densely adherent to the underlying oesophagus, was divided on each side of the oesophagus with a vascular stapler. The upper oesophagus was relatively easy to dissect and was freed up to the root of the neck. It was transected above the top of the stents. The oesophagus below the azygous arch was opened longitudinally, and three stents were extracted to reveal the fistula above the carina (Figs. 22.4 and 22.5). The hole in the trachea was closed transversely with interrupted 4/0 PDS sutures (Figs. 22.6, 22.7, 22.8 and 22.9). An intercostal flap was raised from the fifth interspace and used to buttress the repair by suturing it around the tracheal closure (Fig. 22.10). As the oesophagus distal to the fistula was densely adherent to the surrounding structures, it was decided to leave it in situ. It was opened longitudinally, the mucosa was obliterated with diathermy, and the oesophagus closed after laying a piece of Surgicel within the lumen. After closing the chest with a chest drain in place, the patient was positioned supine, and an end oesophagostomy was performed through a collar incision.

The patient made an uneventful recovery, and a CT scan three months later showed the tracheal fistula firmly closed without associated collections. A reconstruction was carried out four months after the first operation using the transverse colon which was brought up to the neck through a substernal tunnel. The proximal end was anastomosed to the cervical oesophagus and the distal end to the body of the stomach (Figs. 22.12, 22.13 and 22.14). The proximal stomach was unusable because of the previous fundoplication and mediastinal sepsis and this part of the stomach was excised.

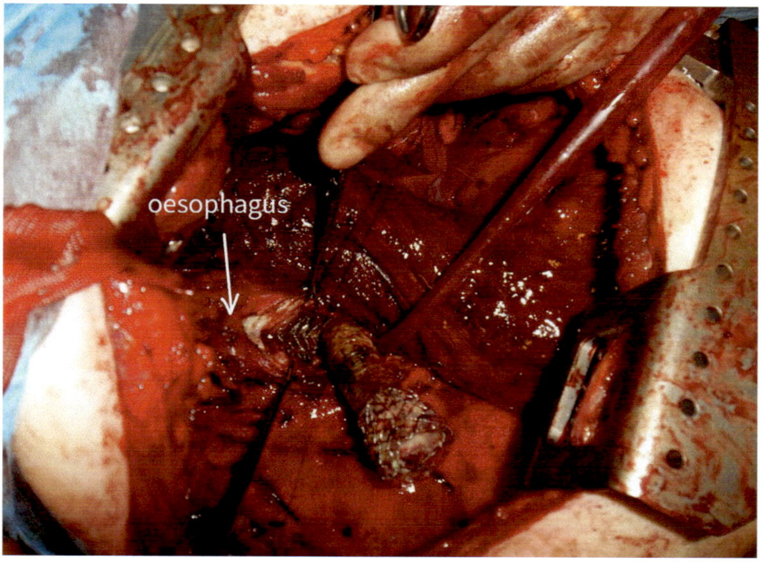

Fig. 22.4 Oesophageal stents being extracted through a longitudinal incision in the oesophagus

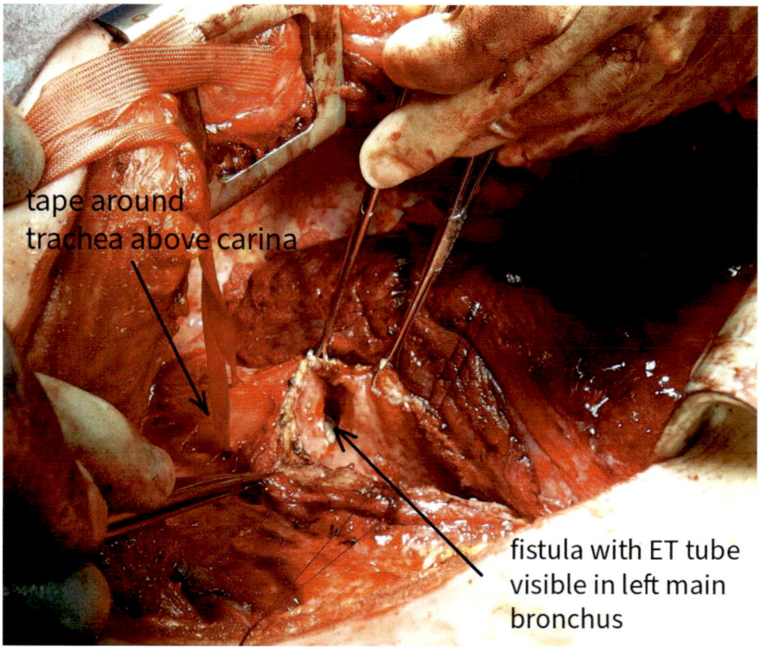

Fig. 22.5 Fistula seen through opened oesophagus which was densely adherent to the airways around the fistula

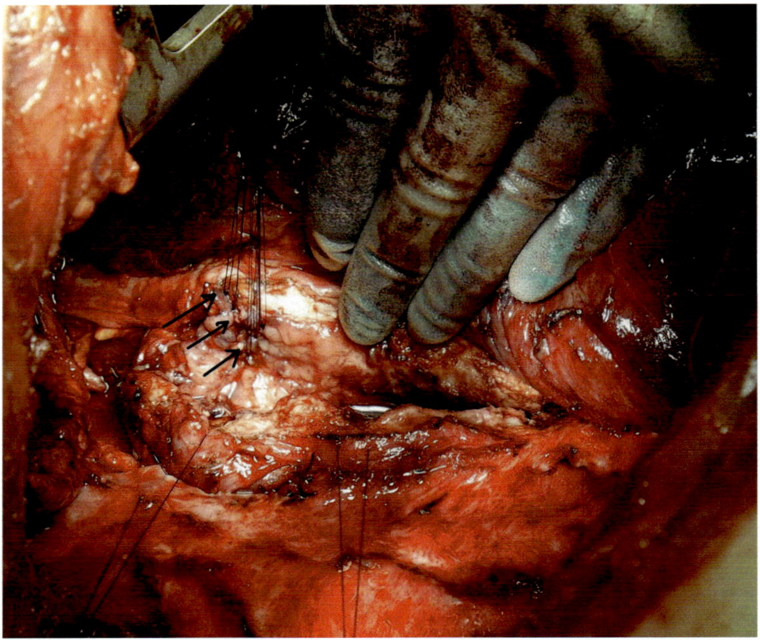

Fig. 22.6 Fistula closed with interrupted 4/0 PDS incorporating the adherent oesophagus

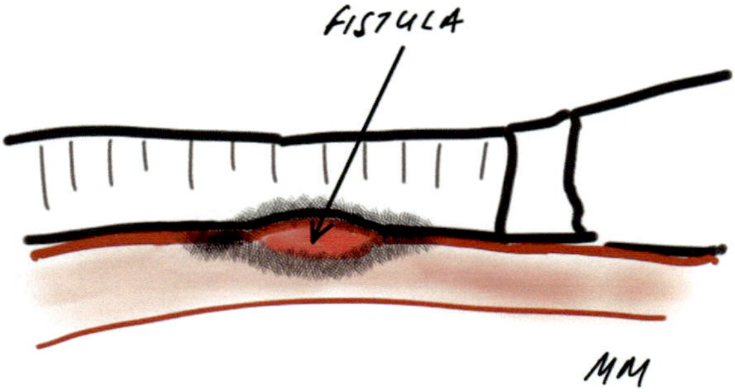

Fig. 22.7 Diagram showing dense adhesion between the trachea and the oesophagus around the fistula

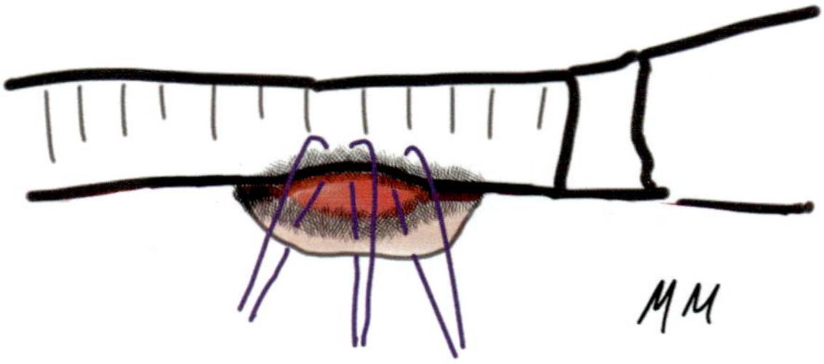

Fig. 22.8 Diagram showing retention of the adherent portion of the oesophagus around the fistula, used for placing the closure sutures

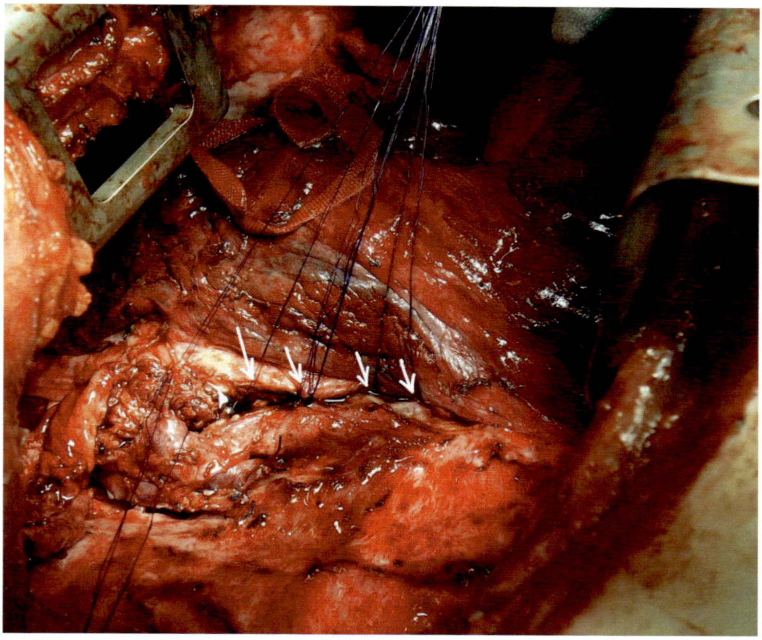

Fig. 22.9 Flange of oesophagus attached to the fistula closed over repair after ablation of the mucosa with diathermy

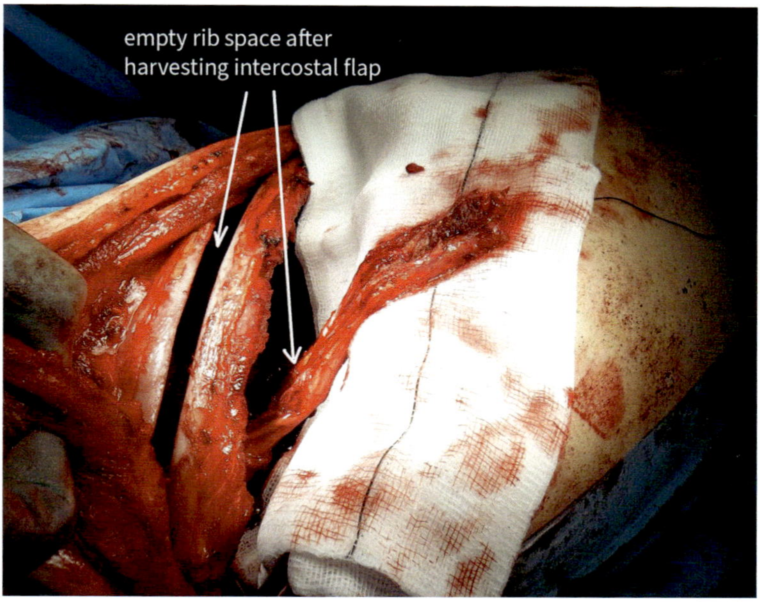

Fig. 22.10 Intercostal flap harvested from the space above thoracotomy and used to buttress the tracheal repair

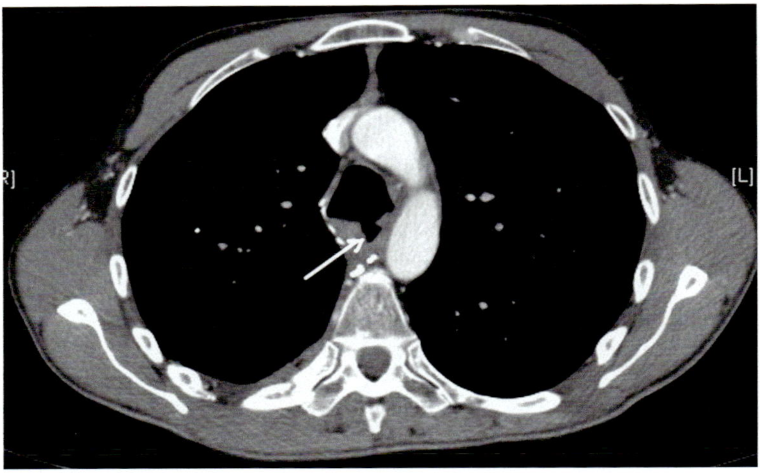

Fig. 22.11 Post-operative CT section showing the closed fistula adjacent to the obliterated oesophagus

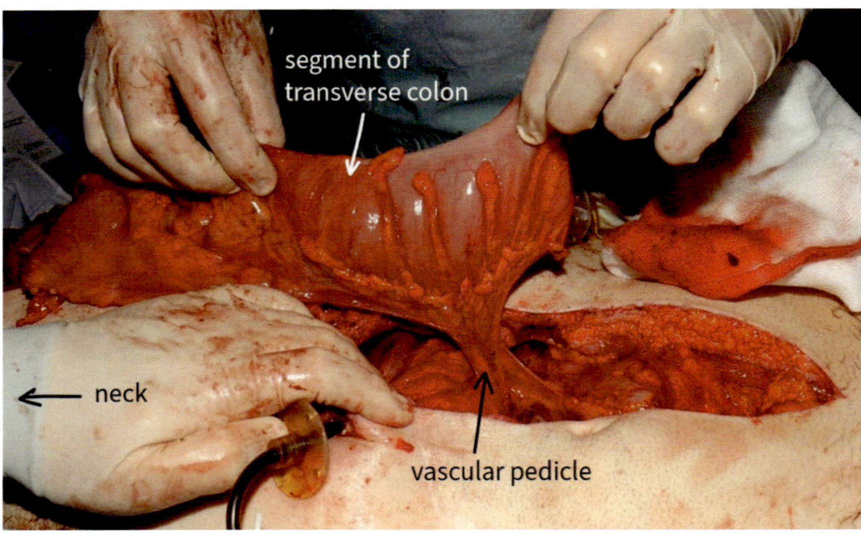

Fig. 22.12 Transverse colon conduit ready for transposition

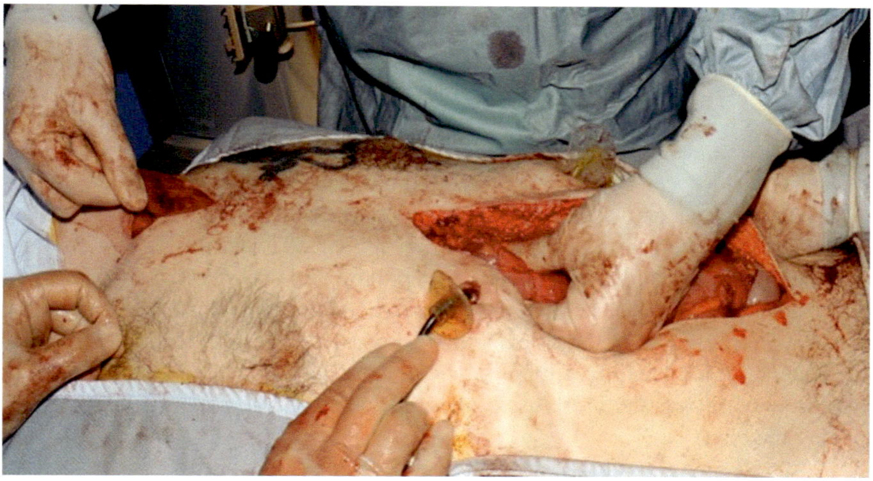

Fig. 22.13 Creating the retrosternal tunnel

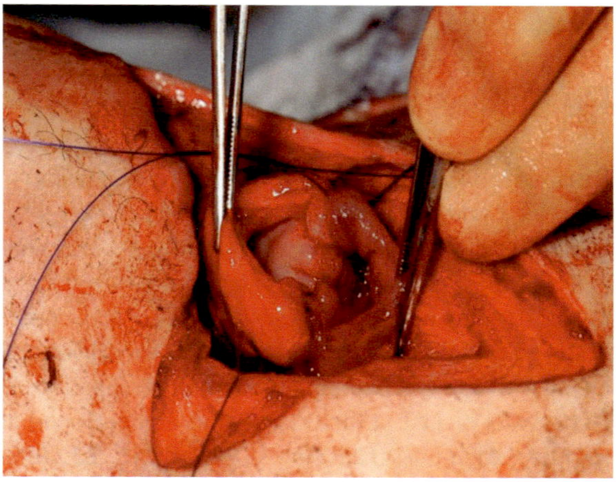

Fig. 22.14 Completed posterior layer of the cervical anastomosis

22.1.2 Learning Points

Oesophageal stents are useful for dealing with perforations and strictures but can cause complications, such as in this case, most likely due to pressure necrosis. In my experience, stent-related fistulae commonly occur at the level of the stent flange, as in this case.

The decision was made in this case to carry out staged surgery, repairing the tracheoesophageal fistula first and carrying out a reconstruction later. This allowed the repair to heal without the added complexity of a reconstruction. If the tracheal repair had not healed properly and had been complicated by serious chest sepsis or a prolonged air leak, this could have jeopardised a concomitant reconstruction. Sepsis in itself could have delayed the healing of the anastomoses, and if the patient had required support with inotropes, this would have compromised the circulation in the conduit.

After the repair of the airways, it is important to avoid post-operative ventilation if possible, which can result in a prolonged air leak. This is part of the planning of the surgery and peri-operative care. The chances of post-operative extubation are significantly increased, and the risk of re-intubation is minimised by achieving optimum pain relief with a combination of epidural and parenteral analgesia.

The stomach would have been the preferred conduit reconstruction, but, in this case, the proximal part of the stomach had been used up for the fundoplication and was unsuitable for creating a long gastric conduit to reach the neck comfortably. A colon conduit was therefore used, and a retrosternal route was chosen to avoid opening the chest.

22.1.3 TOF Complicating Stenting of an Anastomotic Leak After Oesophagectomy

22.1.4 Case Summary

A man in his 40s developed an anastomotic leak after an Ivor Lewis oesophagectomy for a GOJ adenocarcinoma. It was treated with a series of covered stents, which resulted in a tracheo-oesophageal fistula. At that stage, it was decided to pursue a conservative approach rather than put him through another major operation because he had developed a brain metastasis. This was successfully treated with chemoradiotherapy, and he remained recurrence-free 18 months later but continued to have episodes of aspiration pneumonia as the oesophageal stent did not seal the fistula. A Y-stent was placed in the trachea, but he developed another fistula at the top of the oesophageal and tracheal stents (Figs. 22.15, 22.16, 22.17 and 22.18).

The continued aspiration of saliva and gastric contents resulted in frequent admissions to hospital for intravenous antibiotics and physiotherapy. Repeat imaging with CT and PET scans showed no evidence of recurrent or metastatic disease. It was therefore decided to carry out a defunctioning oesophagostomy. This was performed through a collar incision, mobilising the cervical oesophagus, which was transected, the distal end closed and the proximal end brought out as an oesophagostomy. Unfortunately, he continued to aspirate from the reflux of gastric contents into the airways through the fistula. It was envisaged that the fistula was being kept open by the flange of the metal stent embedded in the oesophagus, and removal was not feasible (Fig. 22.17).

After an MDT discussion, to consider all practical options, it was decided to disconnect the conduit from the duodenum to stop bile refluxing into the gastric conduit and causing aspiration through the fistula. At the same time, it was decided

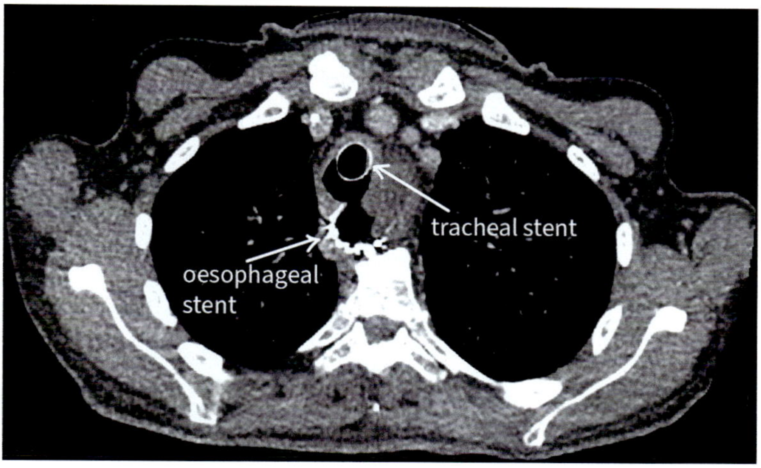

Fig. 22.15 Axial CT section showing tracheal and conduit stents at the level of the fistula

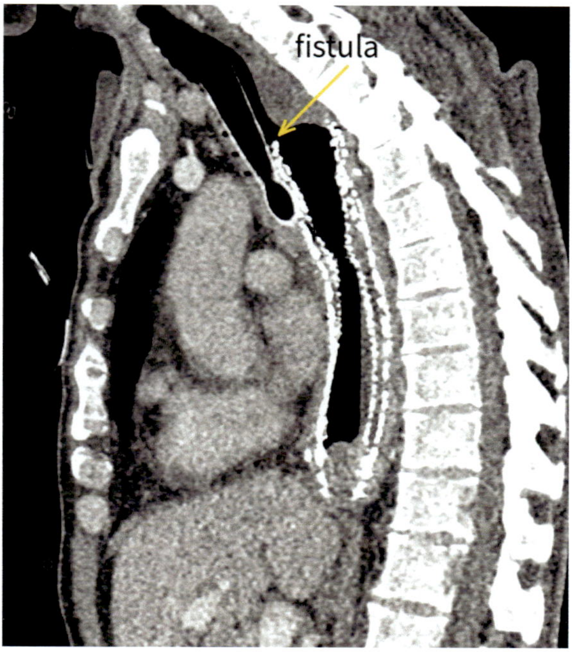

Fig. 22.16 Sagittal CT section showing overlapping stents and fistula

to create an access loop to the conduit, which could be used for the drainage of mucus and saliva in the first instance and later to deploy the EsoSponge device from below to treat the fistula. The position of the fistula relative to the oesophageal and tracheal stents is shown in Fig. 22.18. A laparotomy was carried out, and the antrum and pylorus were mobilised and encircled (Fig. 22.19). Taking care not to damage the

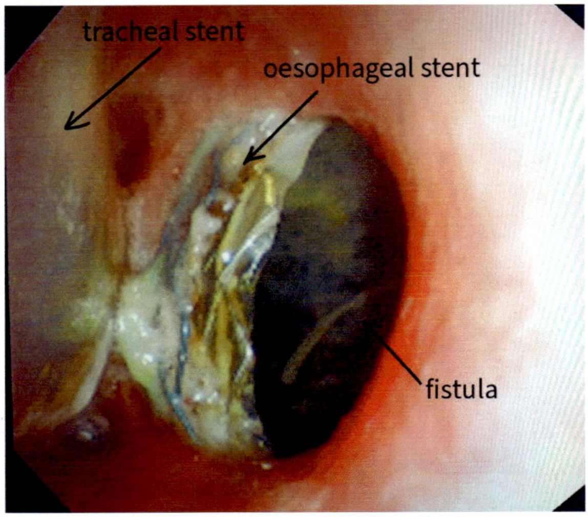

Fig. 22.17 Bronchoscopic view showing the tracheal stent, top of the oesophageal stent and the fistula

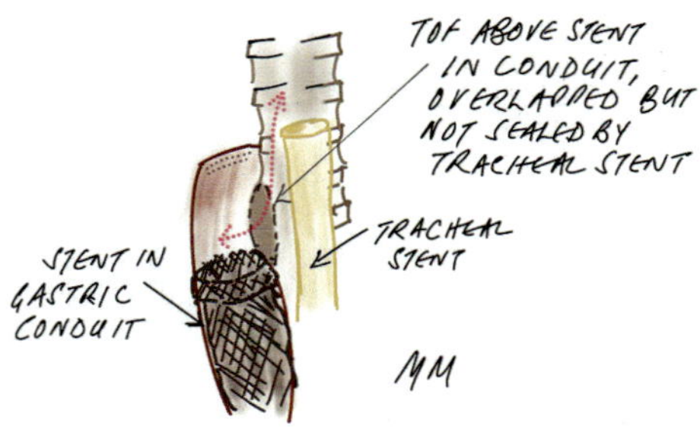

Fig. 22.18 Diagram showing relationship of oesophageal and tracheal stents to the TOF

gastroepiploeic vessels, the stomach was transected with a cutting linear stapler just proximal to the pylorus (Fig. 22.20). A short gastrotomy was made in the antrum just below the hiatus (Fig. 22.21), and a paediatric gastroscope was passed up through the stent in the gastric conduit and the fistula was visible at the top of the stent (Fig. 22.22). The scope could be passed into the trachea, showing a gap between the tracheal wall and the tracheal stent (Fig. 22.23). Mucus and gastric contents were sucked out.

A 30 cm loop of proximal jejunum was isolated on its blood supply (Fig. 22.24), its proximal end anastomosed to the gastrotomy in the antrum (Fig. 22.25) and the distal end brought out as a flush stoma in the left upper quadrant of the abdomen. A 22 French Robinson drain was placed through the stoma across the antrum to reach the fistula (Figs. 22.26 and 22.27). The drain was removed 10 days later.

An EsoSponge was been placed across the fistula via the stoma into the top of the oesophagus to keep the airways clear of secretions.

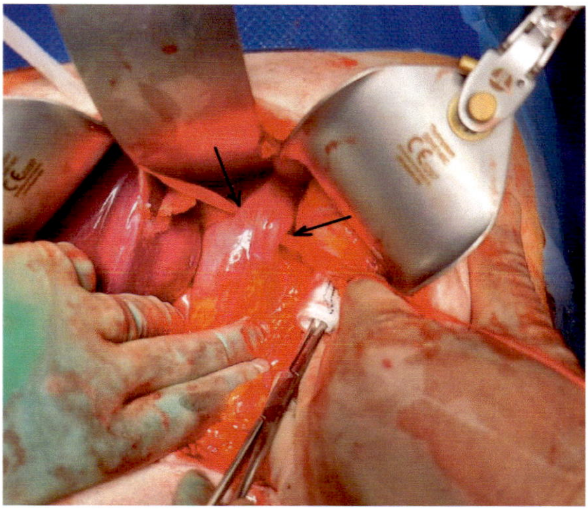

Fig. 22.19 Operative picture showing antrum encircled by nylon tape ready for transection. Dissection kept close to the stomach to safeguard the gastroepiploeic vessels

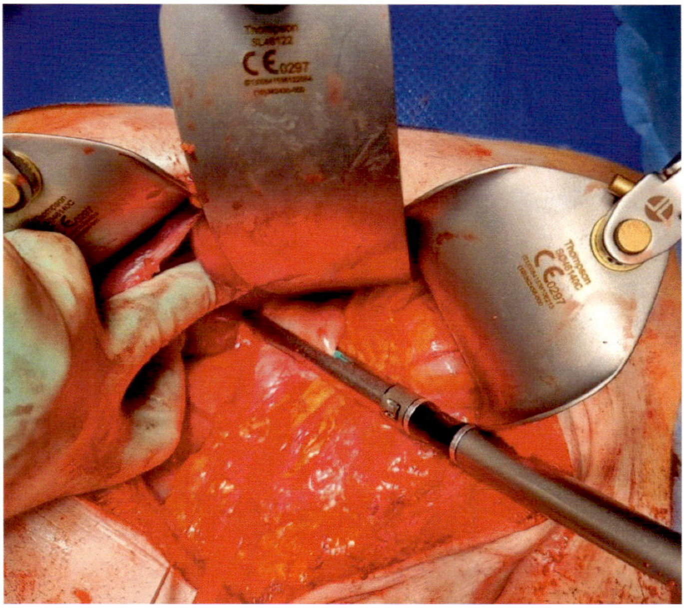

Fig. 22.20 Transection of the antrum with stapler

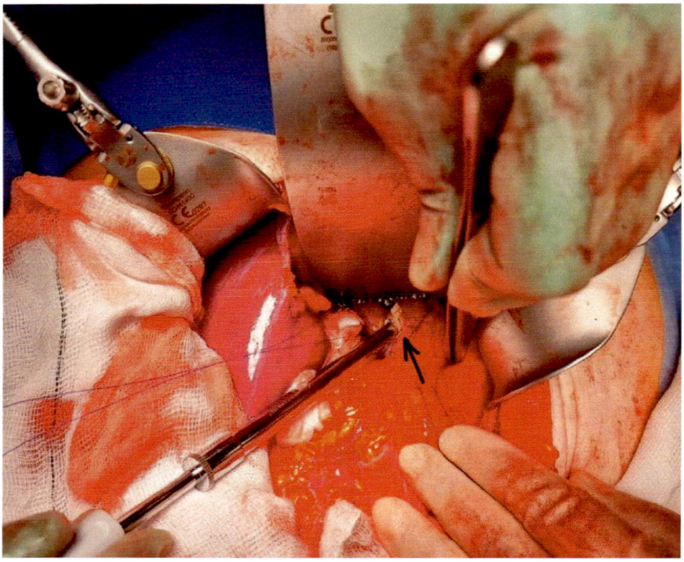

Fig. 22.21 Gastrotomy in the transected antrum to suck out secretions from conduit, prior to inspection with scope and anastomosis to access loop

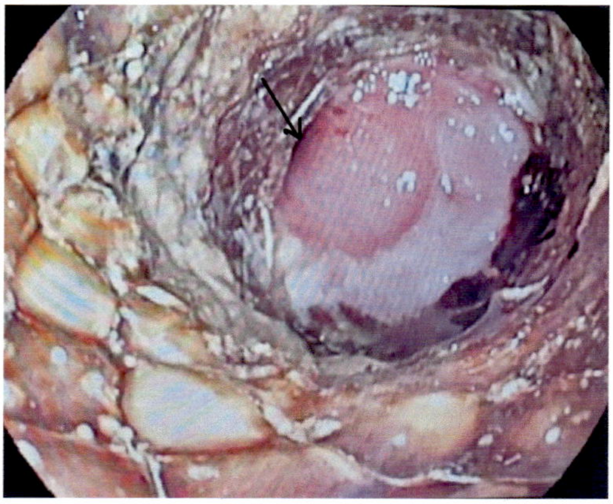

Fig. 22.22 View through endoscope passed up the conduit through gastronomy showing the top of the conduit stent and the tracheal defect just visible at 10 o'clock position

Fig. 22.23 View through scope passed through the fistula into the trachea showing tracheal stent

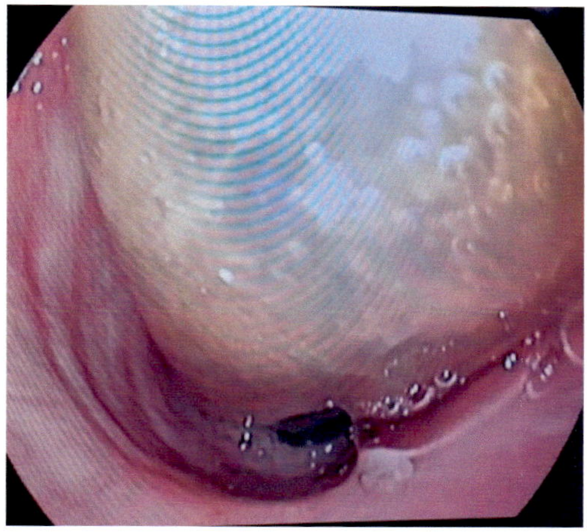

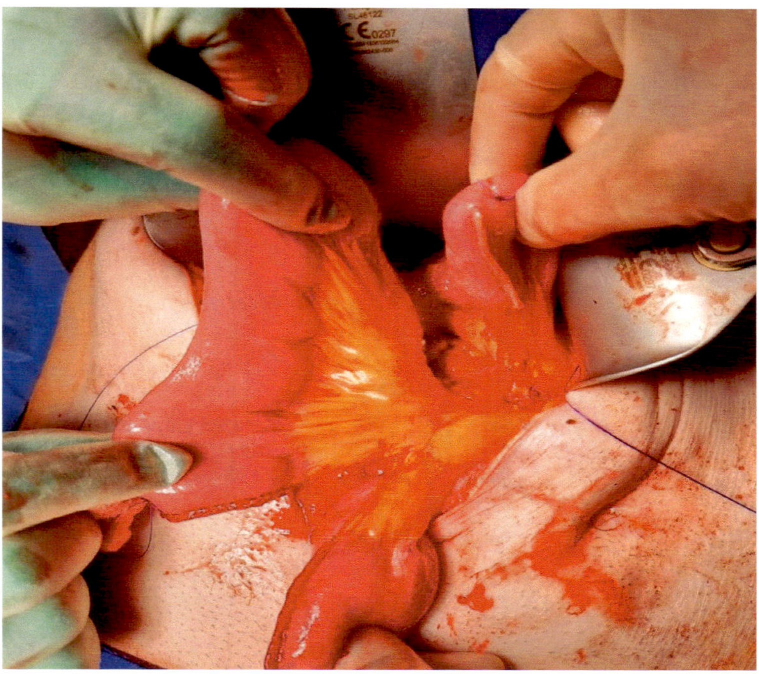

Fig. 22.24 Jejunal access loop prepared

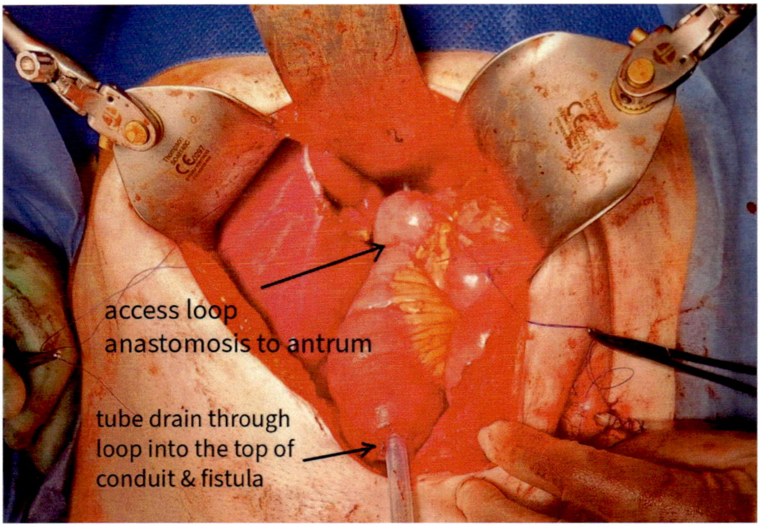

Fig. 22.25 Access loop anastomosed to antrum and 28 Fr drain passed up into the conduit to the level of the fistula

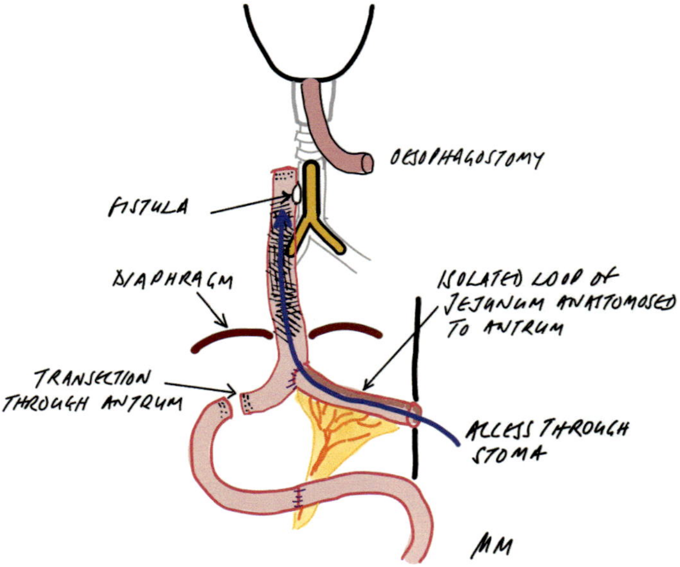

Fig. 22.26 Diagram showing the conduit disconnected from the duodenum and attached to the access loop

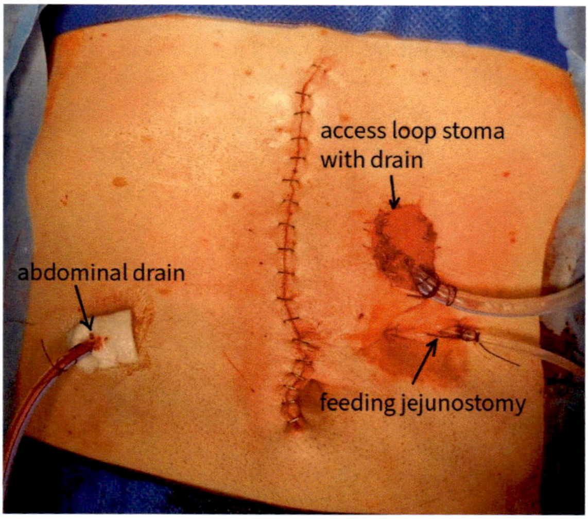

Fig. 22.27 Operation completed with drain passing through the access stoma to the fistula at the top of the gastric conduit

22.1.5 Learning Points

Stents can be useful for managing anastomotic leaks following oesophagectomy, but must be used for as short a time as possible to avoid the risk of pressure necrosis resulting in a fistula to the airways. In this case, the treating team continued to deploy stents rather than put him through major surgery for definitive treatment of the fistula, as he had developed metastatic disease, and his prognosis was considered to be poor. But, contrary to expectations, his brain metastasis showed a complete response to chemoradiotherapy. Nearly five years after the oesophagectomy and two years after the treatment of metastatic disease, he had already undergone the deployment of permanent metal stents into the conduit, and it was decided to place a Y-stent into the airways to try and occlude the fistula from the tracheal side and protect his lungs. It was felt that the removal of the gastric conduit with the embedded stent could result in irreparable damage to the trachea. The treating team decided to perform an end oesophagostomy to minimise aspiration by diverting swallowed fluids and secretions. Unfortunately, the patient continued to have aspiration from reflux up the conduit. We decided to create an access loop as described above after an MDT discussion and counselling with the patient and his family.

References

1. Shin JH, Song HY, Ko GY, Lim JO, Yoon HY, Sung KB. Esophagorespiratory fistula: long-term results of palliative treatment with covered expandable metallic stents in 61 Patients. Radiology. 2004;232(1):252–59. https://doi.org/10.1148/radiol.2321030733.

2. Song, HY, Do, YS, Han YM, Sung KB, Choi EK, Sohn KH, Kim HR, Kim SH, Min YI. Covered, expandable esophageal metallic stent tubes: experiences in 119 patients. Radiology. 1994;193(3):689–95. https://doi.org/10.1148/radiology.193.3.7526414.

Chapter 23
Miscellaneous Tracheo-Oesophageal Fistulas

Abstract This chapter presents diverse cases of tracheo-oesophageal fistulae highlighting the diagnostic and therapeutic challenges posed by these conditions. Case summaries include instances such as a 57-year-old male with a chronic cough and vomiting found to have a fistula between the oesophagus and right lower lobe bronchus, successfully managed through thoracotomy and ligation. Another case involves a 34-year-old female with a history of TB presenting with a fistula from the oesophagus to the right lower lobe, necessitating lobe resection. Additionally, cervical tracheo-oesophageal fistulas, often secondary to medical interventions, are discussed, with emphasis on meticulous surgical planning and techniques, as seen in cases involving a 32-year-old female with a congenital fistula and a 75-year-old male with a longstanding fistula complicated by recurrent aspiration pneumonia. These cases underscore the importance of tailored management strategies and multidisciplinary collaboration in addressing the varied presentations of tracheo-oesophageal fistulas.

Keywords Miscellaneous tracheo-oesophageal fistula · Oesophagus · Thoracotomy · Fistula management · Surgical ligation · Respiratory complications · Multidisciplinary approach · Surgical planning · Case summaries

23.1 Right Main Bronchus Fistula to the Oesophagus

23.1.1 Case Summary

A man in his 50s with a long-standing cough and vomiting underwent a gastroscopy, which showed a fistula between the oesophagus and the airways at 35 cm. This was confirmed on a gastrografin swallow and appeared to be to the right lower lobe bronchus (Fig. 23.1).

M. Mughal, *Reconstructive Surgery of the Oesophagus and Stomach*,
https://doi.org/10.1007/978-3-031-66846-3_23

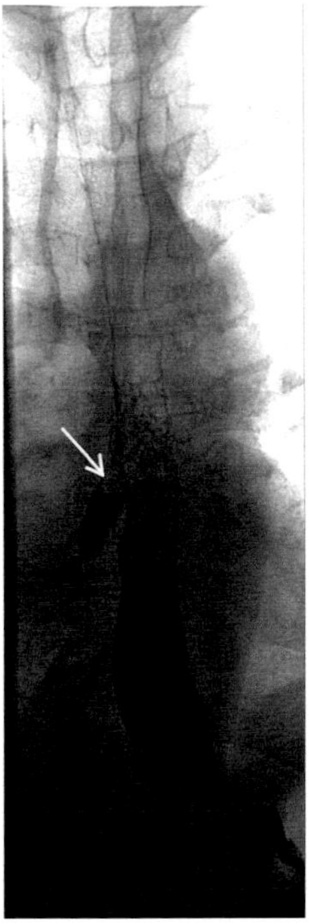

Fig. 23.1 Contrast swallow showing the fistula with a broader base at the oesophageal end

A CT scan showed pre-tracheal adenopathy with calcification of some nodes and volume loss of the right lower lobe with an area of pleurally based consolidation containing foci of coarse calcification. There was associated bronchiectasis and communication between the oesophagus and the right lower lobe segment. The lung changes were considered to be typical of a chronic infection such as TB. The patient gave a history of TB in childhood, but tests showed no active TB at the time of presentation. A bronchoscopy showed a small fistula from the bronchus intermedius of the segmental bronchus to the superior segment of the right lobe. The patient underwent a right thoracotomy, and the fistula was easily identified and noted to have a 5 mm base on the oesophageal side but narrowing to almost 2–3 mm at its attachment with the airways. It was simply ligated at the oesophageal and bronchial ends (Fig. 23.2). The patient made an uneventful post-operative recovery.

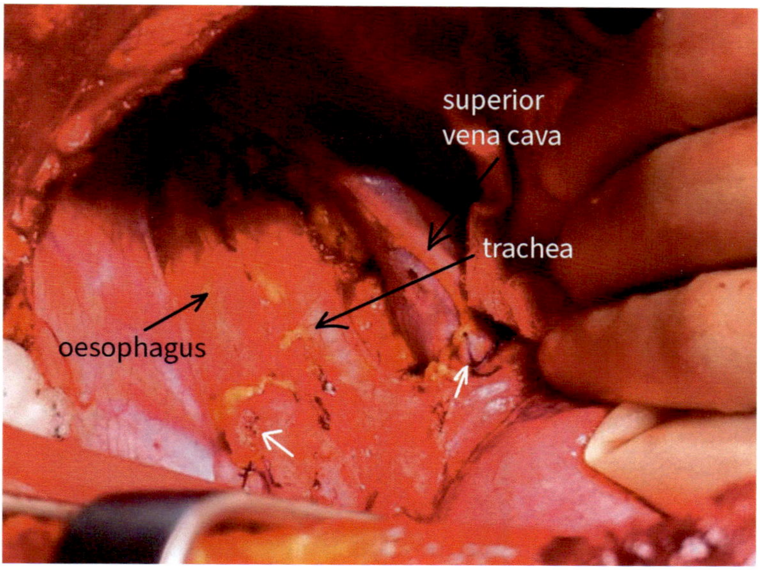

Fig. 23.2 Operative picture with arrows showing ligated ends of fistula tract

23.1.2 Learning Points

Oesophageal fistulation to the airways is not uncommon sequelae of TB and can present many years later, as in this case. As there is often no associated inflammation, the track is usually easy to dissect. The fistula can be treated very easily, as in this case, by simply ligating the tract. However, a lung resection may also be required depending on the degree of associated lung changes.

23.2 Fistula from Right Lower Lobe Bronchus to the Oesophagus

23.2.1 Case Summary

A woman in her 30s with a history of TB, and a past episode of severe haemoptysis treated with a pulmonary coil, underwent investigations for a persistent cough related to eating or drinking. A barium swallow showed a fistula arising from the lower third of the oesophagus to the right lower lobe (Fig. 23.3). CT scan showed an area of dense consolidation at the apex of the right lower lobe and a suggestion of a fistula to the oesophagus.

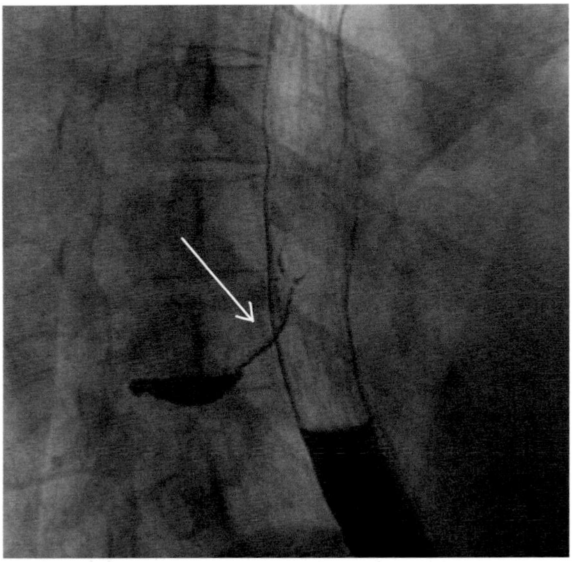

Fig. 23.3 Contrast swallow showing fistula tract from the oesophagus

She underwent a right thoracotomy through the fifth intercostal space. The lower lobe was densely consolidated, and it was decided to resect it along with the fistula. The inferior pulmonary vein and the branch of the pulmonary artery to the lower lobe were divided with a stapler. The fistula to the oesophagus was then isolated and divided after ligation, and the right lower lobe was excised (Fig. 23.4).

A gastrografin swallow four days later showed free flow without a leak (Fig. 23.5). The chest drain was removed, and the patient was discharged 48 hours later on a liquid diet.

The patient made an uneventful post-operative recovery. She was well and reported no gastrointestinal or respiratory symptoms at her last planned review six months later.

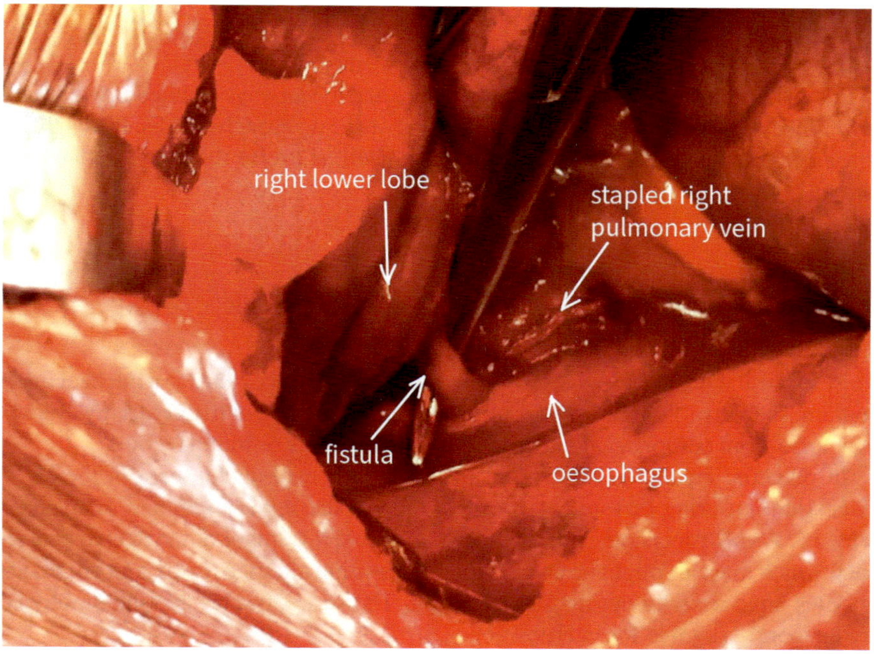

Fig. 23.4 Operative picture showing the fistula dissected out and ready for excision

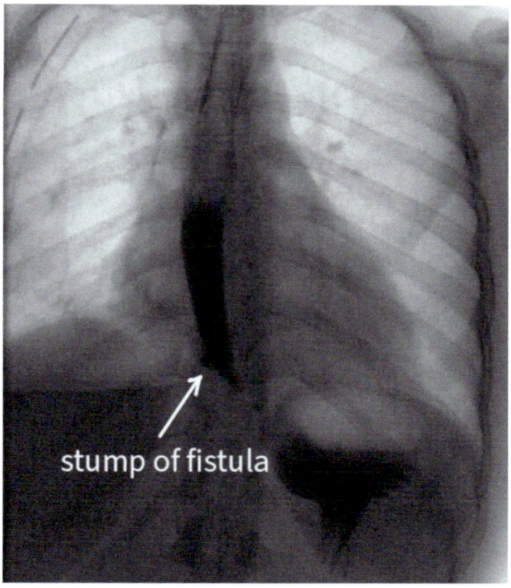

Fig. 23.5 Contrast swallow four days after surgery

23.2.2 Learning Points

In this case, the fistula between the oesophagus and the airways resulted in a diseased lower lobe of the right lung in addition to long-standing bronchiectasis. It was therefore necessary to resect the diseased lobe, as well as excise the fistula rather than simply dividing the connection.

23.3 Tracheo-Oesophageal Fistulas in the Neck

Most cervical tracheo-oesophageal fistulae in adults are secondary to a tracheal intervention, such as prolonged use of a cuffed endotracheal tube or tracheostomy. Rarely, they arise from oesophageal interventions such as stents or trauma.

In planning repair, it is important to include the anaesthetic team in the MDT discussion, ensuring that an endotracheal tube of the right length and diameter is selected. A collar incision gives the best access, and it is important to decide beforehand which muscles might be needed for interposition after the repair, and not divide muscles unnecessarily during the dissection. The strap muscles and the omohyoid are eminently suitable for interposition.

23.4 Cervical TOF 1

23.4.1 Case Summary

A woman in her 30s with a 10-year history of asthma underwent investigations for worsening respiratory symptoms. CT scan of the chest showed a fistula between the trachea and the cervical oesophagus at the level of the root of the neck (Fig. 23.6).

Bronchoscopy confirmed the fistula with the tracheal opening measuring 5 mm in diameter and without any visual evidence of inflammatory or neoplastic pathology. Biopsies from the edge of the fistula showed normal mucosa. OGD showed the fistula and an otherwise normal oesophagus. A detailed history failed to reveal anything to suggest the aetiology of the fistula.

The fistula was approached through a collar incision in the neck. The right lobe of the thyroid was mobilised after dividing the middle thyroid veins, and the recurrent laryngeal nerve was identified and carefully dissected free over a 2 cm length so that it could be displaced anteriorly using a silastic loop. The oesophagus was then carefully separated from the trachea above and below the fistula, which was then looped and dissected out (Fig. 23.7). It was ligated with 3/0 PDS at the oesophageal side. On the tracheal side, it was friable, and it was therefore transected, and the small tracheal defect was closed with interrupted 3/0 PDS. A drain was placed adjacent to the repair before closing the neck. A contrast swallow 48 hours later showed free flow without

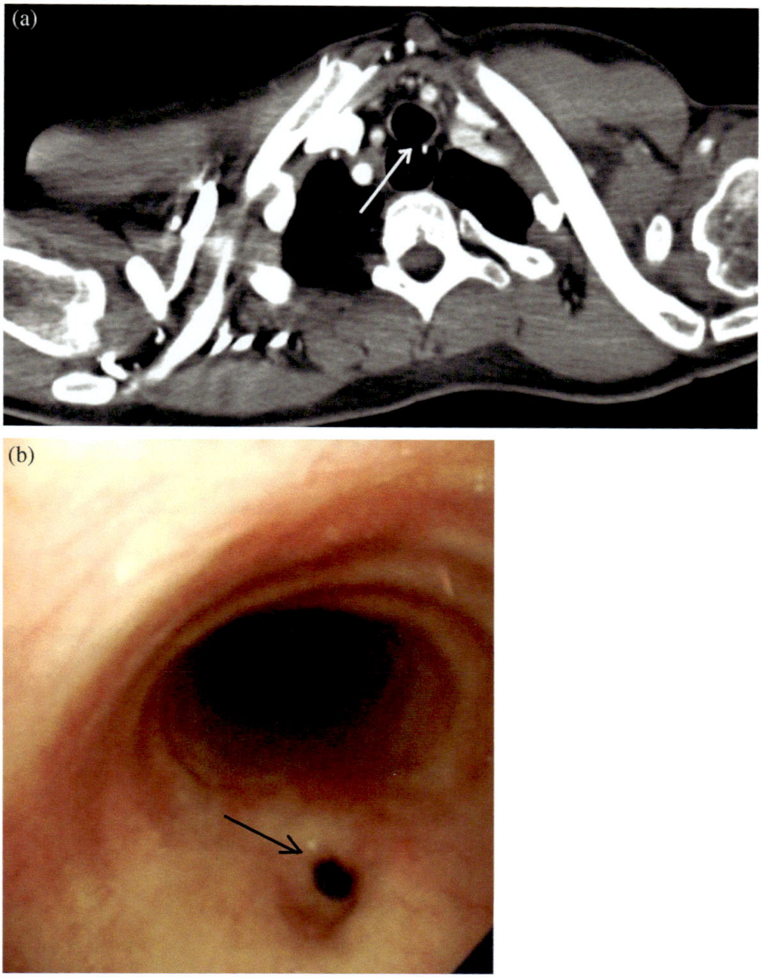

Fig. 23.6 Transverse CT section (**a**) and bronchoscopy (**b**) showing a TOF in the neck

stenosis or a leak (Fig. 23.8). The patient was started on free fluids, progressing to a liquid diet, and the drain was removed two days later. The patient made an uneventful post-operative recovery, and her respiratory symptoms had resolved when she was followed up six weeks later.

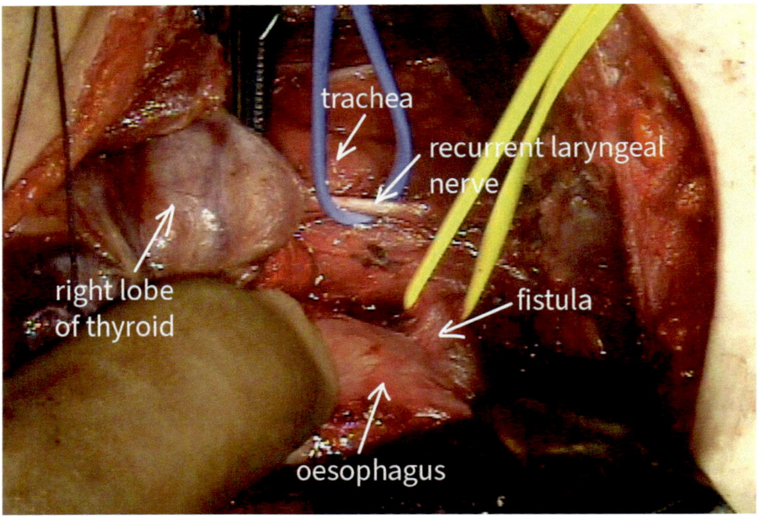

Fig. 23.7 Operative picture showing inferior pole of the thyroid above the finger, the recurrent laryngeal nerve and fistula tract

Fig. 23.8 Contrast swallow 5 days after surgery showing no leak

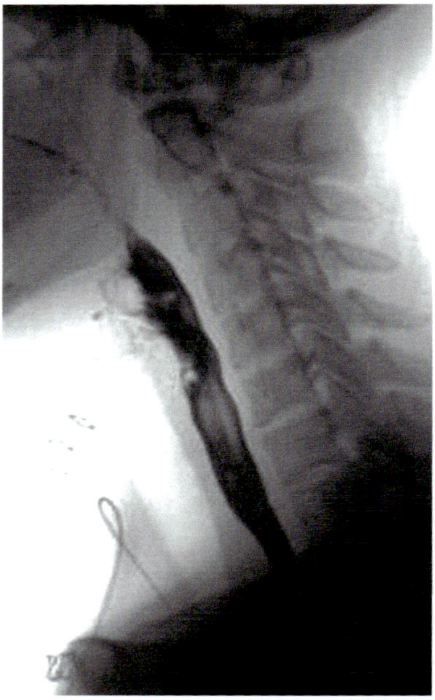

23.4.2 Learning Points

This is an unusual case in that the fistula appeared to be congenital as no other cause could be found. OGD showed the fistula to be at 17 cm from the incisors, about 12 cm below the cricopharynx. The rest of the examination was normal, apart from showing Barrett's C1 M1. The technical point to emphasise in the neck exploration is to identify the recurrent laryngeal nerve and carefully dissect it so that it can be displaced out of the way before starting dissection of the fistula. Unless this is done, the nerve could be damaged or indeed incorporated in some of the sutures, as it commonly lies in the tracheao-oesophageal groove, which is exactly the plane that needs to be dissected. With this in mind, if the use of a nerve stimulator is planned, this needs to be discussed with the anaesthetist in the planning and briefing for the operation.

23.5 Cervical TOF 2

23.5.1 Case Summary

A man in his 70s was referred with a tracheo-oesophageal fistula that had been diagnosed six years previously. Over the previous three years, he had suffered repeated chest infections. CT scan showed a 5 mm diameter tracheo-oesophageal fistula at the level of T1 (Fig. 23.9). Gastrografin swallow showed a small amount of contrast passing through the fistula into the airways.

He had a previous history of a VSD repair performed abroad followed by a prolonged stay in ITU. He had poor exercise tolerance due to diminished cardiac reserve and also suffered from respiratory impairment due to bronchiectasis, presumed to be related to his fistula. While undergoing an assessment of the fistula, he presented with aspiration pneumonia and was admitted to the intensive care unit for ventilatory support. He had a history of previous ICU admissions for similar reasons. He was treated with antibiotics, and extubation was tried but was unsuccessful.

Following an MDT discussion, it was decided to repair the fistula if this could be performed without accessing the chest or abdomen. Because of his poor nutritional state, a feeding jejunostomy was first placed through a mini-laparotomy. He remained reliant on ventilatory support, and four weeks later, it was decided to close the fistula.

Through a collar incision in the neck, the strap muscles were separated, and both thyroid lobes were mobilised by dividing the middle thyroid veins. The proximal oesophagus and trachea were mobilised after identifying both recurrent laryngeal nerves. The fistula was identified and divided, leaving a cuff of oesophagus on the tracheal side. The defects in the oesophagus and trachea were closed with interrupted 4/0 PDS. The left-sided strap muscles were mobilised after detaching them from the

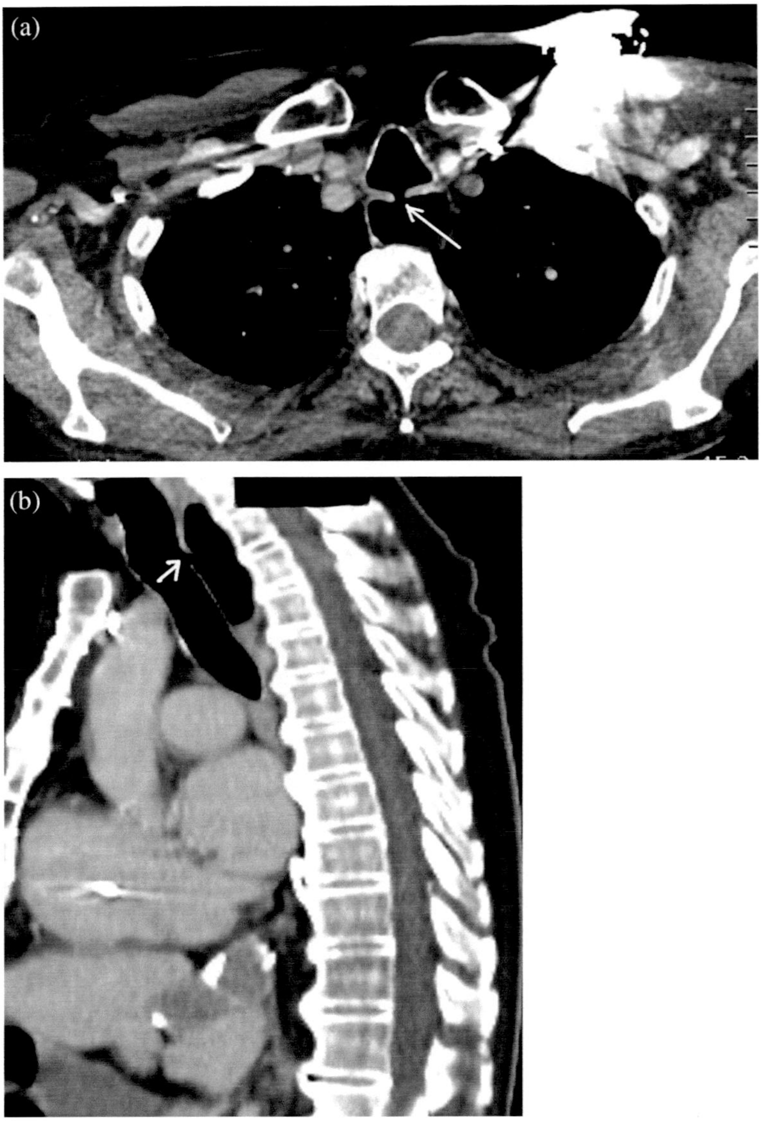

Fig. 23.9 Axial (a) and sagittal (b) CT sections showing a small TOF at the level of T1

hyoid and interposed between the trachea and the oesophagus at the level of repair. A tracheostomy was also performed. His general condition improved, but it proved impossible to wean him off the ventilator, and he passed away two months later.

23.5.2 Learning Points

The patient had been known to have a tracheo-oesophageal fistula for six years and had suffered previous admissions to the ITU for aspiration pneumonia. The cause of his TOF was not clear but it could have resulted from prolonged endotracheal intubation at the time of his VSD repair. When first referred with the fistula, it was not clear that the fistula was the main cause of his recurrent aspiration. While undergoing assessment of the fistula, he was admitted with a severe chest infection requiring ventilation. An MDT discussion was held, including the ITU team and involving him and his family. The ITU team felt that even if the fistula had a minor contribution to the episodes of aspiration, its closure was justified at the same time as a tracheostomy to help wean him off the ventilator.

A feeding jejunostomy was first placed to improve nutrition and, as it was not possible to wean him off the ventilator two weeks later, the fistula was repaired with a surgical tracheostomy. The procedure was carefully planned with the anaesthetists to ensure that the endotracheal tube was long enough, with the cuff placed well beyond the TOF, almost at the level of the trachea.

Mobilisation of both lobes of the thyroid allowed the tracheo-pharyngeal complex to be 'lifted' up and facilitated access to the fistula, which was distant from the cervical access. The tracheostomy tube had also to be chosen and placed with care, ensuring the cuff was below the repair. The procedure was uneventful, without any technical complications, but it was still impossible to wean the patient off the ventilator.

Chapter 24
Anastomotic Leaks and Conduit Necrosis After Oesophagectomy

Abstract Anastomotic leaks following oesophagectomy remain a significant postoperative concern, with incidence rates varying between 5 and 20%, influenced by surgical expertise, patient selection, and leak definition. Improved patient selection and perioperative care have reduced leak rates in high-volume centres. Clinical presentation varies, ranging from subtle signs to sepsis, necessitating early diagnosis through imaging, primarily CT scan with contrast. Management depends on severity and patient condition, with conservative measures often effective for minor leaks. Endoscopic interventions aim to seal leaks and promote healing, while surgery is reserved for complete dehiscence. A case study illustrates complex decision-making, highlighting technical challenges and patient factors influencing outcomes, such as immunosuppression and vascular compromise. Conduit necrosis is uncommon and requires careful assessment and timely interventions. A case study describes the management of conduit necrosis and staged reconstruction using colon.

Keywords Anastomotic leaks · Conduit necrosis · Oesophagectomy · Surgical expertise · Patient selection · Perioperative care · Clinical presentation · Conservative management · Endoscopic interventions · Technical challenges

Anastomotic leaks following oesophagectomy remain a significant postoperative complication, with incidence rates varying between 5 and 20% depending on the study and the surgical technique [1, 2]. The high variability in reported incidence can be attributed to surgical expertise, patient selection, and the definition of anastomotic leak.

Improvements in patient selection, pre-optimisation, and a better understanding of the causes of leaks have resulted in most large-volume centres reporting diminishing anastomotic rates. When leaks do occur, it is now rare to see a complete disruption of the anastomosis, and such leaks can often be treated conservatively as long as the conduit has not become ischaemic. However, from time to time, conduit ischaemia occurs to the extent that it is necessary to take down the anastomosis to deal with the emergency and reconstruct later.

M. Mughal, *Reconstructive Surgery of the Oesophagus and Stomach*,
https://doi.org/10.1007/978-3-031-66846-3_24

The aetiology of anastomotic leaks is multifactorial and can be broadly categorised into technical and patient-related factors. Technical factors include the quality of surgical technique, tension on the anastomosis, and adequacy of blood supply to the anastomotic site. Patient-related factors include pre-existing comorbidities such as diabetes, malnutrition, and vascular diseases that compromise tissue healing. Furthermore, neoadjuvant therapies such as chemotherapy and radiation can affect the vascularity of the tissues, increasing the risk of leaks.

Clinical presentation of anastomotic leaks can vary from subtle signs to overt sepsis. Early signs often include fever, tachycardia, and localized pain. With a major leak, patients may present with signs of sepsis or septic shock. Having a high index of suspicion is crucial, as delayed diagnosis can lead to catastrophic outcomes, including multi-organ failure and death.

Diagnosis is primarily based on clinical presentation and is confirmed through imaging studies. CT scan with oral and intravenous contrast is the most useful and practical way to diagnose an anastomotic leak. In addition to identifying a leak, it provides other valuable information, such as associated collections, the state of the lungs, emptying from the conduit, and its vascularity. CT is more sensitive, but less specific than fluoroscopy [3]. Endoscopy is valuable for direct visualisation of the anastomosis and, in particular, to assess the vascularity of the conduit. It is even more accurate than fluoroscopy [4].

Management depends on the severity of the leak and the general condition of the patient. Conservative management, including antibiotics and nutritional support, may suffice for minor leaks. Additionally, drainage of associated collections may be needed either percutaneously or thoracoscopically, and this can most often be achieved percutaneously [5].

Endoscopic treatment options for anastomotic leaks include the placement of self-expandable stents, endoscopic clips, or vacuum-assisted closure devices [6–8]. These interventions aim to seal the leak, promote healing, and prevent further contamination of the surrounding tissues. Surgery is rarely required nowadays and is reserved for complete anastomotic dehiscence, particularly associated with conduit necrosis.

I will describe a case of anastomotic leak with an unusual background to illustrate the complexities of the decision-making process starting with the planning for surgery.

24.1 Anastomotic Leak After Oesophagectomy

24.1.1 Case Summary

A man in his 70s who had undergone a liver transplant 11 years previously for HCC was found to have an adenocarcinoma at the GOJ on gastroscopy to investigate anaemia. He had otherwise been well on immunosuppression with Cyclosporin A and Tacrolimus. Staging investigations, including EUS, showed a T2 N1 M0 tumour

(Figs. 24.1, 24.2 and 24.3). He underwent two cycles of neoadjuvant chemotherapy, and repeat CT showed minimal response.

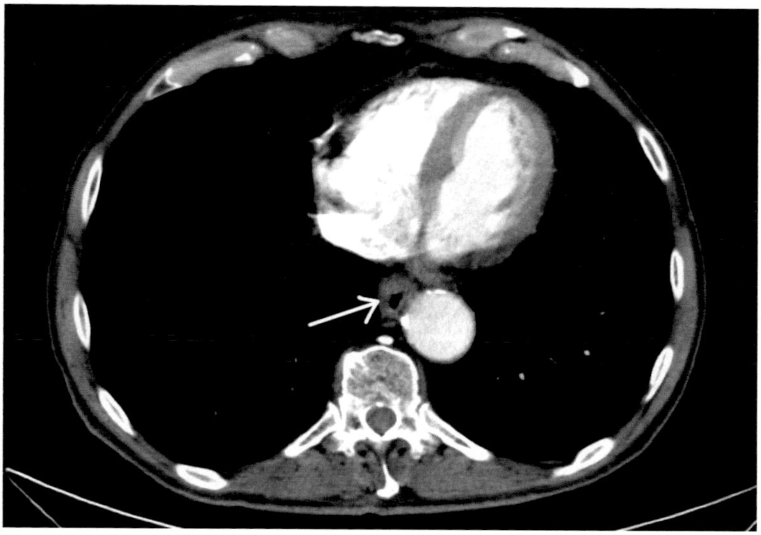

Fig. 24.1 Pre-treatment CT section showing tumour at the GOJ

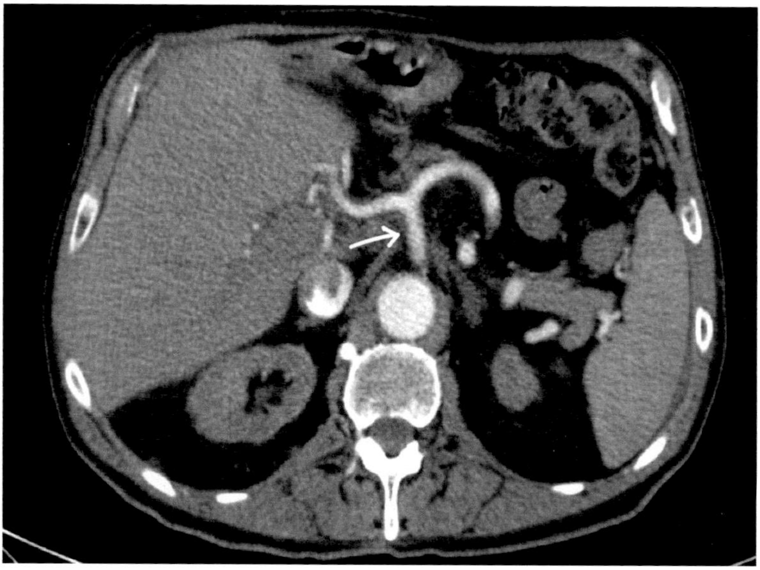

Fig. 24.2 Pre-op CT showing the coeliac axis with its branches and arterial circulation to the liver

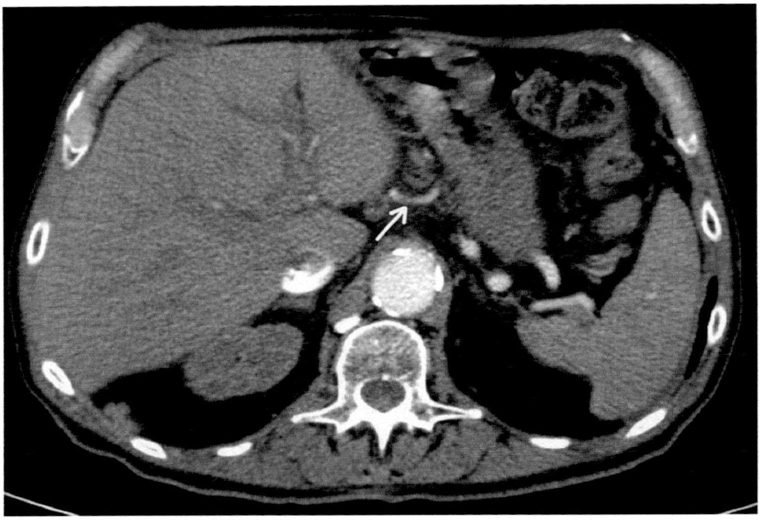

Fig. 24.3 Pre-op CT showing a normal left gastric artery

The MDT recommendation was to offer oesophagectomy, which was carried out with a liver transplant surgeon. Prior to surgery, his immunosuppression was reduced, and treatment was supervised by a hepatologist in the perioperative period.

At laparotomy, there were dense adhesions around the liver, and dissection was performed taking into account the altered vascular anatomy associated with the liver transplant. The gastroepiploeic arch was maintained and, although the mobilised stomach appeared to have reasonable perfusion, there was barely perceptible pulsation in the gastroepiploeic artery. A pyloroplasty was performed and feeding jejunostomy was placed. A routine thoracic dissection was carried out, the tumour resected, the gastric conduit created in the usual way and anastomosed to the oesophagus with a circular stapler.

The patient started draining bile from the chest drain 48 hours later, and fluoroscopy confirmed a large anastomotic leak (Fig. 24.4). Endoscopy showed an intact anastomosis and a dusky but viable gastric tube with a 4 mm punched-out perforation in the gastric staple line, 2 cm below the anastomosis. The pylorus was widely patent. He was kept nil by mouth, administered antibiotics, and fed via his jejunostomy. Immunosuppression was reduced, but drainage through the chest drain remained at 500–600 mL a day for two weeks. Fluoroscopy confirmed a persistent leak (Fig. 24.5). A repeat endoscopy showed a 3–4 mm defect as before. It was closed with three Resolution Boston mucosal clips (Fig. 24.6).

The leak continued but the volume of reduced to 100–300 mL per day, and healed after two weeks (Fig. 24.7). Oral feeding was commenced a week later, five weeks after surgery.

Resection histology was T3 N1 R0. No adjuvant chemotherapy was given, and the patient survived 10 years.

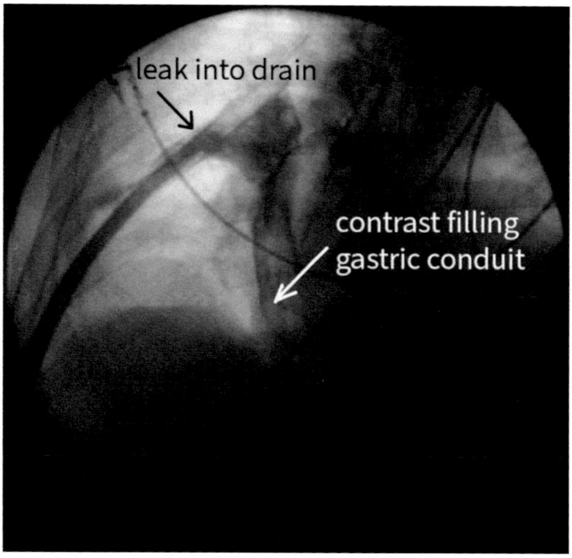

Fig. 24.4 Fluoroscopy 2 days post-op showing a large leak finding its way out through an optimally sited chest drain

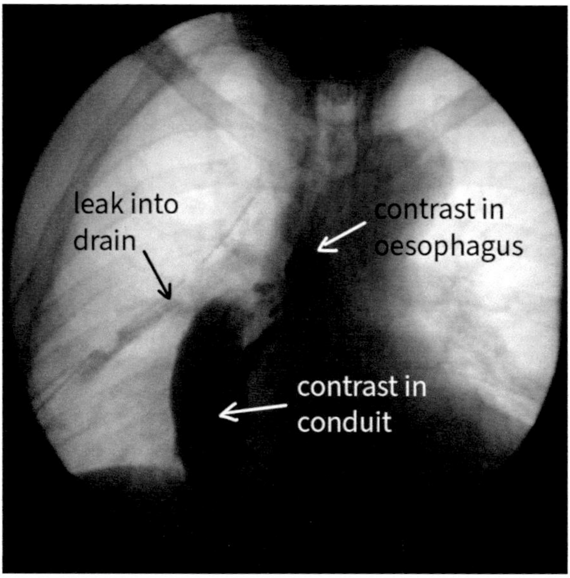

Fig. 24.5 Fluoroscopy 2 weeks post-op showing an improvement but a persistent leak

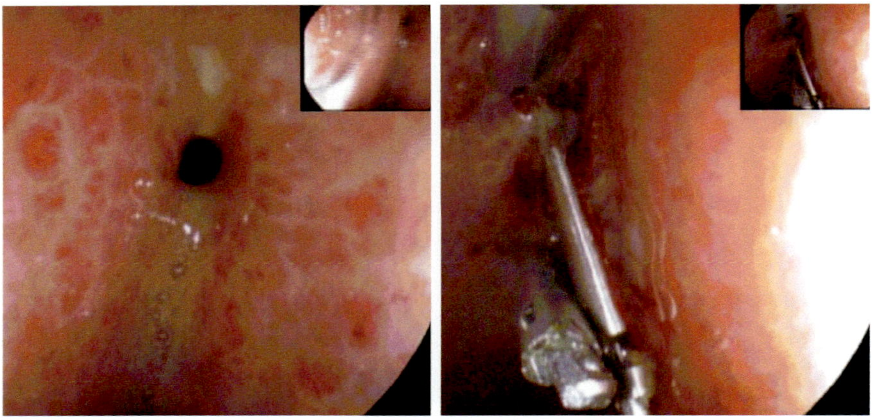

Fig. 24.6 Endoscopic views of the leak and occlusion with clips

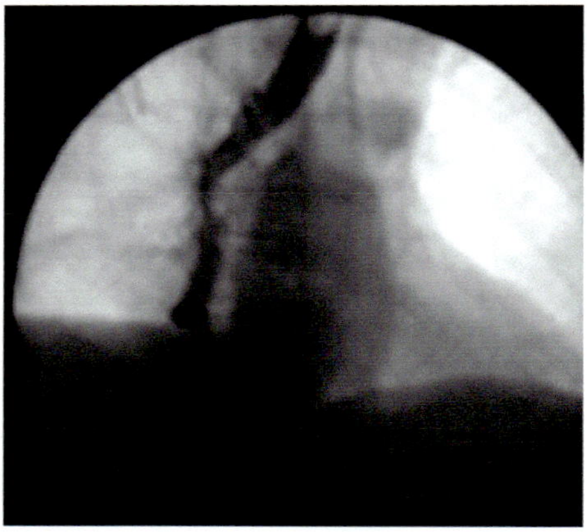

Fig. 24.7 Contrast swallow 4 weeks post-op showing healing of leak

24.1.2 Learning Points

This was a complex case for technical and other reasons. The patient was known to have Barrett's oesophagus but was not on a surveillance programme, as there was no evidence of dysplasia. An increased likelihood of progression of Barrett's to cancer has been reported in liver transplant patients [9]. The case for neoadjuvant treatment was debated at the MDT meeting, particularly in view of the liver transplant and immunosuppression. However, the consensus was to give neoadjuvant EOX, but only two instead of three cycles. As the CT scan after two cycles showed no radiological response, the decision was taken to proceed with a resection. The abdominal part of the operation was performed with a transplant surgeon to ensure that the necessary mobilisation of the stomach did not jeopardise the circulation to the liver. The stomach was successfully mobilised, maintaining the gastroepiploeic arch, and remained vascularised after division of the left gastric pedicle and the short gastric vessels, but there was barely discernible pulsation in the gastroepiploeic vessels. It is likely that in the preparation to receive the new liver, the common hepatic artery had been mobilised and the native gastroduodenal artery divided, as is usually the case for arterial anastomosis in a liver transplant recipient. As the gastroepiploeic artery is a branch of the gastroduodenal, this would have affected the blood supply to the stomach. Although the gastroepiploeic arch is likely to have been perfused through connections from the superior mesenteric artery around the head of the pancreas, there may have been a compromised blood supply to the gastric conduit, which resulted in the staple line leak. Although the patient developed an early, large-volume leak and could potentially have been re-explored to repair the leak, it was decided to treat him conservatively since the leak was fully drained through the chest drain, and he remained systemically well. Ultimately, however, he required closure of the leak with clips, which was successful.

24.2 Gastric Conduit Necrosis Following Oesophagectomy

Gastric conduit necrosis (GCN) is a rare but devastating complication that can occur following oesophagectomy. The incidence of gastric necrosis varies, partly because of a lack of standardisation in the definition and investigations used to diagnose conduit necrosis. A systematic review has shown the incidence to be between 0 and 21%.

It is important to make the distinction between ischaemia and necrosis. Veramootoo and colleagues have proposed a grading of gastric conduit necrosis—Type I being a simple anastomotic leak, Type II focal necrosis and Type III being extensive necrosis requiring excision of the conduit [10].

Endoscopy is the gold standard to diagnose and assess conduit necrosis as some patients with partial necrosis will have a normal CT scan. Page and colleagues have proposed routine OGD evaluation of the anastomosis within a week of oesophagectomy and shown this to be both safe and useful [11]. I think this is unnecessary. Even if the endoscopy shows a tiny leak, most are likely to heal with minimal intervention.

Risk factors for a leak relate to the patient, technique and post-operative circumstances. Arterial disease affecting the visceral circulation, diabetes, and impaired cardiac output are important patient factors that should be looked for in the preoperative assessment. Technical factors are perhaps the most important contributors to leaks. It is important to safeguard the gastroepiploic vessels by careful handling of the stomach during mobilisation. This is particularly important during laparoscopic mobilisation to avoid the application of instruments near the greater curvature of the stomach. A tight hiatus can cause vascular compromise once the conduit has been transposed. It is also important to carry out the transposition with care to avoid tearing the blood vessels. Intraoperative and postoperative factors include the use of vasoconstrictors and prolonged hypertension.

Intraoperative monitoring of gastric circulation has been described and used by some surgeons. The techniques used include Doppler ultrasound, and ICG (indocyanine green) fluorescence imaging. There is some evidence that the use of ICG fluorescence can be helpful in assessing the conduit and ensuring that the part of the conduit chosen for the anastomosis is well vascularised. However, there have been no randomised trials in this area and I, like most surgeons, continue to follow surgical principles and use clinical judgement in the assessment of the vascularity of the conduit.

24.3 Conduit Necrosis After Oesophagectomy

24.3.1 Case Summary

A man in his 70s was referred for oesophageal reconstruction. He had undergone a minimally invasive two-stage oesophagectomy four years previously. Histology showed high-grade dysplasia only. He developed a significant anastomotic leak, necessitating a thoracotomy eight days later. There was a complete breakdown of the anastomosis with necrosis of the distal 2–3 cm of the conduit. The anastomosis was taken down, the necrotic part of the conduit excised, and the gastric conduit returned to the abdomen. An end cervical oesophagostomy and feeding jejunostomy were performed. He had a prolonged stay in the hospital and required a left thoracotomy for decortication of the lung and drainage of an empyema two months later. He made a slow and steady recovery and lived with his oesophagostomy and feeding jejunostomy for three years before enquiring about the possibility of reconstruction.

After referral for oesophageal reconstruction, he underwent an assessment including an up-to-date CT of the chest, abdomen and pelvis. In view of the previous bilateral thoracotomies and mediastinal sepsis, it was decided to use a retrosternal route for the conduit. Laparotomy showed modest adhesions and the defunctioned gastric conduit was dissected out but was not long enough to reach the neck. The colon was mobilised, and the right side was found to be suitable as a conduit (Fig. 24.8). After preparation of the vascular pedicle, the right hemicolon was disconnected and brought up to the neck through a retrosternal tunnel. The caecum was anastomosed to the cervical oesophagus (Fig. 24.9) and the distal end of the conduit to the jejunum 25 cm distal to the DJ flexure. The patient made an uneventful post-operative recovery and a contrast swallow a week after surgery showed no leak (Fig. 24.10).

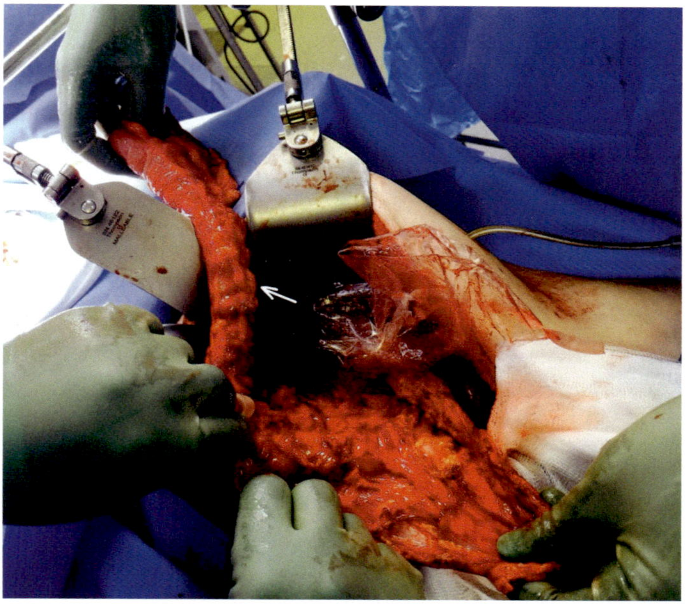

Fig. 24.8 Right colon conduit ready for transposition

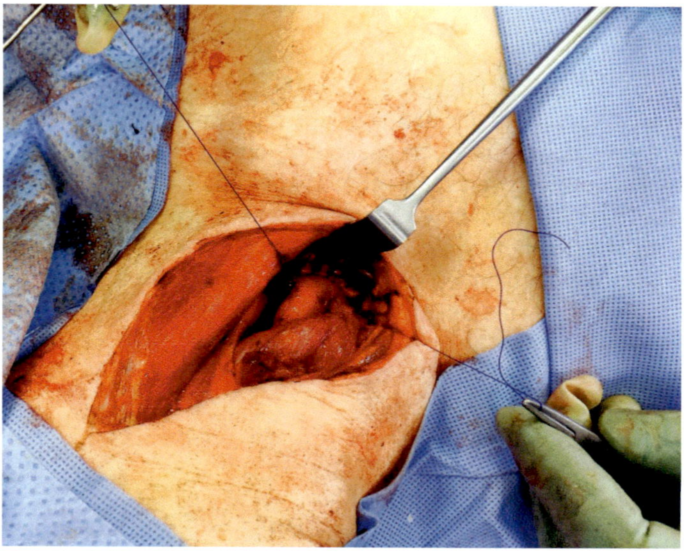

Fig. 24.9 Anastomosis of the caecum to the oesophageal stump

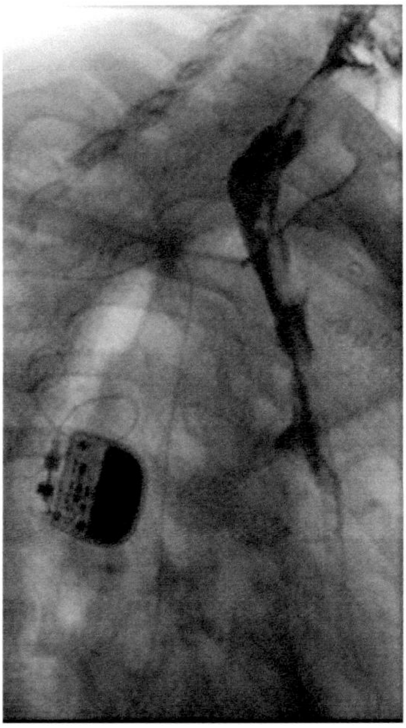

Fig. 24.10 Contrast swallow 7 days after surgery showing no leak

24.3.2 Learning Points

In this case, the resection histology showed high-grade dysplasia only. If it had been an invasive adenocarcinoma, the timing of the reconstruction would have needed to be carefully considered based on the chances of tumour recurrence. Reconstruction is a major operation with significant comorbidity and should only be considered when the risk of recurrence is low and the patient's general condition is good with a complete recovery from the initial surgery. Because of the extensive mediastinal sepsis and bilateral thoracotomies, it was decided to use a retrosternal route. Avoiding a thoracotomy also meant the patient was less prone to chest complications following the reconstruction.

References

1. Markar SR, Karthikesalingam A, Thrumurthy S, Low DE. Volume-outcome relationship in surgery for esophageal malignancy: systematic review and meta-analysis 2000–2011. J Gastrointest Surg. 2012;16(5):1055–63. https://doi.org/10.1007/s11605-011-1731-3.
2. Biere SSAY, Maas KW, Cuesta A, van der Peet DL. Cervical or thoracic anastomosis after esophagectomy for cancer: a systematic review and meta-analysis. Digestive Surg. 2011;281:29–35. https://doi.org/10.1159/000322014.
3. Radiological detection of post-oesophagectomy anastomotic leak—a comparison between multidetector CT and fluoroscopy. Accessed 1 Oct 2023. https://doi.org/10.1259/bjr/30515892.

4. Page, Richard D., Michael J. Shackcloth, Glenn N. Russell, and Stephen H. Pennefather. 'Surgical Treatment of Anastomotic Leaks after Oesophagectomy'. Eur J Cardio-Thorac Surg. 2005;27(2):337–43. https://doi.org/10.1016/j.ejcts.2004.10.053.
5. Low DE. Diagnosis and management of anastomotic leaks after esophagectomy. J Gastrointest Surg. 2011;15(8):1319–22. https://doi.org/10.1007/s11605-011-1511-0.
6. Mala T, Aahlin EK.: Stepping up the management of anastomotic leaks after oesophagectomy: getting a feel through less invasive tentacles. Br J Surg. 2023;110(8):877–79. https://doi.org/10.1093/bjs/znad142.
7. Mandarino FV, Bonura GF, Esposito D, Rosati R, Parise P, Fanti L. A large anastomotic leakage after esophageal surgery treated with endoluminal vacuum-assisted closure: a case report. J Surg Case Rep. 2020(4):rjaa071. https://doi.org/10.1093/jscr/rjaa071.
8. Kouladouros, K. Applications of endoscopic vacuum therapy in the upper gastrointestinal tract. World J. Gastrointest Endosc. 2023;15(6):420–33. https://doi.org/10.4253/wjge.v15.i6.420.
9. Oezcelik A, Kaiser GM, Dechene A, Treckmann JW, Sotiropoulos GC, Reinhardt R, Saner FH, Paul A. Progression to adenocarcinoma in Barrett's esophagus after liver transplantation. Transplantation 2011;91(11):1250–1253. https://journals.lww.com/transplantjournal/toc/2011/06150
10. Veeramootoo D, Parameswaran R, Krishnadas R, Froeschle P, Cooper M, Berrisford RG, Wajed SA. Classification and early recognition of gastric conduit failure after minimally invasive esophagectomy. Surg Endosc. 2009;23(9):2110–16. https://doi.org/10.1007/s00464-008-0233-1.
11. Page RD, Asmat A, McShane J, Russell GN, Pennefather SH (2013) Routine endoscopy to detect anastomotic leakage after esophagectomy. Ann Thorac Surg. 2013;95(1):292–98. https://doi.org/10.1016/j.athoracsur.2012.09.048.

Chapter 25
Delayed Gastric Emptying After Oesophagectomy

Abstract Delayed gastric emptying (DGE) after oesophagectomy and gastric conduit reconstruction is a prevalent complication affecting 15–39% of patients, primarily attributed to pyloric spasm and complete vagotomy-induced gastric motility dysfunction. Temporary in nature for most, DGE's mechanisms include vagal dysfunction, adverse pressure gradients, conduit torsion, and oesophageal hiatus tightness. Tabularised stomachs demonstrate superior emptying compared to whole stomachs, with the addition of pyloric drainage showing no impact on emptying. Severe cases necessitate revision surgery, often complex and with significant morbidity, yet yielding notable symptomatic improvements. Techniques involve conduit reshaping, hernia reduction, and tabularisation, ensuring careful conduit mobilization to preserve vascularity. A case study is presented illustrating the reshaping of a gastric conduit to improve emptying.

Keywords Delayed gastric emptying (DGE) · Oesophagectomy · Gastric conduit reconstruction · Pyloric spasm · Vagotomy · Tabularised stomach · Revision surgery · Symptomatic improvement · Conduit reshaping · Hernia reduction

Delayed gastric emptying (DGE) after oesophagectomy and reconstruction with a gastric conduit is a common complication that occurs in 15–39% of patients.

The main cause is pyloric spasm and dysfunction of gastric motility due to a complete vagotomy. In most patients, this is a temporary phenomenon which resolves or at least diminishes to a degree that it is virtually asymptomatic. Bin Li and colleagues have proposed several mechanisms, including an adverse pressure gradient (negative thoracic pressure, positive abdominal pressure), torsion or angulation of the conduit, conduit redundancy and a tight oesophageal hiatus [1]. In their study, delayed gastric emptying was seen in 15.7% of 356 patients having oesophagectomy without pyloric drainage. Balloon dilatation of the pylorus was effective in improving drainage in most cases.

It has been shown that a tabularised stomach empties better than the whole stomach [2]. A systematic review has also shown that addition of a pyloric drainage procedure

M. Mughal, *Reconstructive Surgery of the Oesophagus and Stomach*,
https://doi.org/10.1007/978-3-031-66846-3_25

and the level of the anastomosis has no bearing on gastric emptying, but a gastric tube drains better than the whole stomach [3].

A small percentage of patients are severely symptomatic or suffer life-threatening complications such as recurrent aspiration with cumulative deterioration of respiratory function. A single institution report of surgery for this group of patients has reported good symptomatic outcomes, including QOL [4]. The authors describe their experience of revision surgery in 125 patients after oesophagectomy, mainly for a redundant conduit or para-conduit hernia. Over 90% of the patients were improved after surgery, but in many cases the operations were complex, involving both abdominal and thoracic access with significant morbidity.

Another group has reported on revision surgery for poor gastric emptying in eight patients out of a group of 400 patients who had undergone an oesophagectomy for cancer over the previous seven years [5]. The average time to reoperation was 3.8 years, and the operations were performed using a combination of thoracotomy and either laparoscopy or laparotomy. The revisions resulted in an improvement in symptoms and patient satisfaction after an average follow-up of 10 months. The authors describe their technique, including dealing with associated para conduit hernias, the reduction of redundant conduits and the tabularisation of dilated conduits. They describe their technique, which involved careful mobilisation of the conduit from the anastomosis to the diaphragm, avoiding injury to its blood supply. Any associated hernias were reduced, and the anastomosis was refashioned if necessary. Dilated conduits were narrowed with a series of silk plication sutures or stapling along the lesser curvature to recreate a 4–5 cm wide tube. Interestingly, the technique of plication to reduce the diameter of a conduit has been described by Kiss and colleagues for end-stage achalasia [6].

25.1 Chronic Dilatation and Delayed Emptying of Gastric Conduit

25.1.1 Case Summary

A 10-year-old boy had undergone initial surgery for oesophageal atresia but had eventually required a gastric pull-up for a resection of a recalcitrant oesophageal stricture. The stomach had been transposed without any resection or tubularisation. Over a period of time, it had become progressively baggy with poor emptying and resultant reflux. Pyloric dilatation had been tried without lasting benefit, and a pyloroplasty had been performed trans-abdominally without any benefit. Contrast studies and CT scans showed a very baggy stomach with a distended contrast-filled antrum, resulting in an acute bend at the level of the oesophageal hiatus. It was felt that this was best managed by reshaping the conduit and reducing redundancy. The gastric conduit was dissected carefully through a right thoracotomy to preserve its

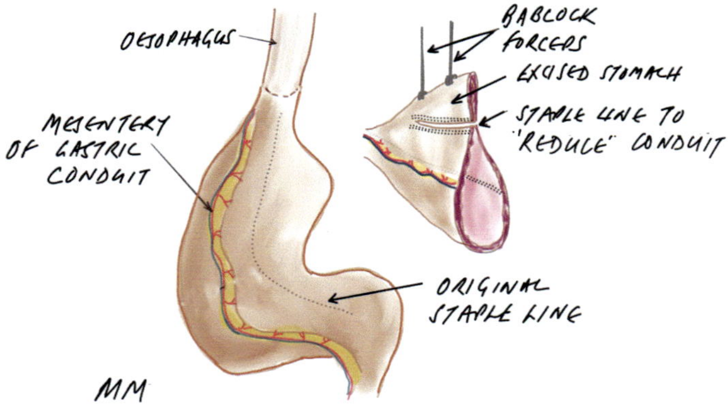

Fig. 25.1 Diagrammatic depiction of tabularisation of a baggy conduit. It is important to mobilise the conduit fully and ensure that the vascular supply is well away from the staple line

blood supply. It was mobilised circumferentially from the oesophagogastric anastomosis to the diaphragm. It was then tubularised by excising a 2 cm wide strip of the stomach between the lesser and greater curvature with a stapler (Fig. 25.1). The patient made an uneventful post-operative recovery with a considerable improvement in symptoms.

25.1.2 Learning Points

A baggy, poorly emptying gastric conduit is much more commonly seen following an oesophagectomy for cancer than in paediatric patients. Reconstruction and tubularisation of the conduit, as in this case is an effective treatment. It does, however, require a thoracotomy and great care must be taken to ensure that the blood supply to the conduit is not damaged during either mobilisation or tabularisation.

References

1. Li B, et al. Delayed gastric emptying after esophagectomy for malignancy. J Laparoendoscopic Adv Surg Tech. 2014;24(5):306–11. https://doi.org/10.1089/lap.2013.0416.
2. Bemelman WA, et al. Delayed postoperative emptying after esophageal resection is dependent on the size of the gastric substitute. J Am Coll Surg. 1995;180(4):461–4.
3. Ronald DLA, et al. Surgical techniques to prevent delayed gastric emptying after esophagectomy with gastric interposition: a systematic review. Ann. Thorac. Surg. 2014;98(4):1512–19. https://doi.org/10.1016/j.athoracsur.2014.06.057.
4. Schaheen LW, Joubert KD, Luketich JD. Revising a gastric conduitxe "gastric conduits" after esophagectomy: How do we get it right? J Thorac Cardiovasc Surg. 2017;154(4):1461–2. https://doi.org/10.1016/j.jtcvs.2017.05.092.

5. Rove JY, Sasha Krupnick A, Baciewicz FA, Meyers BF. Gastric conduit revision postesophagectomy: management for a rare complication. J Thorac Cardiovasc Surg. 2017;154(4):1450–58. https://doi.org/10.1016/j.jtcvs.2017.04.012.
6. Kiss J, Vörös A, Szirányi E, Altorjay Á, Bohák Á. Management of failed Heller's operations. Surg. Today. 1996;26(7):541–45. https://doi.org/10.1007/BF00311564.

Chapter 26
Oesophageal Involvement in Head and Neck Pathology

Abstract This chapter delves into the intricate relationship between head and neck pathology and the cervical oesophagus, emphasizing the potential extension of laryngeal or pharyngeal cancer into the oesophagus, often necessitating complex surgical interventions such as laryngopharyngectomy with oesophageal reconstruction, typically utilizing a gastric pull-up. The text presents illustrative cases, including a thyroid mass infiltrating the oesophagus and a recurrent parathyroid cancer involving pharyngeal muscles and the oesophagus. Preoperative imaging plays a crucial role in assessing the extent of tumoral infiltration and guiding surgical management to achieve optimal outcomes. Surgical approaches involve meticulous dissection to achieve clear margins while preserving vital structures, highlighting the understanding of the surgical anatomy and collaborative efforts between various surgical specialties in addressing these challenging cases.

Keywords Head and neck pathology · Cervical oesophagus · Pharyngeal constrictors · Laryngopharyngectomy · Oesophageal reconstruction · Gastric pull-up · Thyroid cancer · Parathyroid cancer · Oesophageal Schwannoma · Extra-oesophageal pathology · Tumour infiltration · Surgical approach · Preoperative imaging

Head and neck pathology can involve the cervical oesophagus and pharyngeal constrictors. Laryngeal or pharyngeal cancer can extend into the oesophagus and may require a laryngopharyngectomy with oesophageal reconstruction, usually a gastric pull-up. Upper GI surgeons are usually asked to assist with the reconstruction, to fashion a gastric conduit after 'blind' extraction of the normal thoracic oesophagus transhiatally. As the resection of the disease and the anastomosis in the neck are done by the Head and Neck surgeons, I have not covered the creation of the gastric conduit here because it is usually straightforward.

This section will show two examples of extra-oesophageal pathology involving the oesophagus. Various head and neck conditions can involve the cervical oesophagus, but my experience has been mainly with thyroid and parathyroid disease. It is often difficult to know from the imaging whether a large mass in the neck is simply abutting

M. Mughal, *Reconstructive Surgery of the Oesophagus and Stomach*,
https://doi.org/10.1007/978-3-031-66846-3_26

the oesophagus and the constrictor muscles or is infiltrating them, as there is often not a fat plane to be able to make the distinction. However, in the cases that I have managed, as long as radiological imaging indicates that the mass is not demonstrably involving the mucosa, there is a possibility that it is simply abutting or infiltrating the muscles only and is, therefore, technically resectable. Endoscopic ultrasonography can be helpful, although it may be technically difficult [1].

26.1 Thyroid Mass Involving the Oesophagus

26.1.1 Case Summary

A woman in her 50s was referred to the endocrine surgeons with a large mass in the neck, hoarse voice, intermittent stridor and dysphagia to solids. USS showed a large thyroid mass, and core biopsies revealed an anaplastic carcinoma. CT scan showed a $9.7 \times 7.4 \times 7.6$ mass with central necrosis comprising the left thyroid lobe. The trachea was displaced to the right but was patent. There was the suggestion of invasion of the neck strap muscles. The mass appeared to be fused to and compressing the cervical oesophagus and cricopharyngeus. It was intensely avid on PET scan with avid lymph nodes at levels III/IV (Figs. 26.1, 26.2, 26.3). OGD revealed distortion of the cervical oesophagus and normal mucosa.

The MDT recommendation was to perform a total thyroidectomy with lymphadenectomy, followed by adjuvant radiotherapy depending on the resection pathology.

At operation, through a collar incision, the strap muscles were noted to be infiltrated with the mass. They were left attached to the mass and divided well away from it. After the division of the upper pole vessels and the middle thyroid veins, the left lobe of the thyroid was progressively separated from the underlying structures. The left recurrent laryngeal nerve was involved in the tumour and was, therefore, sacrificed. Both parathyroid glands were identified and preserved on the right. The mass almost appeared to be fused to the cricopharyngeus and upper oesophagus. In order to obtain a negative deep resection margin, the cricopharyngeus muscle was excised in continuity with the muscle layer of the involved cervical oesophagus. Dissection was carried medially onto the trachea, separating the mass from it with a knife, working on the surface of the trachea. The right lobe of the thyroid was then mobilised, and a total thyroidectomy was completed (Figs. 26.4, 26.5, 26.6 and 26.7). Level II and IV lymph nodes were cleared on the thoracic duct was identified and ligated.

The patient made an uneventful post-operative recovery with no change in her voice and normal swallowing. Her PTH and calcium levels remained within the normal range. Histology showed an 8 cm, unifocal left lobe anaplastic and papillary thyroid carcinoma with lymphovascular invasion. The tumour extended to the tracheal resection margin. The oesophageal resection margin was clear. She was

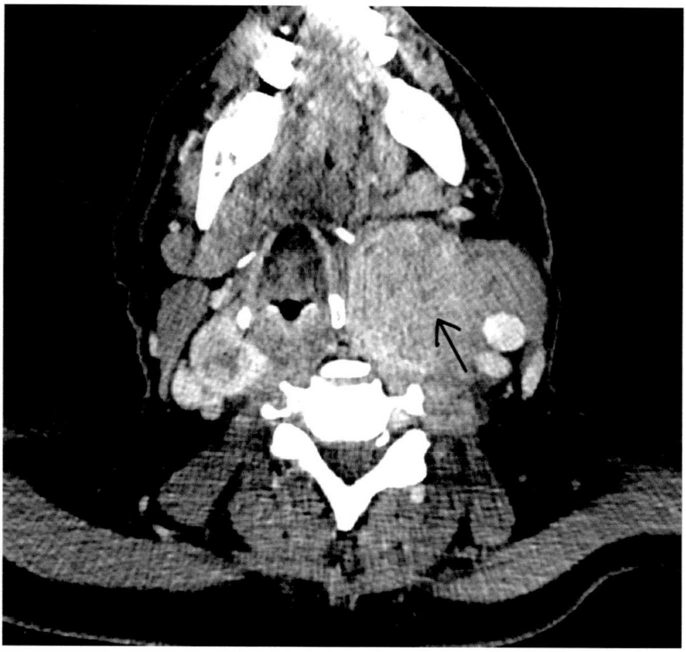

Fig. 26.1 CT section showing large left-sided thyroid mass displacing the larynx to the right

Fig. 26.2 CT section showing displacement and deformity of the trachea. The oesophagus cannot be seen separate from the mass

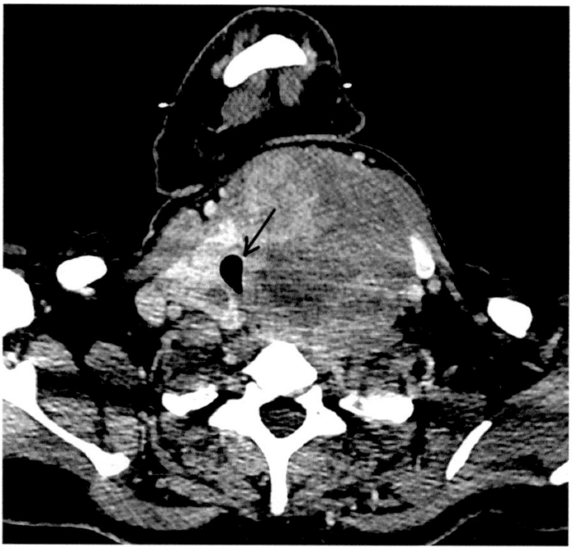

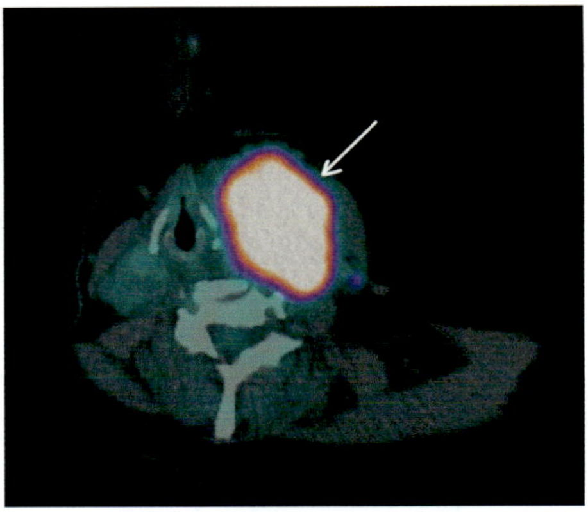

Fig. 26.3 PET scan showing intense activity in the left lobe of the thyroid

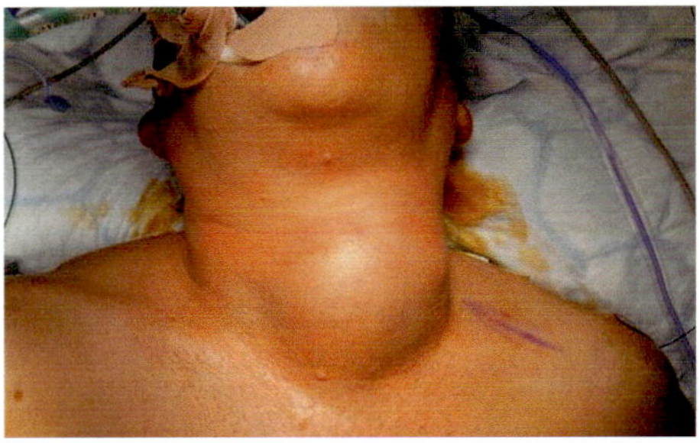

Fig. 26.4 Picture of the neck at the start of the operation

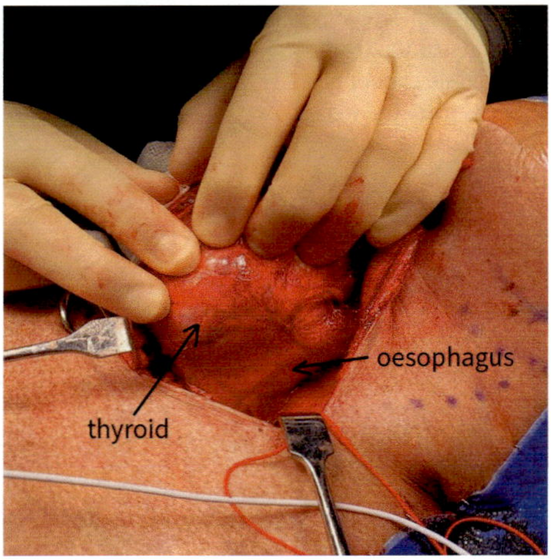

Fig. 26.5 The left lobe of the thyroid is retracted medially. The impression of the nasogastric tube can be seen in the oesophagus, but at this stage, there is no apparent plane between the oesophagus and the thyroid

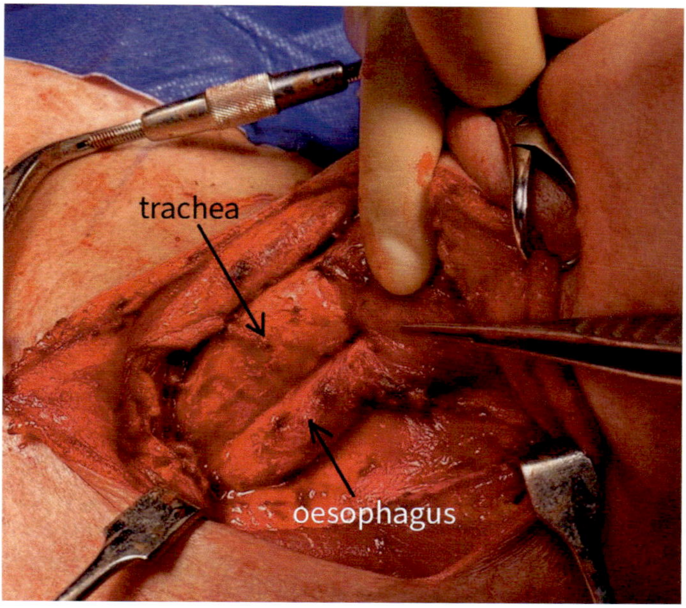

Fig. 26.6 Thyroidectomy completed with en bloc excision of the strap muscles. The forceps are pointing to the cricopharyngeus. The oesophagus below has been denuded of most of its muscle

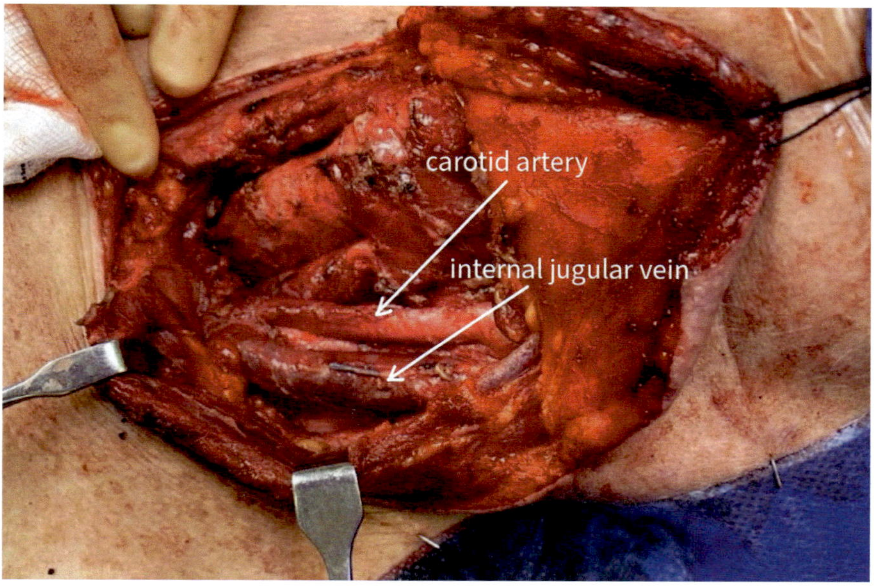

Fig. 26.7 Picture after completing the lymphadenectomy. The carotid artery and internal jugular veins can be seen lateral to the trachea and oesophagus

administered 60 Gr of adjuvant radiotherapy in 30 fractions. Three months following this, she was well, swallowing normally, and an MRI of the head and neck showed no recurrent disease.

26.1.2 Learning Points

Preoperative imaging showed compression of the oesophagus by the thyroid mass with no visible plane between the two structures. In such a case, it is still worth proceeding with a resection if recommended by the MDT. In such a situation, only trial dissection can determine whether an R0 resection is achievable. Concerning the involvement of the oesophagus in thyroid malignancy, my experience is that the oesophagus is usually compressed rather than infiltrated. However, even when there is infiltration, this is rarely full thickness. If necessary, it is possible to excise the oesophagus muscles in the affected area, along with the inferior constrictor. The mucosa in the pharynx and upper oesophagus is quite thick and can be left denuded without a risk of leakage. Swallowing may be affected, and this often results in an outpouching of the mucosa or a pharyngeal pseudodiverticulum. It is important to be aware of the anatomy of the thoracic duct in the neck and attempt to identify and ligate it as part of a radical resection as in this case. Damage to the duct can result in a prolonged chyle leak.

26.2 Recurrent Parathyroid Cancer Infiltrating the Pharyngeal Muscles and Oesophagus

26.2.1 Case Summary

A woman in her 60s with a history of total thyroidectomy for parathyroid cancer was referred with recurrent disease. At the time of the original surgery, there was a fleshy mass at the upper pole of the left lobe of the thyroid associated with a severe desmoplastic reaction. The patient was symptomatic with very high calcium levels associated with markedly raised (34 pmol/l) PTH levels. CT and MRI of the head and neck showed features of parathyroidomatosis with at least 20 visible foci of disease with the most cranial focus lying behind and on the left side of the hypopharynx at the level of the thyroid cartilage (Fig. 26.8). Some foci were located in the strap muscles and the medial aspect of the left sternomastoid. Her case was discussed at the endocrine cancer MDT meeting, and it was recommended that the recurrent tumours be resected with the primary aim of controlling the hypercalcaemia and the possibility of adjuvant treatment for any residual disease.

At operation, the left side of the neck was approached through a collar incision. Multiple parathyroid nodules were found dispersed all over the strap muscles and part

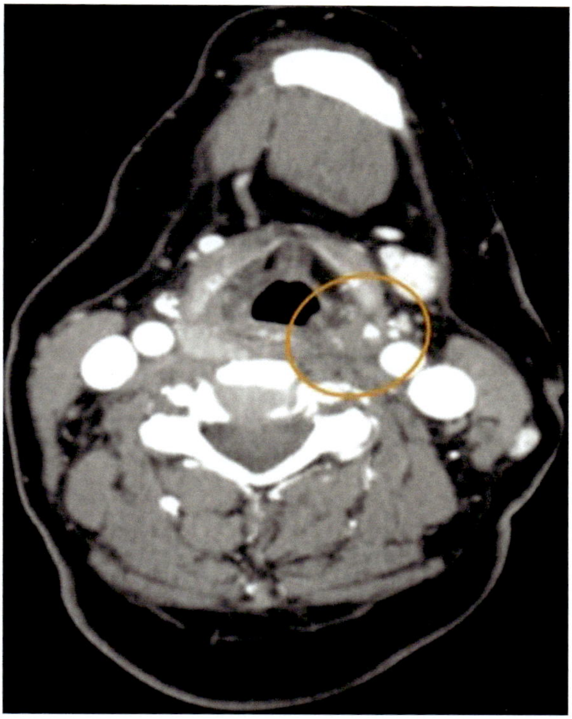

Fig. 26.8 CT section of the neck, with ellipse outlining tumour mass involving the hypopharynx on the left

of the sternocleidomastoid, the left thyroid bed and the inferior pharyngeal muscles. The left recurrent laryngeal nerve was identified within the fibrotic tissue related to previous surgery. It was not infiltrated by tumour and was left undisturbed. The strap muscles were excised, and a retro-pharyngeal mass of tumour was mobilised and removed en bloc with the inferior constrictor muscle (Figs. 26.9 and 26.10). A lymphadenectomy of the level VI lymph nodes was also carried out. Intraoperative PTH monitoring showed the level to be 40 pmol/l before the first incision (normal < 6.9), 10.6 post excision, falling to 6.6 fifteen minutes after completion of surgery. The patient made an uneventful post-operative recovery.

Histology showed multifocal, recurrent parathyroid carcinoma with extensive skeletal muscle invasion and multifocal angioinvasion. The excised lymph nodes were free of tumour. Her PTH and calcium levels returned to normal, and she has had no difficulty swallowing. Adjuvant radiotherapy has been recommended because of the high risk of recurrence.

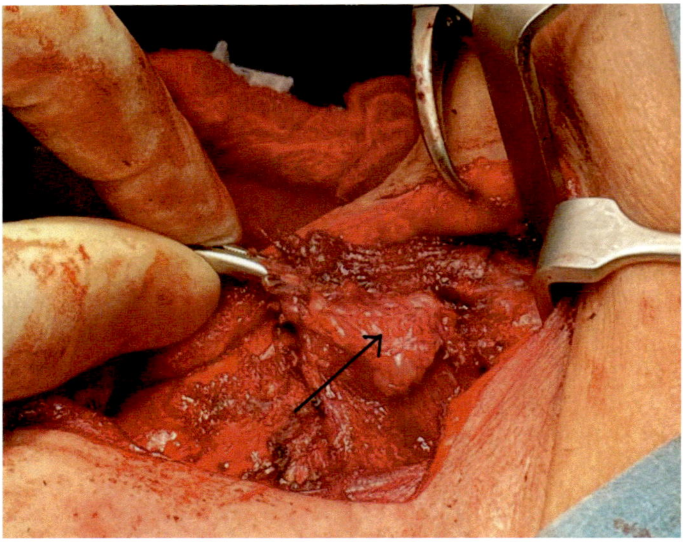

Fig. 26.9 Picture showing the left-sided tumour mass mobilised from the spine but still attached to fibres of the middle constrictor muscle

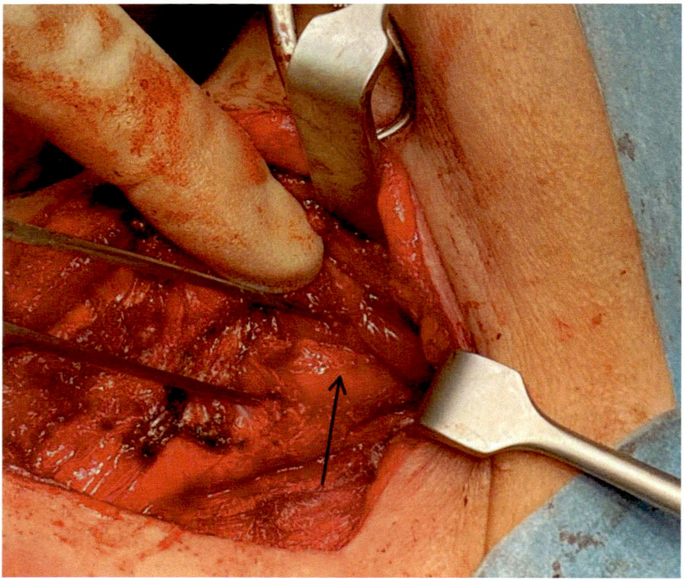

Fig. 26.10 Picture after removing the tumour mass and the attached muscle with the pharyngeal mucosa exposed (arrow), but undamaged

26.2.2 Learning Points

In this case, the preoperative imaging suggested infiltration of the strap and pharyngeal muscles with the tumour. This was confirmed at surgery, but it was possible to excise the tumour with the muscle of the inferior pharyngeal constrictor. The purpose was not necessarily to achieve an R0 resection but to debulk the tumour for better control of the calcium. Although there was a desmoplastic reaction around the tumour deposits, there was a normal plane between the pharyngeal muscle and the thick underlying mucosa.

26.3 Oesophageal Schwannoma

26.3.1 Case Summary

A woman in her 40s presented with a three-month history of swallowing difficulty. She was initially referred for an ENT opinion, and nasoendoscopy was found to be normal. OGD was attempted but the endoscopist was unable to negotiate the scope past an extraluminal swelling in the upper oesophagus. CT and FDG-PET scans showed a 9 × 5 cm mass in the upper mediastinum with an SUV max of 20.7. The mass extended from the thoracic inlet to the level of the carina causing some narrowing of the trachea (Figs. 26.11 and 26.12). EUS with core biopsies showed features of a Schwannoma. The case was discussed in the MDT meeting with the attendance of thoracic and head and neck surgeons. The recommendation was to offer the patient surgery, which was expected to be complex because of the size and position of the lesion despite its presumed benign nature.

OGD before commencing surgery showed bulging of an extraluminal lesion into the oesophagus at 17 cm. from the incisors. After positioning the patient, a right thoracotomy was performed and the azygous vein was ligated and divided. As the upper lobe of the right lung had been completely compressed by the lesion, it was resected. Attempts were made to “shell out” the lesion through an oesophageal myotomy, but it appeared to be fixed to the mucosa and therefore the decision was taken to proceed to a formal resection. The oesophagus and the lesion were separated from

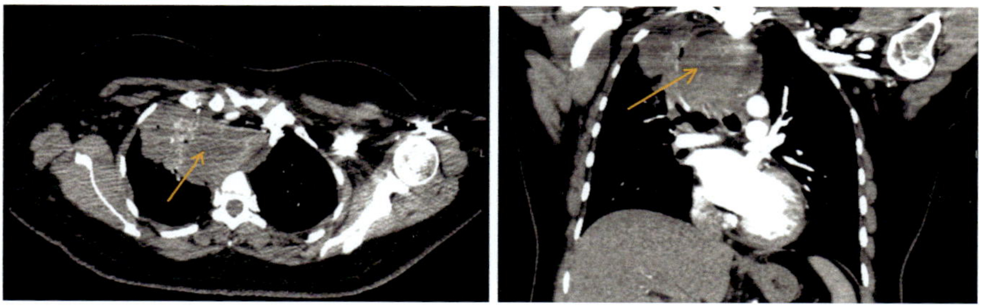

Fig. 26.11 Axial and coronal CT sections, showing a large mass in the superior mediastinum

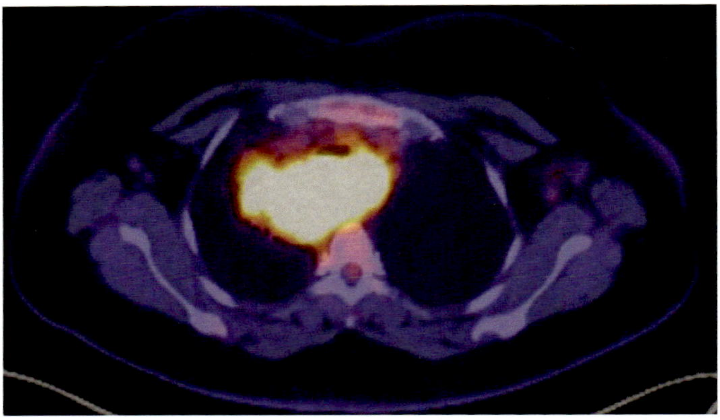

Fig. 26.12 Section from the PET scan, showing the lesion to be intensely FDG avid

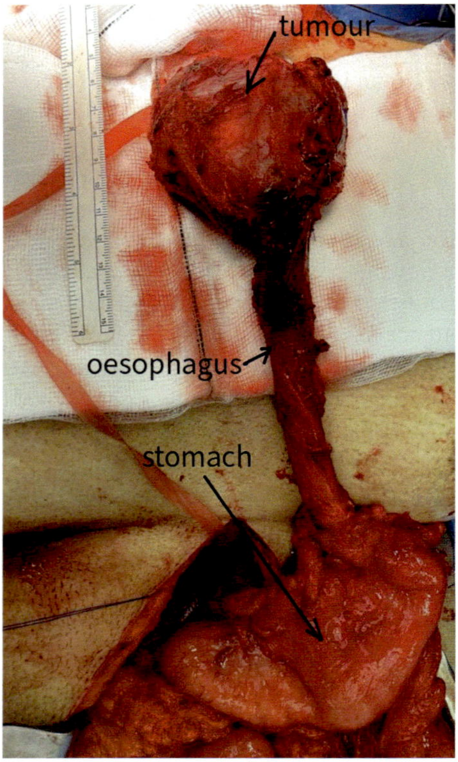

Fig. 26.13 Mass shown with the attached oesophagus and mobilised stomach prior to resection and preparation of gastric conduit

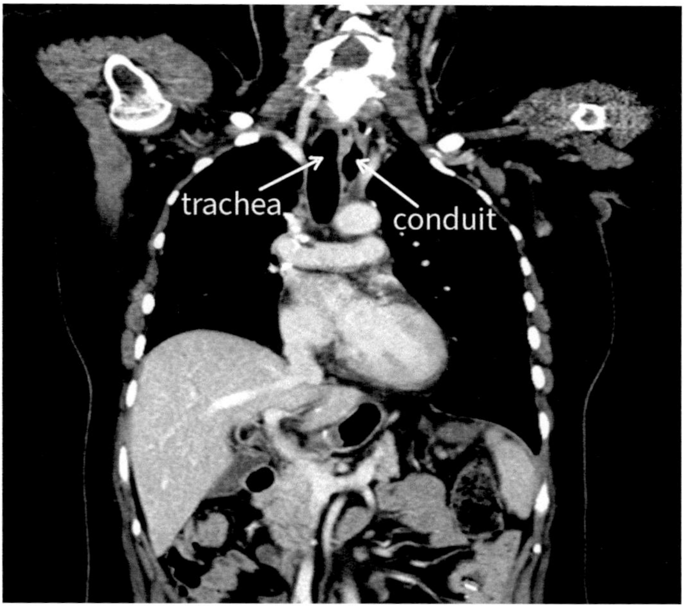

Fig. 26.14 Post-operative coronal CT section

the trachea from the apex of the chest to the diaphragm. The upper lobe of the right lung was found to be attenuated due to compression from the mass and was resected. The chest was closed, and the patient was positioned supine. A laparotomy was carried out and the stomach was mobilised on the right gastric and gastroepiploeic vessels. Through a collar incision, the sternomastoid muscles were mobilised to provide wide access and approach from both sides of the neck. After mobilising the mass, the cervical oesophagus was transected above the mass. The tumour was removed with the mobilised intrathoracic oesophagus (Fig. 26.13). A gastric conduit was prepared in the usual fashion and brought up into the neck through the chest, and anastomosed to the oesophageal stump with interrupted 3/0 PDS. Figure 26.14 shows the postoperative appearances.

The patient made an uneventful post-operative recovery and histology confirmed a Schwannoma.

26.3.2 Learning Points

Schwannoma of the oesophagus is an uncommon but recognised condition with the lesion often getting to a large size before causing any symptoms [2]. In this case, it was important to first establish the nature of the mass to plan treatment, in particular, whether a radical resection and lymphadenectomy were required. Having confirmed that the lesion was a Schwannoma dissection could be kept close to the mass when separating it from the surrounding structures. The position of the mass posed a challenge to access requiring an approach from the neck and the chest in order to mobilise it completely. The prolonged compression of the upper lobe of the right lung also necessitated a lobectomy. The technical challenges posed by this case required the joint working between Head and Neck, thoracic and upper GI surgeons.

References

1. Ohshima A, Yamashita H, Noguchi S. Endoscopic ultrasonography in the evaluation of thyroid cancer invasion into the esophagus. Surgery. 2000;127(4):478–79. https://doi.org/10.1067/msy.2000.105860.
2. Samarasam I, Chandran S, Kurian S, Mathew G. Giant oesophageal schwannomaxe "oesophageal schwannoma." Surg Pract. 2009;13(1):26–9. https://doi.org/10.1111/j.1744-1633.2008.00433.x.

Chapter 27
Complications of Childhood Oesophageal Surgery

Abstract This chapter explores the long-term complications arising from childhood surgeries of the oesophagus, with a focus on sequelae emerging in adult life. It particularly discusses the challenges faced by individuals born with oesophageal atresia and those undergoing surgery for gastro-oesophageal reflux in childhood, who later experience recurrence of symptoms or hiatus hernia. Highlighted cases include issues such as poorly emptying colonic conduits and baggy colonic conduits with distal strictures, stemming from surgeries performed in infancy. The narrative emphasises the importance of meticulous examination and interpretation of investigative findings to guide appropriate management decisions, underscoring the complexity of addressing complications arising from childhood oesophageal surgeries in adulthood.

Keywords Childhood surgery · Oesophageal atresia · Gastro-oesophageal reflux · Long-term sequelae · Colonic conduit · Strictures · Hiatus hernia · Achalasia · Thoracotomy · Surgical management

The sequelae of childhood surgery for conditions of the oesophagus and stomach can present in adult life. This applies particularly to children born with oesophageal atresia, especially long gap atresia [1] but also those who undergo surgery for gastro-oesophageal reflux as children and present with recurrence of symptoms or hiatus hernia in adult life.

Children born with oesophageal atresia show a higher incidence of oesophagitis, both peptic and eosinophilic, as well as Barrett's oesophagus. Recurrent strictures are not uncommon, and there may be late complications of oesophageal reconstruction with colon. Another group of children who may present with conduit related problems in adult life are those who have had oesophageal reconstruction for damage to the oesophagus caused by ingestion of chemicals and batteries.

M. Mughal, *Reconstructive Surgery of the Oesophagus and Stomach*,
https://doi.org/10.1007/978-3-031-66846-3_27

27.1 Poorly Emptying Colonic Conduit

27.1.1 Case Summary

A teenage boy was referred by paediatric surgeons with a history of pharyngolaryngectomy, oesophagectomy, tracheostomy and colonic interposition for caustic ingestion with a hypo-pharyngeal stricture at the age of eight. He had developed normally and was able to communicate using laryngeal speech. He described a feeling of build up of food in the chest when eating. He had undergone several dilatations for his conduit without benefit. No records of the dilatation procedures were available, and therefore the findings and indications for dilatation were unknown. A CT scan showed a non-dilated colonic conduit lying in the bed of the excised oesophagus (Fig. 27.1).

A barium swallow showed that swallowing was initiated normally, and the oropharynx appeared unremarkable. There was a slight pooling of barium at the distal end of the interposition, which cleared within 20–30 seconds. A marshmallow study was performed, and again, these passed freely across the distal anastomosis with only a short delay at the distal end of the colonic interposition (Fig. 27.2).

Endoscopy showed a healthy and relatively straight colonic conduit with no inflammation, stricturing or pooling of fluid. The distal 2 cm of the oesophagus

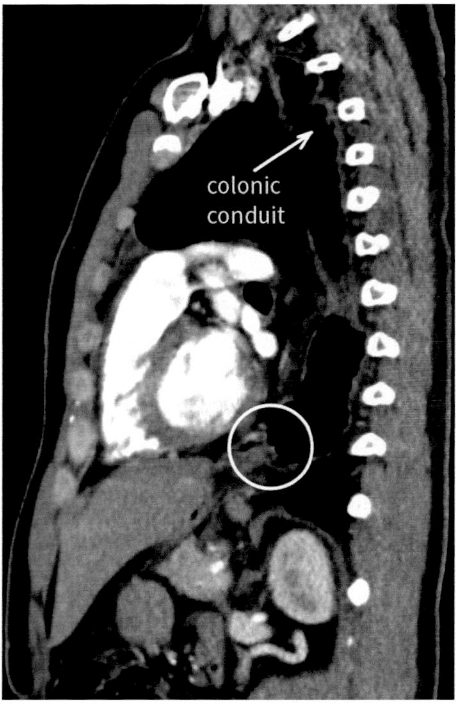

Fig. 27.1 Sagittal CT section, showing the colonic conduit anastomosed to a small length of retained oesophagus above the GOJ

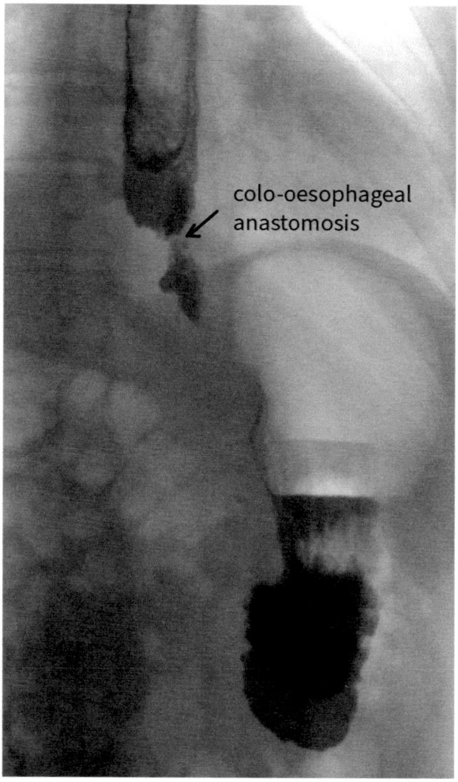

Fig. 27.2 Barium swallow showing a relatively straight colonic conduit anastomosed to the retained oesophagus 2 cm above the GOJ, which is below the diaphragm

appeared to have been retained with the colon anastomosed to it. The gastro-oesophageal junction appeared normal on retroflexion with the appearances of a normally functioning lower oesophageal sphincter gripping the scope (Fig. 27.3). Indeed, reviewing the CT scan (Fig. 27.1) confirmed the endoscopy findings.

The patient was advised to eat slowly and chew his food carefully and was reassured that no surgical intervention was required.

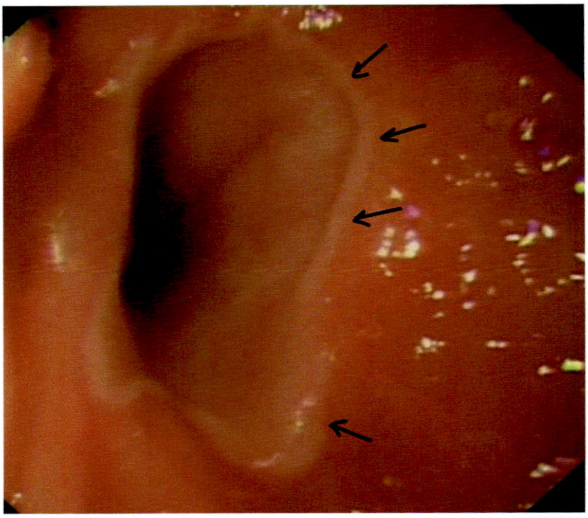

Fig. 27.3 OGD views with arrows indicating demarcation between oesophageal and colonic mucosa

27.1.2 Learning Points

It is unclear what had been dilated previously as there was no stricture at the colo-oesophageal anastomosis. In retrospect, it had not been appreciated that the distal anastomosis of the colonic conduit was to a short stump of the oesophagus with a normal gastro-oesophageal junction. There was no stricture at the anastomosis. The colonic conduit had not become elongated and sigmoid, as is often the case. In all likelihood, the symptoms were due to a normally functioning gastro-oesophageal sphincter joined to a colonic conduit that does not have the same motility as the native oesophagus. High-resolution manometry would have been informative, but the patient refused to have it.

This case highlights the value of careful examination of the different investigations for correct interpretation.

27.2 A Baggy Colonic Conduit with a Distal Stricture

27.2.1 Case Summary

A woman in her 60s was referred with a history of recurrent aspiration and progressive dysphagia. She was born with oesophageal atresia and underwent several operations in infancy, eventually resulting in reconstruction with a colonic conduit. She had gone through most of her adult life without significant problems until three years before referral. Barium swallow showed a distended, baggy colonic conduit with ingested contrast taking 36 hours to clear (Fig. 27.4).

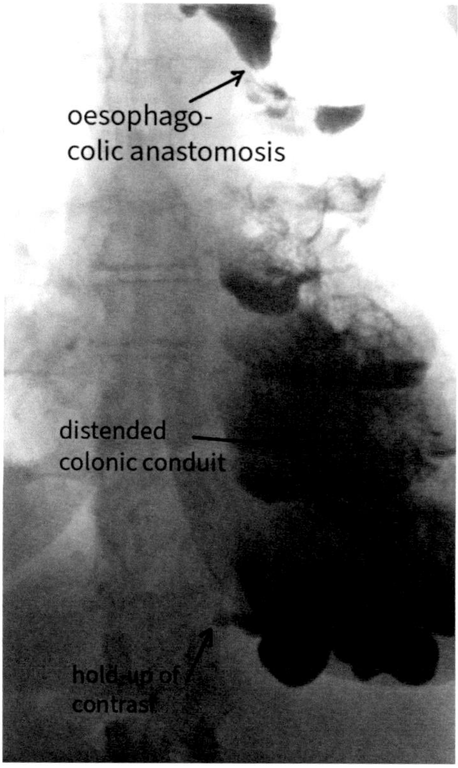

Fig. 27.4 Barium swallow, showing a baggy, distended colonic conduit with retention of contrast two hours after ingestion

OGD showed a stricture at the distal colonic anastomosis. The stricture had been dilated twice with temporary improvement in swallowing, but it became increasingly difficult to traverse with a guide wire (Fig. 27.5).

We attempted a hybrid approach but failed to traverse the stricture through a combined radiological and endoscopic approach. After an MDT discussion, the options considered were replacing the colonic conduit with a gastric conduit, if possible, or, failing that, a stricturoplasty. CT scan of the chest and abdomen with CT angiography was performed to assess the stomach anatomically and its blood supply. The stomach appeared to be intact, with normal anatomy and blood supply. Cardiorespiratory function tests and an anaesthetic assessment indicated that the patient was not fit for thoracotomy due to poor respiratory function from repeated aspiration and bronchiectasis. The decision was therefore made to offer her the lesser procedure of a stricturoplasty.

A laparotomy was performed, and the oesophageal hiatus opened, which revealed a normal gastro-oesophageal junction with what appeared to be a retained short segment of normal oesophagus anastomosed to the colon conduit (Fig. 27.6). The GOJ appeared thickened. These findings suggested that the stricture was not at the distal colonic anastomosis but at the GOJ. A cardioplasty was performed (Fig. 27.6), after which the patient made an uneventful post-operative recovery, with

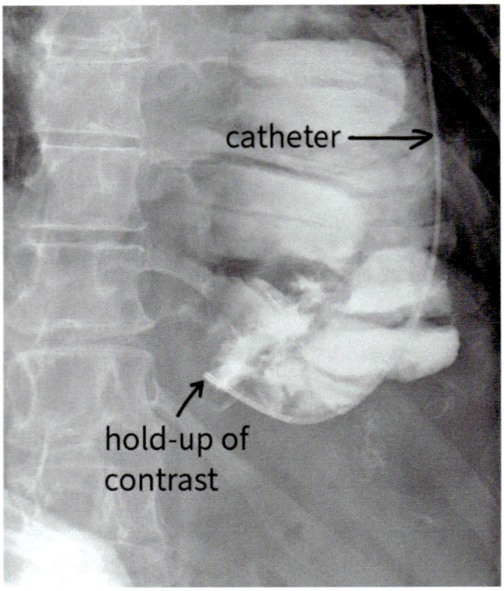

Fig. 27.5 Screening image during combined endoscopy and fluoroscopy, which failed to traverse the stricture

an improvement in her swallowing. Her reflux symptoms worsened, but these were treated medically. An endoscopy two months after the procedure showed a patent cardioplasty.

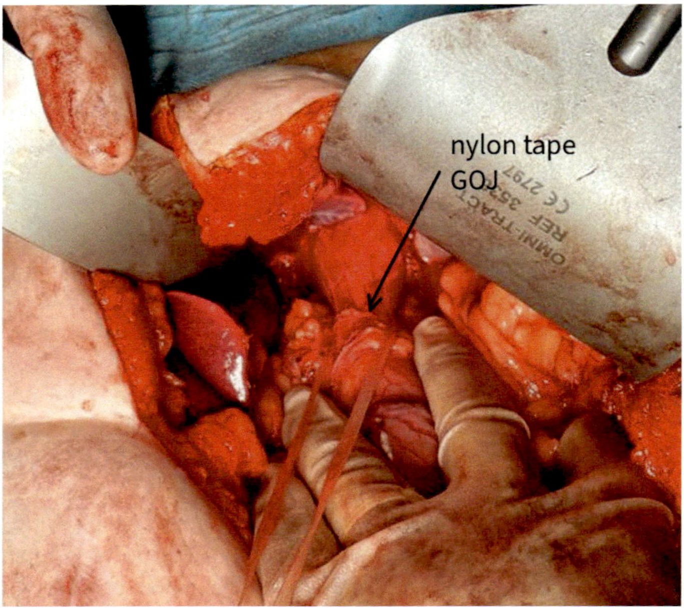

Fig. 27.6 GOJ dissected out and encircled with a nylon tape

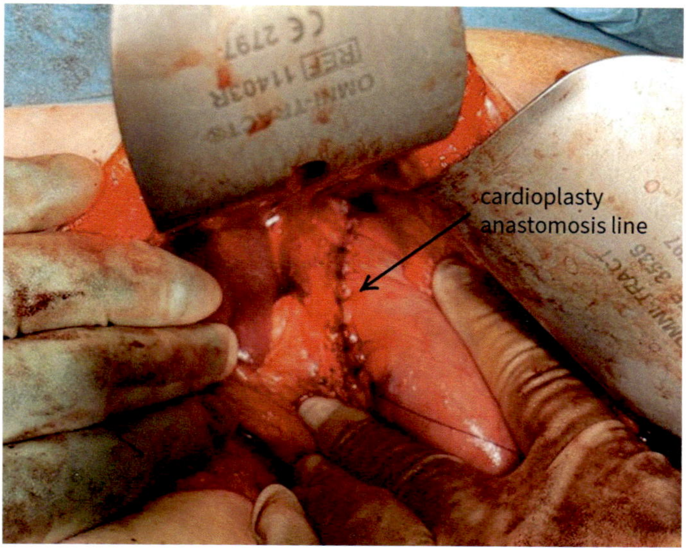

Fig. 27.7 Completed cardioplasty

27.2.2 Learning Points

The original plan for this patient was to excise the colonic conduit and replace it with a gastric conduit. I had done this in two cases previously, and it has been reported by others [2]. Unfortunately, the patient's respiratory function had deteriorated so much that by the time she was referred to me, she was deemed unfit to undergo a thoracotomy. Although transhiatal excision of the colonic conduit could have been performed, I would only have embarked on that if she was fit for a thoracotomy, just in case it was required. We, therefore, decided to perform a cardioplasty instead.

The normal GOJ anatomy found at laparotomy was somewhat of a surprise. Looking back, at endoscopy it had not been appreciated that the colon had been anastomosed to a small length of remnant oesophagus. Review of the endoscopy pictures showed a subtle border between in oesophageal a colonic mucosa (Fig. 27.8). Also, the CT scan performed to examine the anatomy of the stomach and its blood supply reported that "....the colo-gastric anastomosis is in the region of the lower oesophagus and the OG junction". This highlights the importance of careful review and interpretation of investigations. We had failed to appreciate this in the MDT review of the case.

The stricture was, therefore, at the GOJ and not at the anastomosis between the colon and the oesophagus. There was no evidence of peptic oesophagitis, and the mucosa of the GOJ looked normal at cardioplasty. One can speculate that the underlying abnormality was a hypertensive lower oesophageal sphincter of uncertain aetiology.

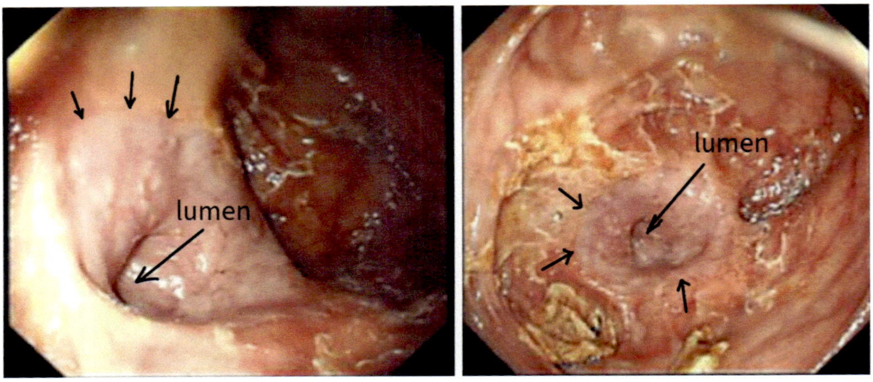

Fig. 27.8 Review of endoscopy images with arrows indicating the demarcation between mucosa of the colon and the short, retained oesophagus and the stricture at the GOJ

References

1. Aumar M, Nicolas A, Sfeir R, Seguy D, Gottrand F. Long term digestive outcome of oesophageal atresia. Best Pract Res Clin Gastroenterol Congenital GI Disorders. 2022;56–57:101771. https://doi.org/10.1016/j.bpg.2021.101771.
2. Baggaley A, Reid T, Davidson J, De Coppi P, Botha A. Late life revision surgery for dilated colonic conduit in long gap oesophageal atresia. Ann. Royal Coll Surg Engl. 2018;100(7):e185–87. https://doi.org/10.1308/rcsann.2018.0120.

Chapter 28
Failed Heller's Myotomy and End-Stage Achalasia

Abstract This chapter highlights the complexities surrounding the management of patients who experience recurrence or persistent symptoms after Heller's myotomy for achalasia. Common causes of failure include inadequate myotomy, fibrosis-induced stenosis, and perforations during the procedure. Various treatment options for recurrent symptoms are explored, ranging from conservative approaches to more invasive interventions like re-myotomy, pneumatic dilatation, and oesophagectomy. Additionally, the chapter discusses the utility of cardioplasty as a technique for addressing failed myotomies, with detailed case summaries highlighting both open and laparoscopic approaches. In cases of end-stage achalasia where other interventions fail, oesophagectomy with gastric conduit reconstruction may be considered, albeit with significant surgical challenges and risks. The importance of multidisciplinary discussion and tailored treatment strategies for individual patients is underscored throughout the chapter.

Keywords Heller's myotomy · Achalasia · Failed myotomy · End-stage achalasia · Recurrence · Cardioplasty · Oesophagectomy · Laparoscopic surgery · Surgical complications · Multidisciplinary approach

The incidence of failed Heller's myotomy varies depending on the study and the definition of failure, but it generally ranges from 10 to 20% [1].

There are several reasons for failure but, in my experience, the most common reason is an inadequate myotomy, usually on the gastric side. It may not have been appreciated at the original operation that the GOJ has not been fully crossed. Also, the plane between the muscle and the mucosa becomes more tenuous as the dissection is carried on to the stomach. Dividing the muscle fibres closely applied to the gastric mucosa requires patience and diligence. Because of the higher risk of perforation on the stomach side of the myotomy, caution may result in inadequate myotomy. Other causes include stenosis due to fibrosis and stricturing due to oesophagitis. I have also seen early failure in cases where a perforation has occurred during the myotomy, which was then abandoned to repair the perforation.

M. Mughal, *Reconstructive Surgery of the Oesophagus and Stomach*,
https://doi.org/10.1007/978-3-031-66846-3_28

Recurrence after cardiomyotomy can be managed in different ways. This includes a conservative approach with the patient accepting their symptoms and making dietary adjustments. They may have noticed a deterioration of swallowing after an initial marked improvement, but even after deterioration the symptoms may be considered to be better than before the operation. In this regard, the Eckardt score and a timed barium swallow are useful metrics of symptomatology and oesophageal anatomy and emptying.

Many different factors have to be taken into account to determine the best course of action after a failed cardiomyotomy and such cases are best discussed by an MDT with the appropriate expertise. Further interventions include a remyotomy, pneumatic dilatation, the POEM procedure, cardioplasty, and, ultimately, an oesophagectomy when all other options have failed.

28.1 Cardioplasty

Cardioplasty is a useful technique after failed cardiomyotomy and in some cases of end-stage achalasia. The principle is to open up the gastroesophageal junction by making a full-thickness incision through it and then performing a plasty of some sort.

Many intriguing and complex techniques of cardioplasty have been described [2]. Some of the procedures described include the creation of an antireflux mechanism. With the advent of laparoscopic surgery, minimally invasive techniques have been described using a stapler applied across the GOJ using the fundus to create the plasty [3].

I describe the technique in two cases. In one case it was performed open because of adhesions from previous surgery and in the other laparoscopically.

28.2 Open Cardioplasty

28.3 Case Summary

A teenage girl was referred with recurrent dysphagia after a laparoscopic cardiomyotomy for achalasia three years previously with good initial symptom relief. OGD showed the GOJ to be tight, although the scope could be passed into the stomach with some pressure. HRM showed features of achalasia with a persistent barrier pressure at the GOJ. She had undergone a pneumatic dilatation and a trial of nifedipine without benefit. As she had undergone multiple open abdominal operations previously, including resiting of gastrostomies, it was decided to offer her a cardioplasty as an open procedure.

At laparotomy, adhesions were found between the liver and the proximal stomach. These were divided to mobilise the distal oesophagus and the GOJ. The fundus of the stomach was also mobilised by dividing the upper short gastric vessels, and the anterior vagus nerve was reflected to the right to ensure that it was not incorporated in the cardioplasty. The fundus was sutured to the side of the oesophagus for a length of about 3 cm before making the incision to start the cardioplasty.

The oesophageal limb of the incision started 3 cm above the GOJ, extending 2 cm below the angle of His and the gastric limb was carried upwards onto the fundus for 5 cm. It is important that the two limbs of the V-incision are of equal length (Fig. 28.1). The cardioplasty is then performed by suturing the layers as shown below (Figs. 28.2 and 28.3).

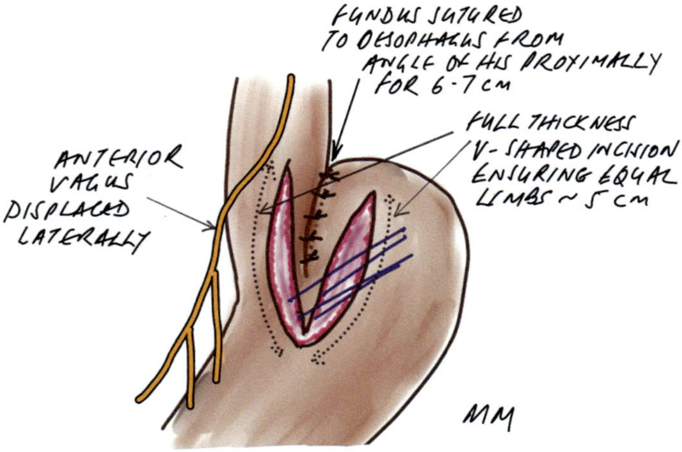

Fig. 28.1 Diagram showing the posterior layer sutures being placed

Fig. 28.2 Posterior layer completed and anterior sutures being placed

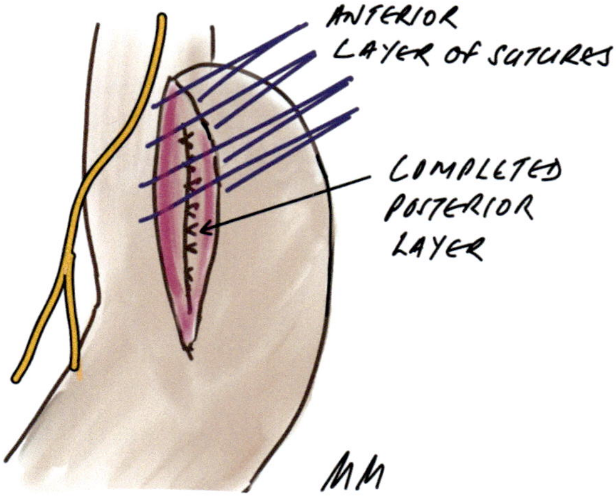

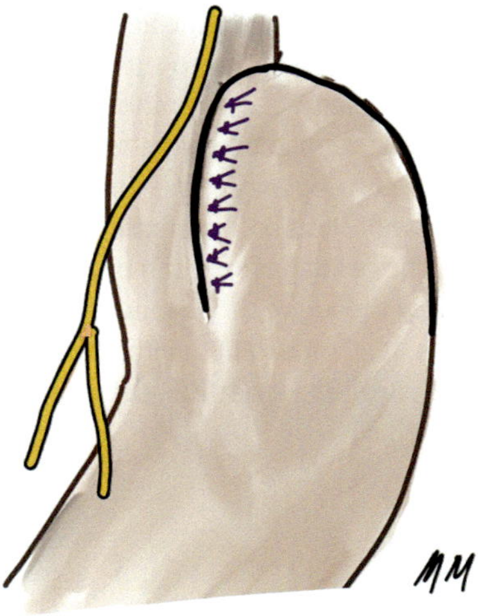

Fig. 28.3 Completed cardioplasty

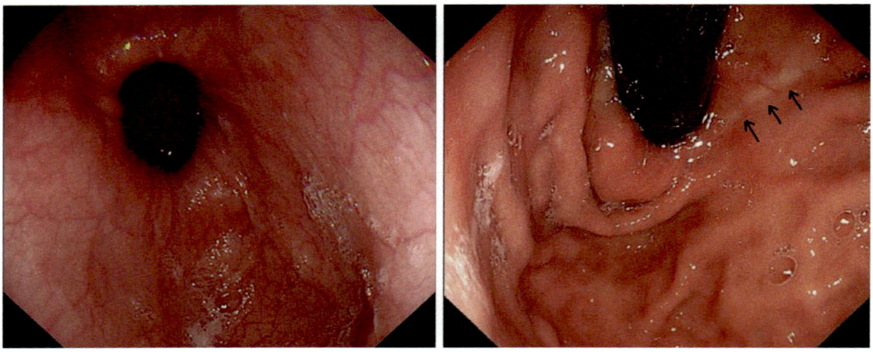

Fig. 28.4 OGD appearances three months after cardioplasty, showing a widely open cardia on the forward view, and the scar of the cardioplasty seen on retroflexion

She made an uneventful post-operative recovery with a significant improvement in her symptoms. Contrast swallow and OGD two months after the procedure showed a widely open GOJ and satisfactory emptying of the oesophagus (Figs. 28.4 and 28.5).

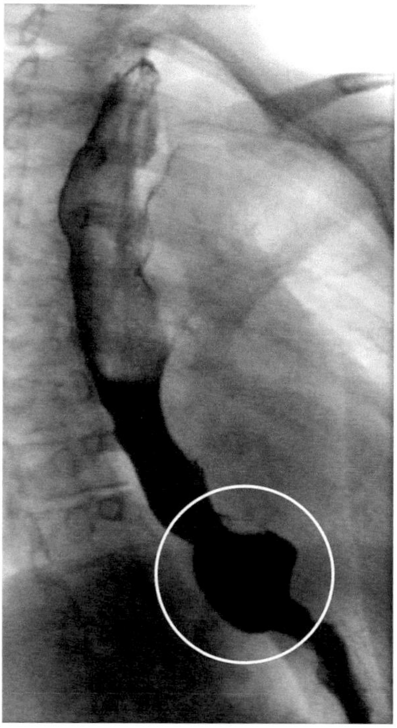

Fig. 28.5 Contrast study, showing widely open GOJ three months after cardioplasty

28.3.1 Learning Points

This patient was offered a further Rigiflex dilatation, but she refused. She was treated nine years previously, and the alternative treatment today would have been to consider a POEM procedure. A technical point to emphasise for an open cardioplasty is to spend time setting it up before starting the plasty. This includes ensuring at least 6–8 cm of oesophagus is mobilised, the GOJ is clearly displayed by removing or reflecting the fat pad and the anterior vagus is retracted to the right to stop its incorporation in the suture line.

28.4 Laparoscopic Cardioplasty

28.4.1 Case Summary

A woman in her 30s with achalasia underwent a laparoscopic Heller's myotomy which was performed with a combination of scissors, and an ultrasonic energy device. Unfortunately, this was complicated by two 5 mm perforations at the proximal and distal ends of the myotomy. These were repaired with interrupted 2/0 Ethibond.

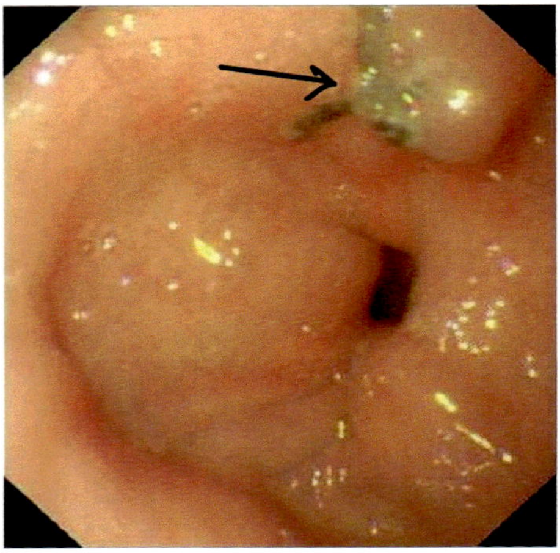

Fig. 28.6 Pre-operative OGD views showing the suture in the oesophagus above the GOJ and a tight sphicter

The patient was kept nil by mouth for two days and resumed oral fluids after a contrast swallow excluded a leak. However, she remained symptomatic with difficulty in swallowing almost to the same degree as before her operation. OGD showed a tight lower oesophageal sphincter (Fig. 28.6) and she underwent a Rigiflex balloon dilatation 18 months later with short-lived improvement in her symptoms. She was then offered a cardioplasty which was performed laparoscopically.

At laparoscopy, dense adhesions were encountered around the cardia which were divided to dissect out the gastro-oesophageal junction. The oesophagus was mobilised to deliver 5 cm into the abdomen, and a cardioplasty was performed by introducing a 60 mm linear stapler through a gastrotomy in the anterior wall of the stomach, 4 cm below the GOJ. The correct positioning of the stapler was checked with endoscopy to ensure that one jaw was properly positioned in the oesophagus. After firing the stapler and closing the gastrotomy, the cardioplasty was inspected with the scope. The patient made an uneventful post-operative recovery and OGD and contrast swallow six weeks later showed a satisfactory cardioplasty with good emptying of the oesophagus (Figs. 28.7 and 28.8).

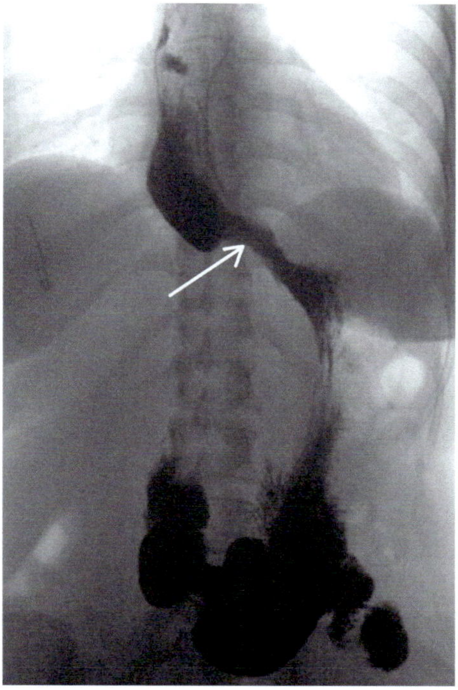

Fig. 28.7 Barium study three months after cardioplasty showing a widely open GOJ

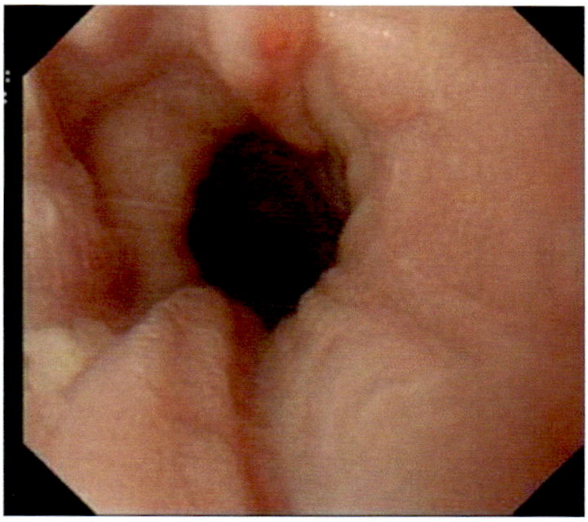

Fig. 28.8 OGD appearances three months after cardioplasty, showing a wide open GOJ and oesophagitis

28.4.2 Learning Points

In this case, suturing of the perforation during the cardiomyotomy was likely to have contributed to the failure of the operation. A Rigiflex dilatation only gave short-term relief but, in view of the previous cardiomyotomy, repeating it was considered to be risky because of the increased risk of perforation. Although the patient had a significant improvement in her swallowing after the cardioplasty, she experienced gastro-oesophageal reflux, and OGD showed oesophagitis. Reflux is unfortunately a complication of cardioplasty, and it is important that this is explained to the patient during the counselling.

This patient was treated six years ago. Now, a POEM procedure would have been considered.

28.5 End-Stage Achalasia

End-stage achalasia is defined as the most severe decompensated state of the condition. A review by Duranceau suggested that despite treatment with pneumatic dilatation and cardiomyotomy, 10–15% of patients will go on to have progressive deterioration, and up to 5% may eventually require an oesophagectomy [4]. Some experts believe that even with a dilated tortuous oesophagus, a cardiomyotomy should be the first option, reserving oesophagectomy for patients who end up with a dilated tortuous oesophagus after multiple failed treatments.

Various operations have been described, including oesophagectomy with gastric transposition to the apex of the chest or neck, as well as colonic and jejunal interposition. Jejunal interposition using the Merendino technique has been described with mixed results and some experts advocate just a cardioplasty because it is relatively straightforward, and does not carry the morbidity of a resection and bowel interposition. Kiss has reported on the use of oesophagoplication to abolish the sigmoid dilatation of the oesophagus in 14 patients with good results [5] (Fig. 28.9).

Oesophagectomy with colon interposition has been reported by several authors, with Peters describing good results in the majority of 15 patients followed up for 1–14 years [6].

With the progress in interventional endoscopic procedures, such as endoscopic plication of the stomach, a similar approach has been used in a small series of patients with a megaoesophagus. Hedberg and Ujiki have reported good symptomatic outcomes with the technique they described as POPE (per oral plication of the oesophagus) [7].

Because of the heterogeneity of cases reported, there is a lack of evidence on how best to treat this condition. However, it is important to discuss such cases in an MDT and recommend interventions tailored to the patient's symptoms and co-morbidity, as well as carefully taking the risks and benefits into account.

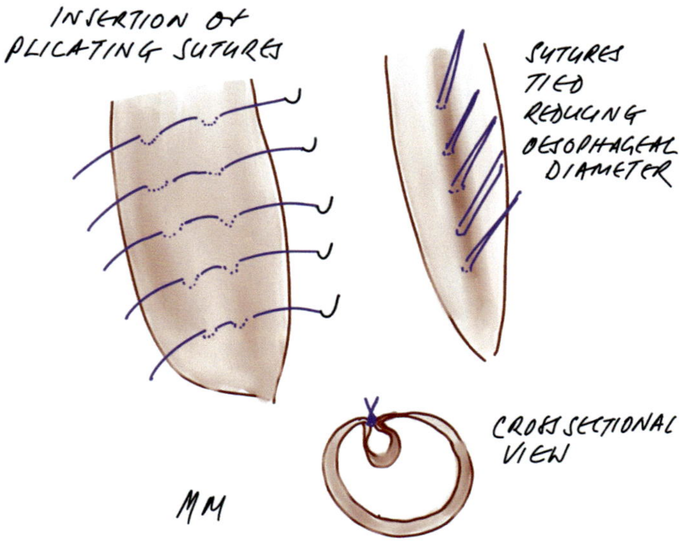

Fig. 28.9 Illustration of suture oesophagoplasty as described by Kiss et al.

28.6 Oesophagectomy for End-Stage Achalasia

28.6.1 Case Summary

A man in his 40s with a long history of swallowing difficulties had a barium swallow that showed a massively dilated oesophagus with the typical GOJ appearance of achalasia. OGD confirmed a dilated oesophagus containing food residue with a tight lower oesophageal sphincter. HRM was unsuccessful as the catheter could not be positioned across the GOJ. CT scan showed a massively dilated oesophagus (Fig. 28.10). He had not undergone any previous treatment and had managed his symptoms as best as possible by adjusting his diet and lifestyle. His case was discussed at the MDT, and it was considered that for such a dilated oesophagus an oesophagectomy would be the best option.

After detailed counselling, the patient underwent an oesophagectomy. The abdominal phase to mobilise the stomach was carried out laparoscopically, preserving the right gastric and gastroepiploeic vessels and a feeding jejunostomy was placed at the same time. After closure of the abdomen, the patient was repositioned, and a right thoracotomy was performed. After dividing the azygos vein, the oesophagus was mobilised to the apex of the chest. Dissection was kept in the peri-oesophageal plane. The oesophagus was 8 cm wide at the level chosen for transection in the upper chest. The stomach conduit was 4 cm in width. To avoid a sump in the retained upper oesophagus, it was decided to staple the oesophagus obliquely, thereby creating a funnel-like configuration (Fig. 28.11).

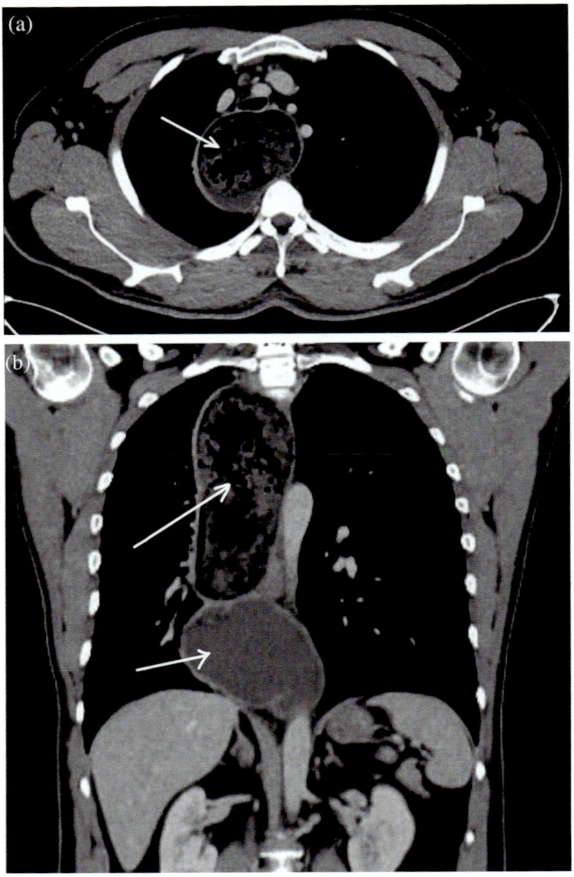

Fig. 28.10 Axial (a) and coronal (b) CT sections showing a massively dilated oesophagus, full of fluid and food

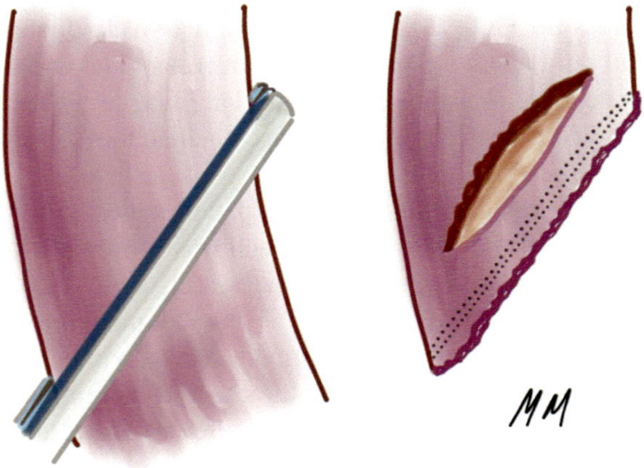

Fig. 28.11 Diagram showing oblique transection of the oesophagus using a stapler and the oesophagotomy parallel to the staple line, ready for anastomosis

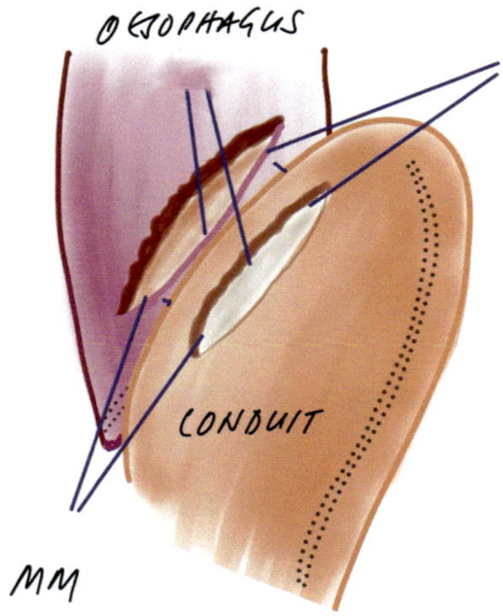

Fig. 28.12 Anastomosis of the gastric conduit commencing with interrupted sutures posteriorly

The gastric conduit was then anastomosed with interrupted 3/0 PDS sutures across a 4 cm oesophagostomy parallel to the oesophageal staple line (Fig. 28.12). The resected oesophagus and cardia are shown in Fig. 28.13. A nasogastric tube was positioned across the anastomosis into the conduit, and the chest was closed with two drains.

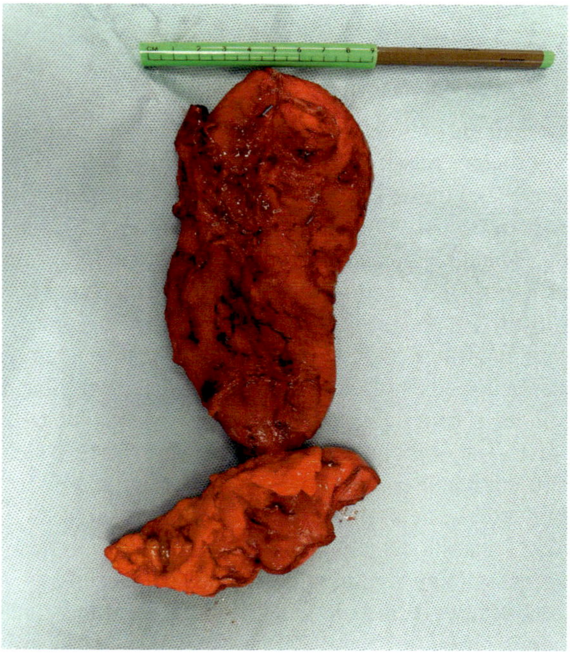

Fig. 28.13 Resected oesophagus with attached cardia

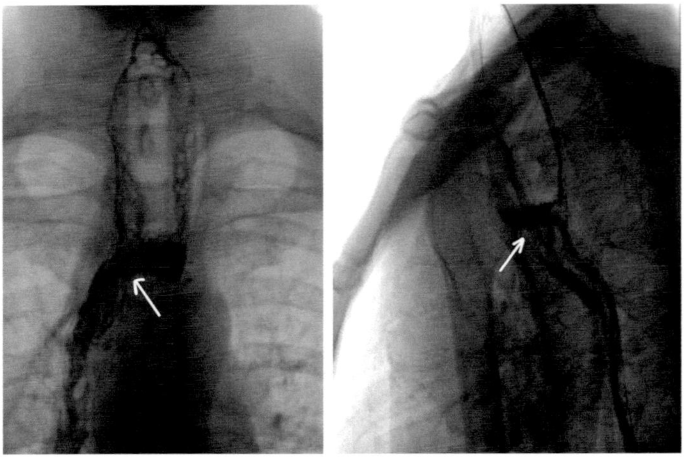

Fig. 28.14 Contrast swallow six weeks after surgery

The patient made an uneventful post-operative recovery and had near-normal swallowing when he eventually progressed to solids. A post-operative gastrografin swallow showed a satisfactory appearance of the anastomosis and good emptying of the oesophagus (Fig. 28.14).

28.6.2 Learning Points

This patient presented very late in the development of his condition, by which time the oesophagus was grossly dilated. Although less invasive procedures such as cardiomyotomy and POEM and Rigiflex were considered, it was felt that the outcome would be poor because of the capacious oesophagus. Oesophagectomy is a procedure with significant risks and complications, and therefore careful counselling was carried out with the patient, and he was given time to consider his options. He chose to go ahead with an oesophagectomy. In my experience, oesophagectomy for end-stage achalasia is more difficult than that for cancer. The distended oesophagus causes distortion of the anatomy, displacing structures away from their usual position. There is therefore the risk of damage to the airways, the thoracic duct and the recurrent laryngeal nerve. The oesophagus is often also very vascular due to neovascularisation. Therefore particular care has to be taken during the dissection to minimise bleeding by meticulous attention to haemostasis. This includes dividing the segmental vessels from the aorta, which, in my experience, tend to be larger than usual, and are better ligated or clipped rather than divided with an energy device. The mismatch between the diameter of the oesophagus (8 cm) and the conduit (4 cm) also posed a challenge. An end-to-end anastomosis would not have been feasible, and transecting the oesophagus transversely with a side-to-side anastomosis above the staple line would have resulted in an oesophageal sump with a depth of at least 2 cm. To avoid this, it was decided to staple off the oesophagus obliquely, thus avoiding or, at least, minimising the volume of the sump. This is apparent on the gastrografin swallow.

References

1. Dempsey DT. Endoscopic and surgical treatments for achalasia: a systematic review and meta-analysis. Yearbook Gastroenterol. 2009;2009:155–6. https://doi.org/10.1016/S0739-5930(09)79328-6.
2. Braghetto I, Korn O, Cardemil G, Coddou E, Valladares H, Henriquez A. Inversed Y Cardioplasty plus a Truncal Vagotomy-Antrectomy and a Roux-En-Y Gastrojejunostomy Performed in Patients with Stricture of the Esophagogastric Junction after a Failed Cardiomyotomy or endoscopic procedure in patients with achalasia of the esophagus. Dis Esophagus. 2010;23(3):208–15. https://doi.org/10.1111/j.1442-2050.2009.01021.x.
3. Griffiths EA, Devitt PG, Jamieson GG, Myers JC, Thompson SK. Laparoscopic stapled cardioplasty for end-stage achalasia. J Gastrointest Surg. 2013;17(5):997–1001. https://doi.org/10.1007/s11605-012-2111-3.
4. Duranceau A, et al. End-stage achalasia: end-stage achalasia. Dis Esophagus. 2012;25(4):319–30. https://doi.org/10.1111/j.1442-2050.2010.01157.x.
5. Kiss J, Vörös A, Szirányi E, Altorjay Á, Bohák Á (1996) Management of failed Heller's operations. Surg Today. 1996;26(7):541–45. https://doi.org/10.1007/BF00311564.
6. Peters JH. Esophageal resection with colon interposition for end-stage achalasia. Arch Surg. 1995;130(6):632. https://doi.org/10.1001/archsurg.1995.01430060070013.
7. Hedberg HM, Attaar M, McCormack MS, Ujiki MB (2023) Per-oral plication of (neo)esophagus: technical feasibility and early outcomes. J. Gastrointest. Surg. 2023;27(8):1531–38. https://doi.org/10.1007/s11605-021-05205-9.

Chapter 29
Miscellaneous Conditions

Abstract This chapter discusses three distinct cases of miscellaneous conditions affecting the upper gastrointestinal tract. The first case presents a challenging scenario of unresectable leiomyosarcoma at the gastroesophageal junction (GOJ), leading to rapid progression of dysphagia and necessitating oesophageal bypass surgery. The second case involves a complex situation of enterocutaneous fistulae alongside oesophageal perforation, requiring a combined surgical approach for repair. Lastly, chronic gastric volvulus secondary to a prior gastroenterostomy is explored, highlighting the importance of thorough investigation and surgical intervention to alleviate symptoms and restore normal anatomy. These cases underscore the need for multidisciplinary collaboration and tailored management strategies in addressing uncommon upper GI pathologies.

Keywords Leiomyosarcoma · Gastroesophageal junction · Dysphagia · Oesophageal bypass · Enterocutaneous fistulae · Oesophageal perforation · Gastric volvulus · Gastroenterostomy · Upper gastrointestinal tract · Multidisciplinary collaboration

29.1 Unresectable GOJ Leiomyosarcoma

29.1.1 Case Summary

A woman in her 40s was referred for further management of an intractable peptic stricture at the GOJ, unresponsive to dilatation. Endoscopy showed a 2.5 cm lesion at the cardia with a central ulcer. Multiple biopsies were initially inconclusive. CT scan showed slight focal thickening of the gastric wall, measuring 3 × 1.6 cm, just below and lateral to the GOJ along the lesser curve. There was no other abnormality on the scan. A repeat endoscopy was carried out and further biopsies were taken from the area of abnormality. These showed features suggestive of a spindle cell tumour. Repeat CT four weeks after the initial examination showed that the thickening had

M. Mughal, *Reconstructive Surgery of the Oesophagus and Stomach*,
https://doi.org/10.1007/978-3-031-66846-3_29

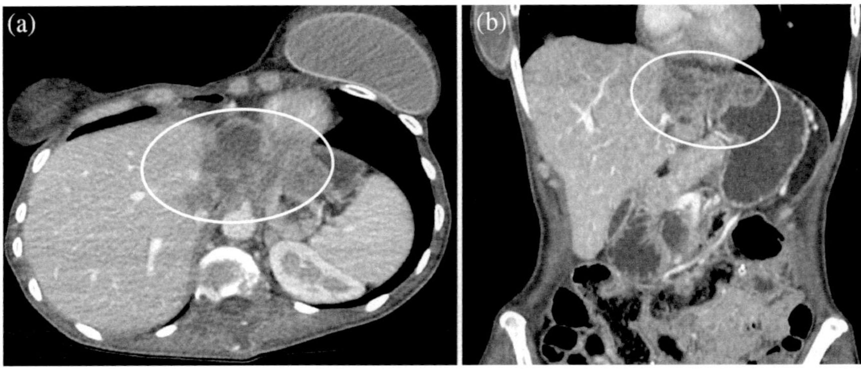

Fig. 29.1 Axial (a) and coronal (b), CT sections showing a large tumour (circled) at the GOJ invading the left lobe of liver

developed into a mass to the left of the GOJ and a tumour deposit had also appeared in the adjacent left lobe of the liver as well as spinal deposits (Fig. 29.1).

Her dysphagia progressed rapidly and became complete within two weeks, such that she was unable to swallow her own saliva. Attempts at stenting the GOJ failed. The oncology team recommended chemotherapy, and because of the complete dysphagia, the decision was made to bypass the oesophagus as well as to place a feeding jejunostomy. The stomach could not be used as a conduit because of the tumour was found to be directly invading the left lobe of the liver.

The cervical oesophagus was dissected out through a collar incision. A laparotomy was performed and a loop of the ascending colon based on the middle colic vessels was used as a conduit. The conduit was brought up to the neck through a retrosternal tunnel. The oesophagus was transected as low as possible in the superior mediastinum, the distal part was ligated, and the proximal part was anastomosed to the conduit with 4/0 PDS. The distal colon was anastomosed to the jejunum 25 cm distal to the DJ flexure. The patient developed a low volume leak from the cervical anastomosis which healed within three weeks. She was able to resume oral feeding and recovered sufficiently to commence chemotherapy. Postoperative appearances six weeks after surgery are shown in Fig. 29.2. Unfortunately the tumour did not respond to treatment and she passed away three months later.

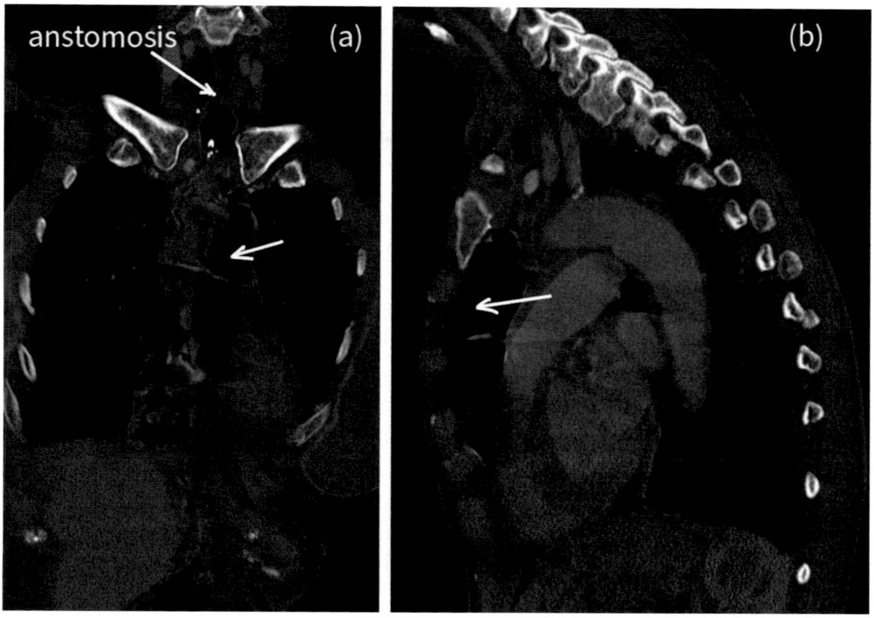

Fig. 29.2 Post-operative coronal (a) and sagittal (b) CT scan sections showing colonic conduit in the retrosternal position

29.1.2 Learning Points

This patient illustrates the aggressive nature of a leiomyosarcoma of the stomach. A subtle lesion on initial endoscopy, enlarged rapidly, infiltrating the left lobe of the liver and metastasising to the spine. I have seen several similar patients whose symptoms of dysphagia are out of proportion to a subtle and seemingly innocuous GOJ nodule on that has turned out to be submucosal adenocarcinoma or a leiomyoma. In some cases, it has been thought that the patient has achalasia, but, like this patient, turned out to have a neoplasm. Stenting of the GOJ failed in the hands of a highly experienced interventional gastroenterologist. However, as will be appreciated on examination of the limited CT sections in Fig. 29.1, the rapid growth in the tumour had virtually completely obliterated the oesophageal lumen.

The decision to carry out an oesophageal bypass was carefully considered with the involvement of the oncologists, gastroenterologists and the wider MDT. As the patient was young and previously fit, the recommendation from the MDT was to do whatever was feasible to improve her swallowing and general condition so that she could have chemotherapy. An oesophageal bypass without a thoracotomy is a relatively low-risk procedure, with the main risk being the possibility of conduit necrosis. The patient was fully informed of the risks and complications of the proposed surgery.

29.2 Combined Oesophageal Reconstruction and Repair of Entero-Cutaneous Fistula

29.2.1 Clinical History

A woman in her 50s had undergone a laparotomy for adhesions which was complicated by multiple enterotomies resulting in multiple enterocutaneous fistulae. Management included leaving the abdomen open, control of sepsis and parenteral nutrition. During her long hospital stay with multiple complications and interventions, she developed an oesophageal perforation, which was treated with a chest drain and antibiotics. The cause of the perforation was unknown. Eventually, an end cervical oesophagostomy was performed to exclude the oesophagus. The prolonged chest sepsis was eventually controlled but she developed an empyema which was treated with a radiologically placed pigtail drain. After she improved sufficiently to be considered for closure of her enterocutaneous fistula her case was discussed at the MDT meeting regarding oesophageal reconstruction. The recommendation was to combine oesophageal reconstruction with closure of the enterocutaneous fistula. It was felt that removing the excluded oesophagus would require a thoracotomy with a difficult dissection. Adding this to a 12–16 hour abdominal operation would greatly increase the morbidity. It was decided, therefore, to leave the defunctioned oesophagus in place and use the stomach as a conduit to join the cervical oesophagus.

The operation started with a laparotomy and a complete adhesiolysis, including an examination of the stomach and its blood supply, which appeared to be normal. The

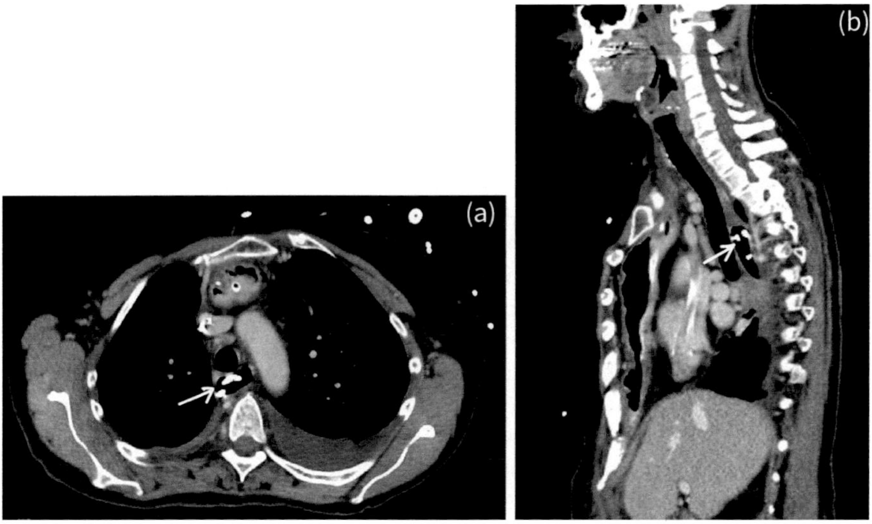

Fig. 29.3 Postoperative axial (a) and sagittal (b) CT sections showing gastric conduit in the retrosternal position and pigtail drain in the excluded oesophagus

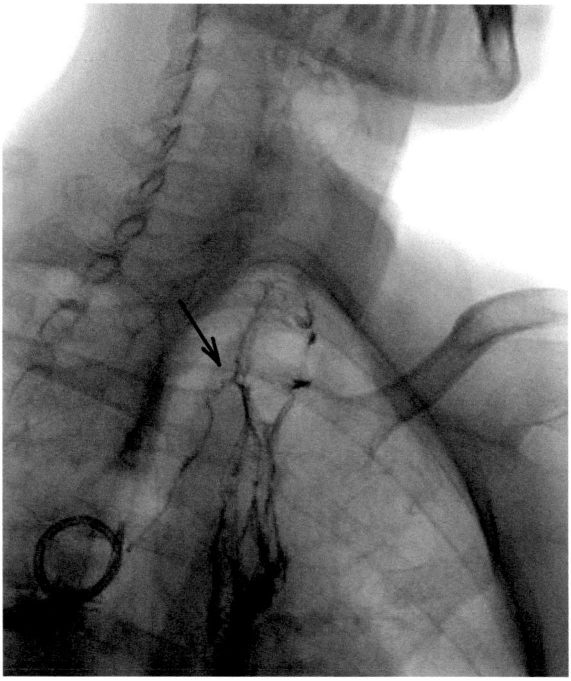

Fig. 29.4 Contrast swallow two weeks after reconstruction, showing a small leak which healed without intervention

enterocutaneous fistula was excised, resulting in a limited small bowel resection, and a primary anastomosis was performed. Through a collar incision, the oesophagostomy was taken down. A conduit was created from the mobilised stomach based on the greater curvature using staplers and retaining the separated strip of the lesser curvature attached to the oesophagus. The gastric conduit was brought up through a retrosternal tunnel and anastomosed to the oesophagus (Fig. 29.3). A Foley catheter was placed into the end of the partitioned lesser curve to provide drainage to the oesophagus, and the lesser curve was hitched up to the abdominal wall at the exit site of the Foley catheter. The patient made a straightforward post-operative recovery. A contrast swallow showed a small leak, which healed after two weeks with antibiotics and nil by mouth (Fig. 29.4).

29.2.2 Learning Points

It is not clear how the oesophageal perforation occurred. It was treated at the initial admitting hospital, where the decision had been made to limit any oesophageal interventions to a minimum, considering that the patient was seriously ill for many weeks due to her abdominal complications. When she was well enough and transferred to the intestinal failure unit, it was decided to defunction the oesophagus with an oesophagostomy. As she was on total parenteral nutrition for her enterocutaneous fistulae, there was no urgency about dealing with the oesophageal problem. However, the closure of the enterocutaneous fistula provided an opportunity for reconstructing the oesophagus, provided this could be done without excessive morbidity. The risks and benefits were carefully weighed and discussed by the MDT and with the patient. Leaving the oesophageal reconstruction to another time would avoid adding morbidity to the risk of complications associated with repair of the enterocutaneous fistula. However, the patient would have derived minimal benefit to her quality of life. She would still be unable to eat even if the enterocutaneous fistulae were successfully repaired and bowel continuity restored. Furthermore, a future attempt at oesophageal reconstruction, requiring a laparotomy, would have carried the risk of inadvertent enterotomies due to a potentially hostile abdomen. Although reconstruction combined with repair of the enterocutaneous fistula added further risk, this was thought to be manageable and the potential benefits to be significant. If both operations were successful, the patient would have a much better general outcome and quality of life. With this in mind, the sequencing of the two operations was important. It was agreed that the primary aim of the operation was to repair the enterocutaneous fistulae, and that the oesophageal reconstruction would only be carried out if the fistulae repair went well, which turned out to be the case.

This case had added layers of complexity and required a detailed plan of the operation and strategy. Also, this was one of the rare occasions when carried out an oesophageal reconstruction concurrently with colleagues who closed an enterocutaneous fistula.

29.3 Chronic Gastric Volvulus with a Complex History

29.3.1 Case Summary

A woman in her 40s was referred with a history of intermittent left upper quadrant pain and abdominal distension ever since having a gastroenterostomy in her late twenties. There were no obvious triggering factors and she had taken to adopting unusual postures to alleviate symptoms, such as lying head down on her right side. She had also experienced symptoms suggestive of dumping.

Twenty-one years previously, she had been admitted to hospital with vomiting and epigastric pain. Investigations showed gastric outlet obstruction from pyloric stenosis due to ulceration. Biopsies from the pyloric channel showed inflammatory changes only, with no evidence of malignancy. She was given a trial of treatment with PPIs, but the pyloric stenosis did not resolve. A laparoscopic anterior gastroenterostomy was therefore performed. The operation notes made no mention of any abnormality of the gastric anatomy. She remained well until developing the symptoms described above three years prior to my meeting her.

Barium studies and small bowel MRI were performed, which showed the stomach to be upside down such that the gastric fundus lay inferiorly, and the pylorus was situated above the GOJ under the left hemidiaphragm (Fig. 29.5). These features were ascribed to a mesenteroaxial volvulus of the stomach. The gastroenterostomy appeared to be at the level of the gastric fundus so that the ingested contrast entered the fundus and passed immediately and preferentially into the dependent portion of the small bowel with hardly any passing beyond the pylorus. OGD showed distortion of the body of the stomach but a healthy gastroenterostomy and a normal pylorus. The first and second parts of the duodenum appeared to be normal.

The patient's symptoms were considered to be due a combination of intermittent gastric volvulus and likely dumping related to the unusually high gastroenterostomy. Correction of the volvulus was planned but it was considered that taking down the gastroenterostomy would be beneficial to resolve possible dumping. However, in order to disconnect the gastroenterostomy, it was important to know that the duodenal loop was normal, as it had not been visualised on the contrast studies, and OGD had only reached the second part of the duodenum. Therefore, a radiological study was performed by passing a catheter into the stomach and positioning its tip beyond the pylorus. Contrast was then injected, which showed normal peristalsis in the second and third parts of the duodenum, with contrast progressing normally to the proximal loops of the jejunum (Fig. 29.6).

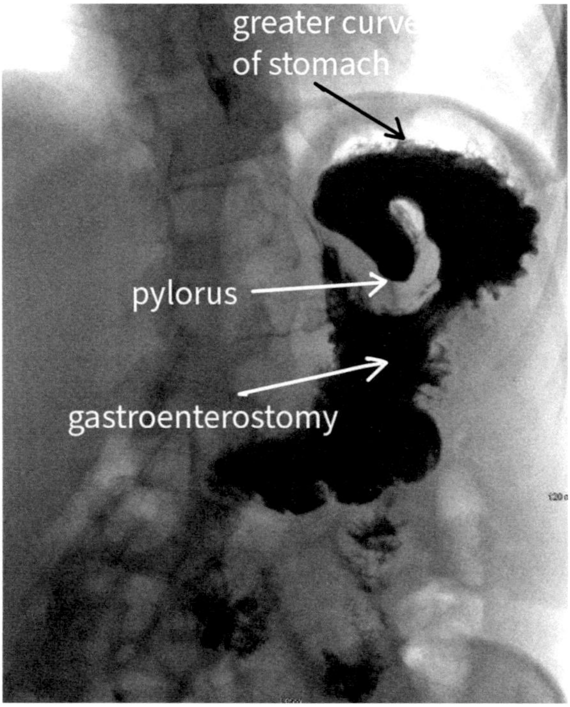

Fig. 29.5 Pre-operative barium meal, showing gastric volvulus with barium exiting the stomach through the gastroenterostomy

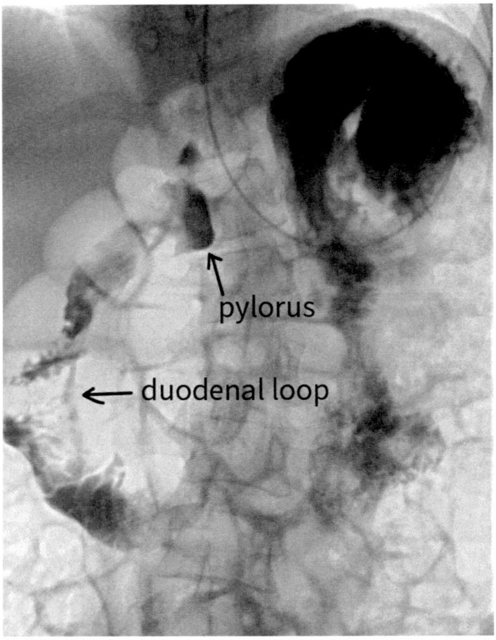

Fig. 29.6 Contrast study through a catheter placed in the pylorus, outlining the duodenal loop and progress of contrast through it and beyond into the jejunum

A laparotomy was performed which showed a very high posterior gastroenterostomy with a mesenteroaxial volvulus. The pylorus and duodenal loop appeared normal. The gastroenterostomy was disconnected using a linear stapler and the stomach was easily restored to a normal anatomical configuration. To keep it in place, a gastropexy was performed with four 2/0 Ethibond sutures attaching the greater curvature the stomach to the anterior abdominal wall.

The patient made an uneventful post-operative recovery, and she reported significant improvement in symptoms until follow-up 18 months later.

29.3.2 Learning Points

Obtaining the original hospital records in this case proved invaluable in understanding the background and interpreting the imaging. It is interesting that no mention was made of a volvulus at the time of the gastroenterostomy. If there had been one, it would have been obvious. It is likely, therefore, that the volvulus was secondary to the gastroenterostomy, perhaps unmasking a propensity as a result of laxity of the attachments of the stomach. Once the decision had been made to offer a correction of the volvulus, it was necessary to determine that the duodenal loop was normal if the gastroenterostomy was to be taken down. This reassurance was provided by the radiological study by selectively injecting contrast beyond the first part of the duodenum.

Chapter 30
Outcomes of Oesophageal Reconstruction

Abstract This chapter considers studies evaluating functional outcomes following oesophagus replacement with various conduits. Gastric conduits have been shown to be associated with dysphagia and reflux, which generally improves with time. Long-term outcomes with colonic interposition are generally favourable, but early satiety is common, and a reoperation rate of about 10% for colonic redundancy. One systematic review has shown better outcomes using the left colon through the retrosternal route. However, individualised conduit selection and route are crucial for optimal outcomes. Limited data exist on jejunal loop reconstruction, with mixed results. Overall, while various conduits offer potential solutions, careful consideration of patient factors is paramount for optimal outcomes.

Keywords Oesophageal reconstruction outcomes · Gastric conduit · Isoperistaltic grafts · Colonic interposition · Dysphagia · Retrosternal route · Jejunal loop reconstruction

A recent systematic review by Irino et al. examined publications from 2006 to 2015 to investigate the functional outcome after oesophagus replacement with different conduits [1]. The quality of the studies was generally poor. They found that gastric conduits were associated with varying levels of dysphagia, which tended to decrease over time. However, many patients still experienced mild to moderate reflux years after surgery. There were few long-term studies on isoperistaltic grafts, and the available data were insufficient to draw meaningful conclusions.

However, in a study by Greene and colleagues, it was reported that patients who underwent colonic interposition surgery had good long-term functional outcomes after a mean follow-up of 13 years. Over 80% of the patients were free of dysphagia, regurgitation, or heartburn, but reported early satiety as the most common symptom. However, almost 10% of the patients required reoperation due to colonic redundancy [2]. Brown and colleagues studied the outcome of the choice of colonic conduit and the placement route [3]. They conducted a systematic review and meta-analysis analysing 27 observational studies that included nearly 2000 patients. The pooled morbidity and mortality of using the right colon were worse than the left colon, and

M. Mughal, *Reconstructive Surgery of the Oesophagus and Stomach*,
https://doi.org/10.1007/978-3-031-66846-3_30

the retrosternal route was associated with better outcomes. Like many systematic reviews, the study has inherent weaknesses, mainly due to the heterogeneity of cases and other factors, such as variations in expertise and experience, and, most importantly, decision-making regarding the choice of the conduit. Although I prefer to use the right colon, I assess each case on its merits and do not hesitate to use other parts of the colon if that would provide a better conduit.

There are very few studies on the long-term outcomes following the use of a jejunal loop to reconstruct the oesophagus. Baker and colleagues [4] reported treating six patients with supercharged pedicled jejunal interposition after gastric and colonic conduits failed. Out of the six patients, three had to undergo surgery due to a leak. After a median follow-up of 6.5 years, five patients were able to resume an oral diet without the need for supplemental nutrition.

References

1. Irino T, Tsekrekos A, Coppola A, Scandavini CM, Shetye A, Lundell L, Rouvelas I. Long-term functional outcomes after replacement of the esophagus with gastric, colonic, or Jejunal conduits: a systematic literature review. Diseases Esophagus. 2017;30(12):1–11. https://doi.org/10.1093/dote/dox083.
2. Greene CL, DeMeester SR, Augustin F, Worrell SG, Oh DS, Hagen JA, DeMeester TR. Long-term quality of life and alimentary satisfaction after esophagectomy with colon interposition. Ann Thorac Surg. 2014;98(5):1713–20. https://doi.org/10.1016/j.athoracsur.2014.06.088.
3. Brown J, Lewis WG, Foliaki A, Clark GWB, Blackshaw GRJC, Chan DSY. Colonic interposition after adult oesophagectomy: systematic review and meta-analysis of conduit choice and outcome. J. Gastrointest. Surg. 2018;22(6):1104–11. https://doi.org/10.1007/s11605-018-3735-8.
4. Baker CR, Forshaw MJ, Gossage JA, Ng R, Mason RC. Long-Term outcome and quality of life after supercharged Jejunal interposition for oesophageal replacement. Surgeon. 2015;13(4):187–93. https://doi.org/10.1016/j.surge.2014.01.004.

Chapter 31
Innovations in Oesophageal Replacement and Repair

Abstract Recent advancements in oesophageal replacement and repair, including transplantation and tissue-engineering techniques, offer promising avenues for improving functional outcomes and reducing complications associated with traditional reconstruction methods. Experimental work in oesophageal transplantation and tissue engineering aims to develop artificial oesophagi, particularly targeting long-gap oesophageal atresia cases. Successful foetal transplantation of the oesophagus in animals has been achieved, showing potential for clinical application. Tissue-engineering approaches involve biomaterials, stem cells, and growth factors to create functional neoesophageal tissue. Studies in animal models demonstrate promising results in terms of graft integration and functionality.

Keywords Innovative oesophageal replacement · Transplantation · Tissue engineering · Artificial oesophagus · Long-gap oesophageal atresia · Graft integration · Graft rejection · Anastomotic leakage · Neoesophageal tissue

31.1 Transplant and Tissue-Engineering

In recent years, significant advancements have been made in oesophageal replacement and repair, including transplantation and tissue-engineering techniques. These innovative approaches hold promise for improving functional outcomes and reducing complications associated with traditional reconstruction techniques.

Experimental work is being carried out on both oesophageal transplantation and tissue engineering to create an artificial oesophagus. This work is mainly being done by research teams working with paediatric surgeons in the hope of finding better ways of treating long gap oesophageal atresia. Successful foetal transplantation of the oesophagus has been reported between syngenetic Lewis rats [1].

Tissue-engineering approaches for oesophageal reconstruction involve the use of biomaterials, stem cells, and growth factors to generate a functional, neoesophageal tissue that can replace or augment the damaged oesophagus. Several studies have demonstrated the feasibility of using such grafts for oesophageal replacement in

M. Mughal, *Reconstructive Surgery of the Oesophagus and Stomach*,
https://doi.org/10.1007/978-3-031-66846-3_31

animal models, with promising results in terms of graft integration, epithelialisation, and functionality [2]. Professor De Coppi's group at Great Ormond Street Hospital in London are at the forefront of research in this area, reporting promising results [3].

Like any innovative surgical technique, oesophageal transplantation and tissue-engineering approaches carry inherent risks and complications. Potential complications include graft rejection, infection, anastomotic leakage, and stricture formation. Moreover, the long-term outcomes of these procedures, particularly regarding their functional results, remain to be fully elucidated.

References

1. Yamataka A, Kato Y, Ohshiro K, Miyazaki E, Wang K, Miyano T. Fetal esophageal transplantation in rats: a treatment option for long-gap esophageal atresia. J Pediatric Surg. 1999;34(11):1638–40. https://doi.org/10.1016/S0022-3468(99)90633-4.
2. Badylak SF, Vorp DA, Spievack AR, et al. Esophageal reconstruction reconstruction with ECM and muscle tissue in a dog model. J Surg Res. 2005;128(1):87–97.
3. Urbani L, Camilli C, Phylactopoulos DE, Crowley C, Natarajan D, Scottoni F, Maghsoudlou P et al. Multi-stage bioengineering of a layered oesophagus with in vitro expanded muscle and epithelial adult progenitors. Nature Commun. 2018;9(1):4286. https://doi.org/10.1038/s41467-018-06385-w.

Chapter 32
The Case for Oesophageal Reconstruction Centres

Abstract This chapter underscores the pressing need for designated centres specialized in oesophageal reconstruction within the UK healthcare system. It highlights the complex challenges involved in managing patients requiring oesophageal reconstruction, ranging from surgical expertise to post-operative care. The scarcity of such centres is emphasized through statistics on the low volume of oesophageal reconstructions performed in individual centres, indicating a potential unmet need. The chapter advocates for the centralisation of expertise to improve patient outcomes, enhance training opportunities for surgeons, and facilitate comprehensive research programs. Key components of proposed centres include multidisciplinary teams, specialized clinics, dedicated operating lists, and a focus on research and innovation. The chapter emphasises the importance of collaboration with professional organisations and sister specialties to advance the field of oesophageal reconstruction.

Keywords Oesophageal reconstruction centres · Multidisciplinary teams · Surgical expertise · Patient outcomes · Training opportunities · Research opportunities · Infrastructure · Post-operative care

There is currently no designated centre for oesophageal reconstruction in the UK. Patients requiring oesophageal reconstruction often present multiple challenges, including management of chest and abdominal sepsis, nutritional support, specialist radiological and endoscopic interventions and complex surgery requiring the skills to operate in the neck, chest and abdomen. Reconstruction requires experience and expertise in choosing the most appropriate conduit, routing and timing of surgery.

Nationally, few colonic interpositions are performed for oesophageal reconstruction in the UK. HES (Health Episode Statistics) data for 2023–24 recorded only 7 colonic interpositions and 25 operations for tracheo-oesophageal fistula in adults [1]. A national audit of colonic interposition for oesophageal replacement between 2001 and 2015 showed that 306 such operations were performed in 58 hospitals over the 14 years studied [2]. The two highest volume hospitals did 42 and 45 operations. Thirteen consultants were responsible for more than five operations each (0.62

M. Mughal, *Reconstructive Surgery of the Oesophagus and Stomach*,
https://doi.org/10.1007/978-3-031-66846-3_32

operations/consultant/year). The remaining 204 operations were carried out by 133 individual consultants (0.11 operations/consultant/year).

There is likely an unmet need, with some clinicians and patients unaware of the possibility of complex oesophageal reconstruction for many of the conditions and examples described in this book. In my own experience, I have had patients contacting me from different parts of the UK to enquire about the possibility of reconstruction because they have not been offered the possibility locally or regionally. Some regions lack the expertise or experience, as I have had referrals from experienced UGI surgeons working in designated oesophagogastric centres in the UK.

The centralisation of OG cancer surgery has resulted in the 'passive' centralisation of emergency benign OG conditions, such as incarcerated paraoesophageal hernia, with improved outcomes, as expected [3]. In my opinion, it is only a matter of time before this happens, and some of these centres could be designated for oesophageal reconstruction.

It is essential to train the next generation of surgeons; that is not achievable if reconstructions are carried out in small volumes across many hospitals.

The need for oesophageal reconstruction is likely to rise because of rising numbers of bariatric operations and, therefore, catastrophic complications requiring complex reconstruction, and young patients having antireflux surgery. Up to 20% may eventually require re-do surgery, of whom about 10% may require complex oesophageal reconstruction

There is a great need for a comprehensive research programme in many areas of complex benign oesophagogastric surgery. There is a steady increase in endoscopic interventions for conditions which have been treated by surgery. It is more important than ever to evaluate new techniques and devices properly to help clinicians to select the best option for their patients.

32.1 Proposed Framework and Infrastructure

32.1.1 Specialist MDT

Cancer MDTs were part of the UK Improving Outcomes Guidance in 2001, which set the framework and standard of cancer care. I believe applying the same principles to decision-making for benign-complex oesophagogastric conditions is long overdue. Arguably, the stakes are even higher in this group of patients, who are often young with a likely normal lifespan. Good decision-making and optimal treatment are likely to deliver a significant impact in terms of Quality Adjusted Life Years.

The proposed core membership is as follows:

Two OG surgeons with specialist expertise in oesophageal reconstruction
Gastroenterologist with OG interventional skills
Radiologist with OG interventional skills
Thoracic surgeon
Dietician
Speech and language therapist
Clinical Nurse Specialist
Clinical Fellow

32.1.2 Specialist Clinic and Dedicated Operating Lists

A specialist clinic dedicated to patients being assessed for or followed up after oesophageal reconstruction goes hand-in-hand with the MDT. Dedicated operating lists are necessary to ensure the staff are experienced in this area. Ideally, these operating lists would take place in an appropriately equipped and dedicated theatre, for instance, accommodating endoscopic and laparoscopic equipment, as well as the standard set-up for open surgery. In many cases, complex reconstruction involves on-table endoscopy and bronchoscopy and the appropriate equipment and skills should be available. Also, hybrid procedures are increasingly used, for instance, laparoscopic and VATS procedures combined with laparotomy and/or thoracotomy.

32.1.3 Surgical Team and Training

It is ideal for these complex cases to be performed jointly by two experienced consultant surgeons, but they would also be joined by senior surgical Fellows being trained in this area. Joint operating should be the standard for complex cases. Intraoperative decision-making is helped by having another experienced colleague by one's side. Also, it helps to share the intense part of the operation with another colleague and not be in a situation where decision-making is being affected by fatigue six or eight hours into an operation.

32.1.4 Research and Innovation

There are many potential areas of research, both clinical and translational:

- Study of current practice, provision of service and outcomes
- Gap analysis to determine the unmet need nationally

- Developing a standardised assessment framework (by the same iterative process that assessment algorithms were developed for intestinal failure patients)
- Studies of techniques of reconstruction and how they are best applied in different situations
- Study and assessment of emerging endoscopic techniques for managing oesophageal leaks and perforations and development of new procedures
- Translational research into materials and tissue engineering for oesophageal repair and replacement.

32.1.5 Developing Partnerships

The centres would develop partnerships with professional organisations, regulators, specialist training organisations, and sister specialities, such as paediatric surgeons with an interest in oesophageal reconstructions. I regularly work with paediatric colleagues, assisting them with oesophageal reconstruction. They tell me that my adult expertise is helpful to them, and I have learnt a lot from their approach to oesophageal reconstruction in the child, as well as picking surgical techniques that I have applied to my adult practice.

References

1. https://digital.nhs.uk/data-and-information/publications/statistical/hospital-admitted-patient-care-activity/2023-24
2. Fisher RA, Griffiths EA, Evison F et al. A national audit of colonic interposition for esophageal replacement. Diseases Esophagus. 2017;0:1–10.
3. Markar SR, Mackenzie H, Wiggins T, et al. Influence of national centralisation of oesophagogastric cancer on management and clinical outcome from emergency upper gastrointestinal conditions. Brit J Surg. 2018;105:113–20.

Chapter 33
Management Algorithms Relevant to Oesophageal Reconstruction

Abstract This chapter includes algorithms to manage some of the most challenging scenarios in oesophagogastric surgery. Early recognition, intervention and effective management of conditions and complications that may ultimately require oesophageal reconstruction is emphasised. While the chapter includes several algorithms addressing common scenarios, it acknowledges the impossibility of covering every potential presentation. Emphasizing the pivotal role of multidisciplinary teams (MDTs) in treatment decisions, the chapter highlights the nuanced approach needed for each case. Furthermore, it anticipates that advances in artificial intelligence (AI) will enable personalised management of many of the scenarios described.

Keywords Boerhaave's syndrome · Instrumental perforation · Corrosive injury · Anastomotic leaks · Sleeve gastrectomy leaks · Aero-digestive fistula · Atrio-oesophageal fistula

I have included some algorithms for managing some of the conditions and complications which can lead to the eventual need for oesophageal reconstruction. Early and effective management of these conditions can avoid the need for reconstruction.

It is impossible to have algorithms for every potential presentation. As I have stated at several places in this book, the most important factor in achieving good outcomes is an MDT. The MDT is best placed to consider treatment options, considering the particular nuances of each case.

I am sure that advances in AI in the coming years will result in the availability of Applications that will assist in planning treatment based on key information and data for a specific patient.

M. Mughal, *Reconstructive Surgery of the Oesophagus and Stomach*,
https://doi.org/10.1007/978-3-031-66846-3_33

33.1 Algorithm for Boerhaave's Syndrome

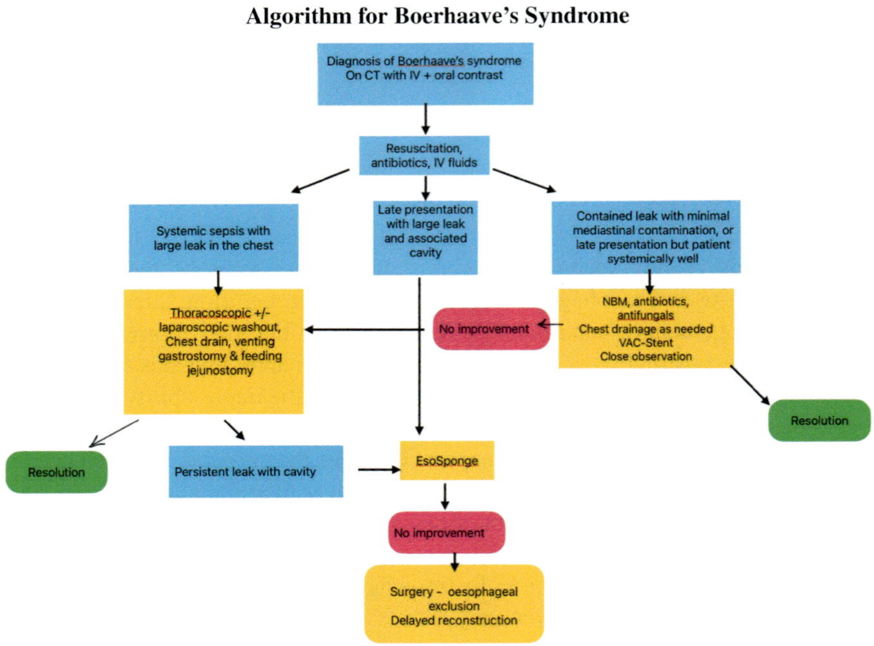

33.2 Algorithm for Instrumental Perforation of the Oesophagus

Algorithm for an Instrumental Perforation of the Oesophagus

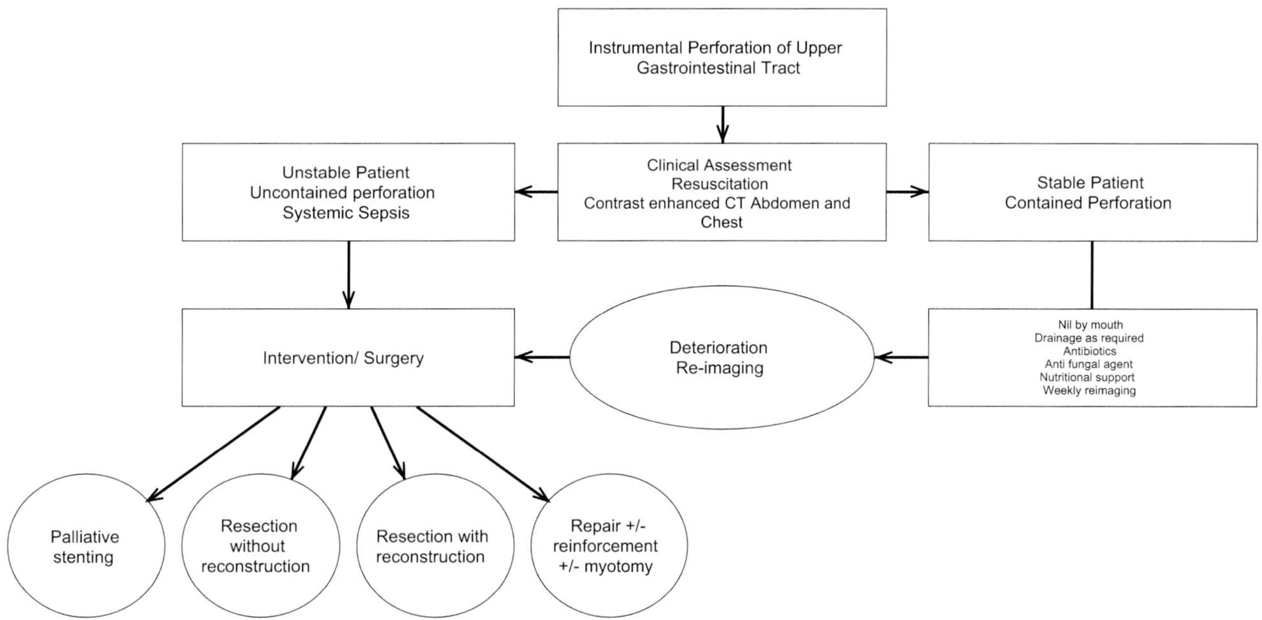

33.3 Algorithm for the Management of Corrosive Ingestion

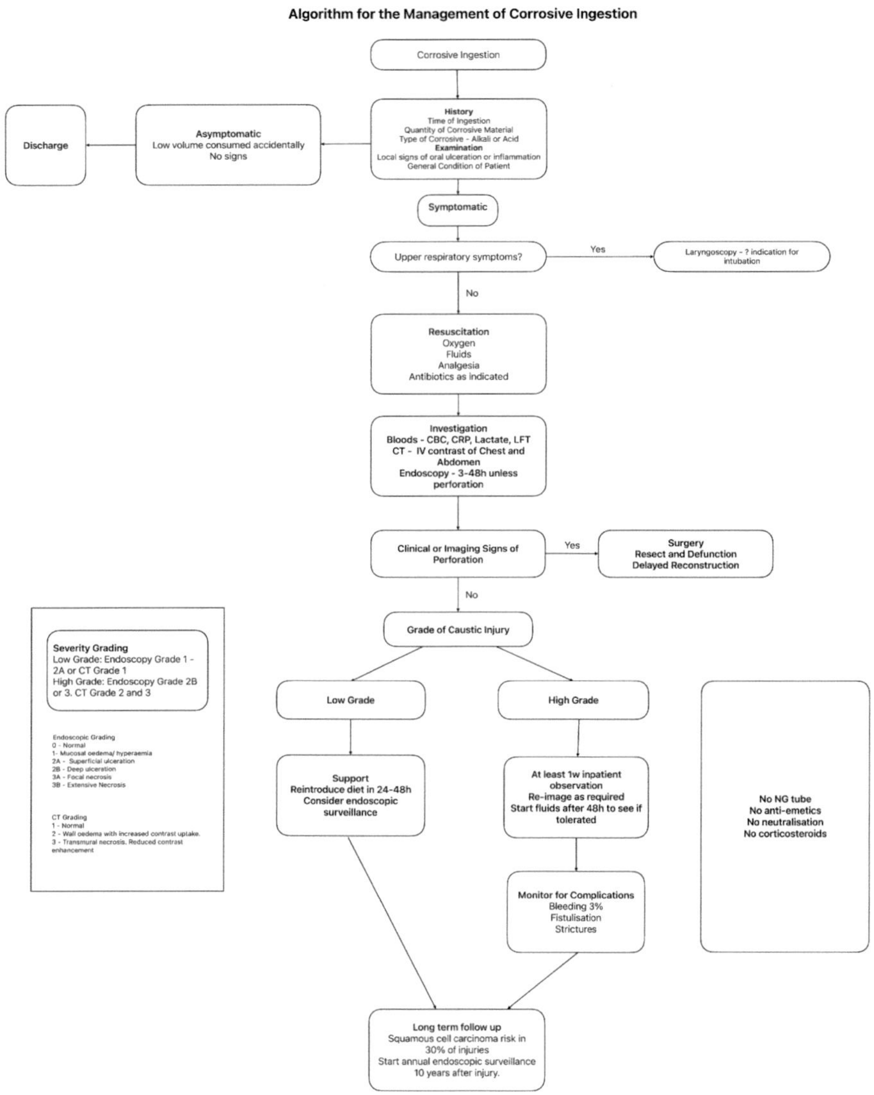

33.4 Management of Anastomotic Leaks After Oesophagectomy

Algorithm for the Management of Anastamotic Leak after Oesophagectomy

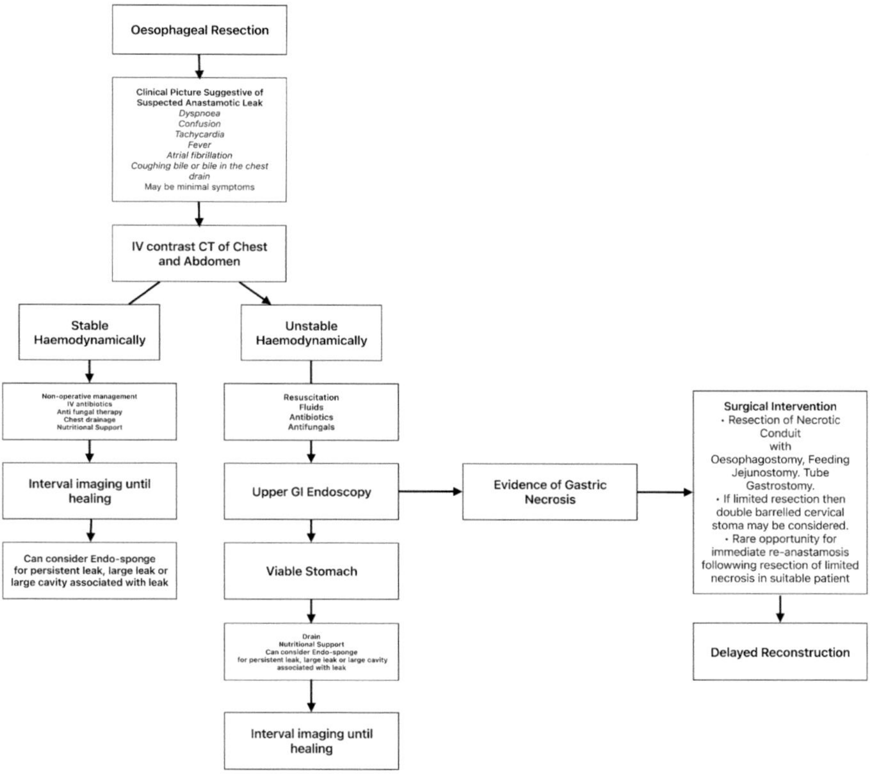

33.5 Algorithm for Treating Sleeve Gastrectomy Leaks

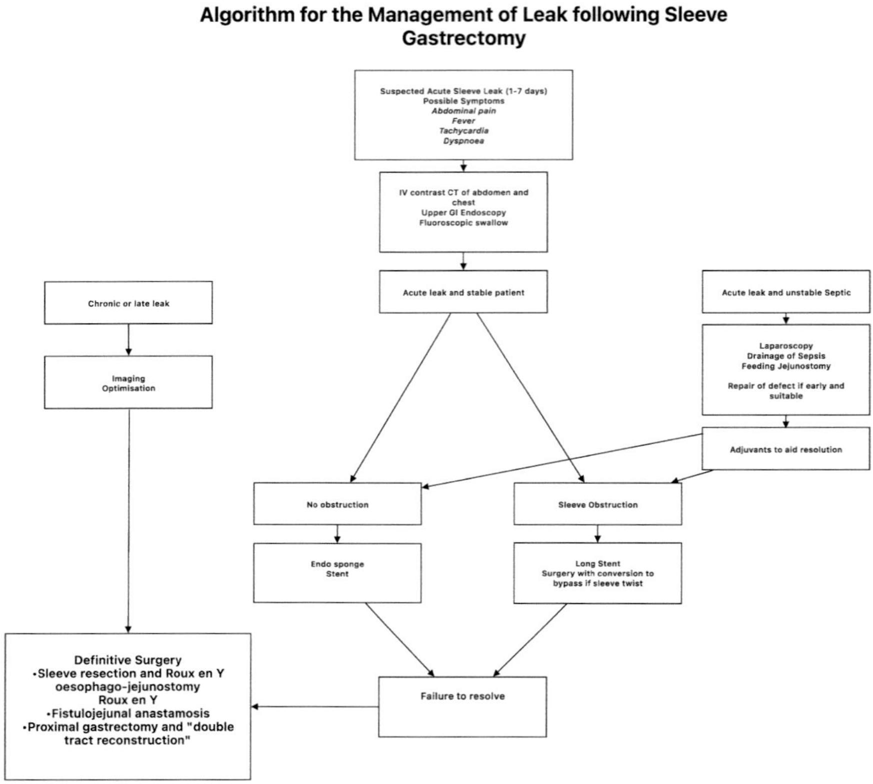

33.6 Algorithm for Aero-Digestive Fistula [1]

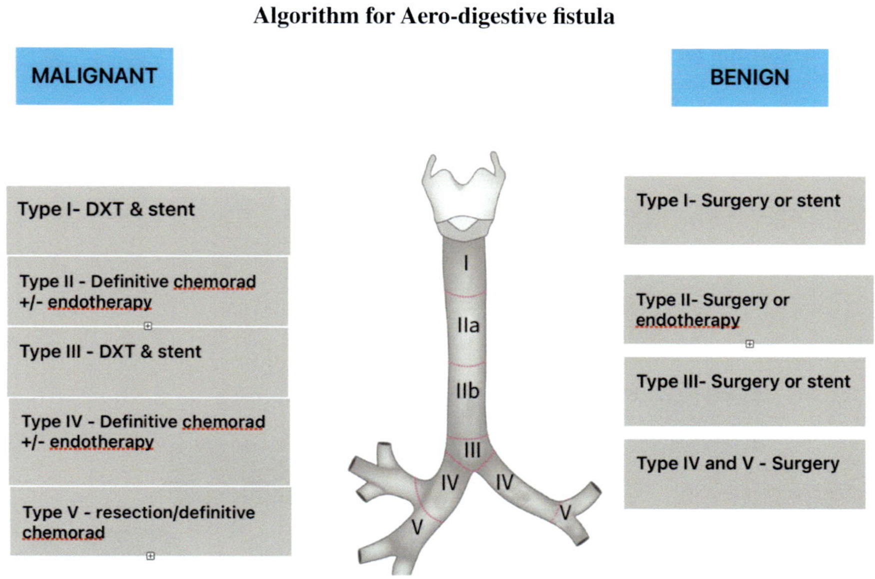

33.7 Algorithm for the Management of Atrio-Oesophageal Fistula [2]

Algorithm for the management of atrio-oesophageal fistula

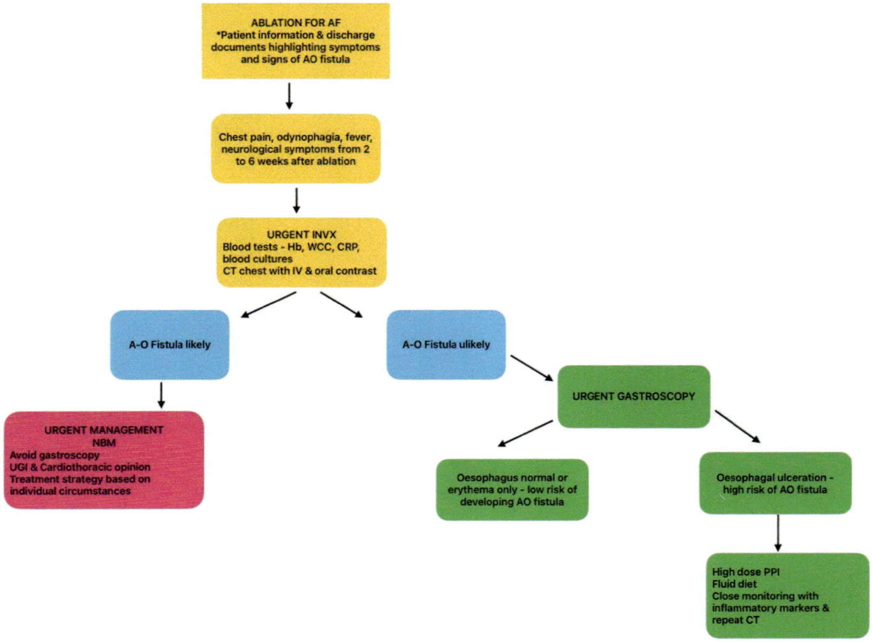

References

1. Qureshi YA, Muntzer Mughal M, Fragkos KC, Lawrence D, George J, Mohammadi B, Dawas K, Booth H (2018) Acquired adult aerodigestive fistula: classification and management. J Gastrointest Surg. 2018;22(10):1785–94. https://doi.org/10.1007/s11605-018-3811-0.
2. Kapur S, Barbhaiya C, Deneke T, Michaud GF (2017) Esophageal Injury and atrioesophageal fistula caused by ablation for atrial fibrillation. Circulation. 2017;136(13):1247–55. https://doi.org/10.1161/CIRCULATIONAHA.117.025827.

Index

M. Mughal, *Reconstructive Surgery of the Oesophagus and Stomach*,
https://doi.org/10.1007/978-3-031-66846-3

MIX
Papier aus verantwortungsvollen Quellen
Paper from responsible sources
FSC® C105338

If you have any concerns about our products,
you can contact us on
ProductSafety@springernature.com

In case Publisher is established outside the EU,
the EU authorized representative is:
Springer Nature Customer Service Center GmbH
Europaplatz 3, 69115 Heidelberg, Germany

Printed by Libri Plureos GmbH
in Hamburg, Germany